Recovery From Disability

Recovery From Disability

MANUAL OF PSYCHIATRIC REHABILITATION

Robert Paul Liberman, M.D.

Distinguished Professor,

Department of Psychiatry and Biobehavioral Sciences;

Director, UCLA Psych REHAB Program,

University of California, Los Angeles

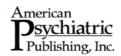

American Psychiatric Publishing, Inc.

WASHINGTON, DC • LONDON, ENGLAND

If you would like to buy between 25 and 99 copies of this or any other APPI title, you are eligible for a 20% discount; please contact APPI Customer Service at appi@psych.org or 800-368-5777. If you wish to buy 100 or more copies of the same title, please e-mail us at bulksales@sales.psych.org for a price quote.

Manufactured in the United States of America on acid-free paper
12 11 10 9 8   5 4 3 2 1
First Edition

Typeset in Adobe Minion.

American Psychiatric Publishing, Inc.
1000 Wilson Boulevard
Arlington, VA 22209-3901
www.appi.org

Library of Congress Cataloging-in-Publication Data
Liberman, Robert Paul, 1937–
    Recovery from disability : manual of psychiatric rehabilitation / by Robert Paul Liberman.
— 1st ed.
        p. ; cm.
    Includes bibliographical references and index.
    ISBN 978-1-58562-205-4 (pbk. : alk. paper) 1. Mentally ill—Rehabilitation. 2. Mentally ill—Services for. I. Title.
    [DNLM: 1. Mental Disorders—rehabilitation. 2. Mentally Disabled Persons—rehabilitation. 3. Rehabilitation, Vocational—methods. 4. Social Adjustment. WM 400 L695r 2008]
RC439.5.L523 2008
616.89′1—dc22
                                                                                                    2007018821

British Library Cataloguing in Publication Data
A CIP record is available from the British Library.

To Janet, my wife and closest friend,
who has steered my ship through seas rough and calm.
My respect and gratitude for her editorial assistance
with this book are beyond words.

Contents

Foreword

JOHN A. TALBOTT, M.D.

Fifty years ago, the patients in our nation's state hospitals began to leave for what was optimistically called "the community," and new admissions to such facilities were curtailed. By the late 1960s, the nation's press had declared this process of callous deinstitutionalization a national scandal. Most psychiatrists working in public mental health settings were overwhelmed with patients for whom they had no effective treatments aside from medications. Medications did help to reduce the severity of symptoms, but medication could not teach patients how to live well in the community. Fortunately, Bob Liberman, then a young psychiatrist brimming over with ideas translated from the laboratories of learning theories, began his quest for evidence-based methods for psychiatric rehabilitation.

Liberman, uniquely among us, saw opportunity where most saw defeat. He assembled a group of talented mental health professionals around him and plunged into the pool of psychiatric rehabilitation where others would not venture a toe. Working with the most severely disabled of the mentally ill, he and his associates made progress in developing psychosocial and behavioral treatments for successful rehabilitation. Together in hospitals and mental health centers, they designed, field-tested, researched, and empirically validated techniques that were utilitarian and effective in improving patients' social and role functioning. Social skills training, behavioral family therapy, and social learning therapy were among the techniques that emerged from their work.

Liberman's genius was in training hosts of clinicians to use his innovative techniques. In disseminating and adapting the new services to fit the needs of a broad spectrum of patients—inpatients and outpatients, patients in forensic hospitals and prisons, developmentally disabled patients as well as patients with serious mental disorders—he was able to demonstrate that practitioners working in ordinary facilities and communities could successfully apply the new techniques. His techniques have been translated into 23 languages and are used on every continent. Only a rare few can invent or discover something of value, fewer still are successful in bringing it to the market, and only a minuscule number succeed in having their innovations bear fruit worldwide.

This book is the culmination of Liberman's efforts. It summarizes the current state of the panoply of evidence-based treatments now entering the field of psychiatric rehabilitation. By embracing the goal of "recovery," Liberman moves his efforts into the contemporary view that, using the current array of effective treatments, it is possible to empower patients to live reasonably normal lives in their communities: working, learning, relating with family and friends, and enjoying longer periods of wellness. This book is not a ponderous and comprehensive textbook; rather it offers practical guidelines for clinicians, patients, and families to work collaboratively as partners in the treatment process. Liberman does not present his techniques as gospel, but as road maps to recovery.

I recall 30 years ago when I began my association with the American Psychiatric Association's journal *Hospital & Community Psychiatry*, now renamed *Psychiatric Services*. I told my colleagues and friends that my goal for the journal was for it to be academically rigorous while maintaining its reputation for readability, relevance to clinical practice, and accessibility. They scoffed at me, but with the help of many scientist-practitioners who participated on the editorial board, we succeeded in achieving my vision for the journal. In a similar vein, you will find this book fascinating as well as practical. Being practical and interesting are not mutually exclusive, just as being scientifically rigorous and useful are not. Follow Liberman's advice; dip in, sample, taste, and try the treatments that he so clearly describes. You will agree with me that this is a manual for serving the needs of clinicians, patients, and families for years to come.

John A. Talbott, M.D.
Professor of Psychiatry, University of Maryland School of Medicine, Baltimore, Maryland

Preface

Today is the best of times in psychiatry. We have available new generations of antipsychotic and antidepressant medications that offer the promise of symptom control and remediation of cognitive impairments in persons with serious and disabling mental disorders. Psychosocial treatments have been developed and been shown to be demonstrably effective for motivating mentally disabled persons to manage their illnesses, establish personally relevant goals, acquire social skills, improve family support, obtain employment, and overcome the ravages of substance abuse. Recovery from serious and persistent mental disorders has never been closer to reality.

Today is also the worst of times for psychiatry. Medications heralded for their superior efficacy in schizophrenia and mood disorders have failed the test of time and are no more effective than those that have been available for more than three decades. Evidence-based psychosocial treatments have not been able to penetrate academic walls into everyday clinical practice. Motivational enhancement, illness management, social skills training, behavioral family therapy, supported employment, and integrated systems of care for dually diagnosed mentally ill substance abusers are flourishing in journals and books but rarely leap from the printed page into regular clinical practice. This book is for practitioners who wish to bridge the gap between what is known and what can be actually used in real-life mental health programs.

Every day, those of us who are clinicians labor together with our patients and their families to reduce disability and speed recovery. With currently available, evidence-based biobehavioral treatments, *disability* no longer needs to be synonymous with *mental illness*. Recovery from disabling mental disorders is a realistic and attainable goal for the twenty-first century. Mental health professionals, patients, relatives, policy makers, and other stakeholders have become familiar with the term *recovery* as it has echoed in reports, commissions, and publications at the national, state, and local levels. But while familiarity may breed "halo effects," it does not yield a clear understanding of the concept. It will be hard to rally around the recovery flag unless there is a consensus on how the term is defined among all those having a stake in the future of psychiatric rehabilitation. Unless we know where we should be heading to foster our patients' recovery, we may never get there.

Recovery can be defined in objective and subjective ways as well as on a continuum of process to outcome. Objectively, persons can be said to have recovered from mental disability if they have no symptoms that seriously intrude on their daily functioning or quality of life and are living independently, managing their own money and medication, working or attending school in normal settings at least half-time, participating in social and recreational activities and events with peers in normal community sites at least once per week, and enjoying reasonably cordial family relations. Subjectively, the recovery experience comprises having hope for a brighter future, taking personal responsibility for one's life, and being empowered with skills, supports, and respect to make decisions that offer satisfaction and meaning in daily living. The process of recovery is set in motion by a collaborative therapeutic relationship that enhances motivation and self-directed choices for mentally disabled persons as they select their personal goals and treatment opportunities.

Optimism and hope for recovery have sprouted from destigmatization of mental illness and the increasing evidence that getting a normal life comes from comprehensive, continuous, coordinated, and consumer-oriented treatment that is delivered competently and compassionately. Practitioners who are equipped with personal qualities that enliven the treatment relationship enable medications, skills, and supports to exert their positive effects. Technical competence in the use of evidence-based treatments is not sufficient for clinicians to mobilize patients and families in their search for recovery.

▶ The Key to Recovery Is Held by the Clinician Who Cares

As clinicians we must be sensitive to our "looking glass selves." Our therapeutic impact is always mediated by how we are viewed by our patients and

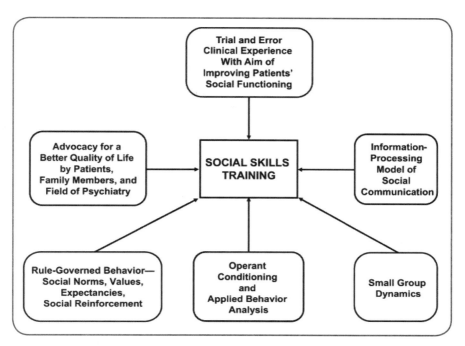

FIGURE 1. Sources of basic and applied contributions to the development of social skills training as a modality of psychiatric rehabilitation.

with randomized, controlled clinical trials as well as through the life stories that we elicit from our patients. Evidence for effective treatments can come legitimately from large-scale research projects that "prove" the value of an intervention by dint of statistically significant mean differences favoring the innovative treatment over customary care. An even more compelling basis for evidence supporting the value of a treatment comes from careful observation, measurement, and replication within the same individual. In their effective application, treatments must be adapted to each individual's unique symptoms and cognitive impairments, functional strengths and deficits, learning capacity, supports, and resources. Knowing that a treatment "on average" is statistically more effective than another offers frail guidance to any clinician whose patient may not fit the average subject in a large clinical trial.

The design, development, validation, and dissemination of best practices for psychiatric rehabilitation constitute a process that, when successful, resembles an interactional sequence of steps starting with formative inspiration. This developmental process is graphically represented in Figure 2. Note that the phases of research, development, and dissemination of rehabilitation modalities are bidirectional. Thus, the design of a treatment, program, or service may be modified on the basis of feedback from clinical experience,

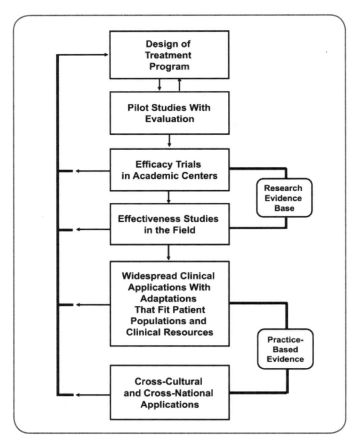

FIGURE 2. Process of designing, validating, and disseminating best practices for psychiatric rehabilitation. The process is dynamic and interactive among the developmental levels, with adaptation, modification, improvement, and reinvention of a treatment to fit the special circumstances of each clinical site.

pilot testing in the field, and efficacy or effectiveness trials. In fact, even after a particular treatment program is thoroughly and empirically validated by research, the program developers may go back to the drawing board as the result of experience with a broad array of patients treated in a wide variety of facilities for varying lengths of time by practitioners of varied disciplines, experience, and competence. The unfolding readjustments of innovations can be viewed as practice-based evidence for their clinical value.

There are several modes of validation for determining the empirical support for any one treatment's efficacy and effectiveness. Efficacy is usually determined by a novel treatment showing superior outcomes (vs. customary treatment) in randomized, controlled studies in academic settings where treatment is delivered by experts and the patients are highly selected to exclude those with very chronic and complicated disorders. In contrast, effectiveness studies are carried out in ordinary mental health settings with regular staff members providing the novel and standard treatments. Social validation is accomplished when professionals, consumers, and other stakeholders endorse the treatment as useful and beneficial in helping patients to reach real-world goals. Cross-cultural validation occurs when a treatment developed in one country is implemented and adapted by professionals in a second country, with documented effectiveness and perceived value by the mental health field in that second country. It is reassuring that many of the current evidence-based modes of treatment and rehabilitation for mentally disabled persons, initially designed and validated in the United States, have been translated, culturally adapted, and empirically supported in other countries.

▶ The End of Ideology Heralds a Future of Empirically Based Treatments

Forty years ago, when I began my work in rehabilitation, I was in a derided minority. Psychoanalytic theories held sway over other treatments, including psychopharmacology, which were viewed as defaults for those patients who did not respond to insight-oriented therapy. Even after my early research showed clearly that behavioral principles could be used to reduce symptoms and teach patients to interact normally, those in ascendance in the academic and clinical worlds denounced the results as trivial. Contemporaries viewed my efforts to apply social learning and other practical approaches to the seriously mentally ill as eccentric, shallow, superficial, or worse. Warnings were issued that improvements in psychosocial functioning achieved through educational procedures would lead to "symptom substitution." Anachronistic hydraulic theories, based on psychic energy being dammed up by any improvement not accompanied by insight, predicted that functional and symptomatic improvements brought about by behavior therapy would elicit even more serious problems when the dam crumbled under a flood of symptoms and behavioral regression.

Only after decades of research demonstrations and replications pushed psychodynamics into retreat did skills training, behavioral family therapy, and supportive interventions become accepted as best practices. The leaders of psychiatric therapeutics initially stated, "Rehabilitative treatments based on behavior therapy were not really effective." When efficacy was documented, the mental health establishment averred that "rehabilitation might be effective but the interventions were not clinically important." The final retrenchment by the "psychiatric powers that be" was capitulation to empirically based services: "Rehabilitation was effective and important, but we've been doing that sort of thing all along." Now, in the twilight of my career, it is enormously satisfying to see behavioral therapies and psychosocial rehabilitation—in league with pharmacotherapy—as the undisputed best practices across the landscape of psychiatric disorders.

How can we prevent psychiatry from relapsing into fascinations for treatments that are based on overvalued and misguided assumptions of etiology of mental disorders? It will be all too easy to fall into the trap of hewing to treatments that have the appeal of intellectually compelling ideology in the guise of science. I harbor misgivings about the ascendance of the biomedical model, with its dominant scientific paradigm in medicine and psychiatry. It is certainly reassuring that psychiatry now is viewed as having a scientific basis by the public and colleagues in other fields of medicine. Psychiatry is slowly climbing from its centuries-old place at the bottom of the totem pole of medical specialties, but the brain will not readily release its mysteries. When we realize that each of the trillion neurons in the brain has hundreds of synaptic connections to other neurons and brain regions, parsing the significance of the neural interconnections for mental disorders becomes a minefield of exploded findings and theories.

Science is fundamentally reductionistic. It seeks answers to complex questions of disease and disability from probabilities of electrons, genes, molecules, and neuroimaginal structures and functions. Defining the tangled diversity of an individual is beyond the current capacity of neuroscience, but the practice of psychiatric rehabilitation is ultimately focused on the individual and his/her struggles to win a satisfying place in the world. The individual who is our patient defies oversimplification by biomedical science and yearns to find practitioners who can offer healing through understanding the sea of uncertainty and unpredictability of an individual's seeking a pathway to recovery. Traditional science cannot accurately predict the trajectory of complex systems such as people with mental disabilities. Lacking a cure and dissatisfied with drug treatments that can attenuate but rarely eliminate intrusive and dysphoric symptoms, our patients hope for restoration of their functional and experiential selves. Psychiatric rehabilitation provided in the context of a collaborative and compassionate relationship, combined with pharmacotherapy, opens new roads to hope and recovery.

On the contemporary scene, the exciting advances of neuroscience have trapped many academic psychiatrists, researchers, mental health professionals, and consumer advocates in a reductionistic belief that mental disorders and their ultimate treatments will eventually be decoded from the complexities of the brain. The brain is undoubtedly host to the neural mechanisms that mediate the symptoms, cognitive impairments, and abnormal psychosocial functioning of persons with mental disabilities. However, the brain is an open system that is influenced by behavior and the environment and is malleable throughout the life span; it does not operate in a unidirectional way to control behavior. Only by gradually deciphering the complex interactions among genes, brain development, environment, and the physiological, social-emotional, and instrumental dimensions of human behavior will our field continue to generate robustly effective treatments that diminish disability and promote recovery for our patients.

Abandoning treatments based on ideological and philosophical assumptions of human behavior for evidence-based treatments will permit the scientific method to spawn new and more effective services in the future. Today's evidence-based treatments will be regularly supplanted by new and innovative practices that research reveals to be based on superior evidence. The need to disseminate the benefits of evidence-based rehabilitation throughout the mental health systems of care is gradually yielding a technology for knowledge transfer. As thousands of mental health professionals increasingly acquire the clinical skills to use evidence-based treatments with fidelity, recovery from disability will go beyond mere slogans.

The future is bright with promise. In the coming decades, upward of half of mentally disabled patients will be able to recover, enjoying fuller, more rewarding, and satisfying lives. I remain tenaciously optimistic that the principles and practices of psychiatric rehabilitation—as described in this manual—will bring symptom remissions, hope, personal responsibility, choices, autonomy, and dignity to hundreds of thousands of mentally disabled persons. It is time for them to come out from the shadows of stigma and take their place with the rest of humanity in the brilliance of daylight.

Acknowledgments

Innumerable mentors, colleagues, trainees, and patients and their family members contributed to my research and clinical work in psychiatric rehabilitation. Some of the more important people whose influence and collaboration have been instrumental to the success of my 40 years of professional activity and productivity are B. F. Skinner, Ph.D., Albert Bandura, Ph.D., Louis Lasagna M.D., Elliot Mishler, Ph.D., Herbert Weiner, Ph.D., Nathan Azrin, Ph.D., Michael Serber, M.D., Gordon Paul, Ph.D., Philip R. A. May, M.D., Jim Mintz, Ph.D., William DeRisi, Ph.D., Larry King, Ph.D., Timothy Kuehnel, Ph.D., Thad Eckman, Ph.D., Alex Kopelowicz, M.D., Ana Wong-McDonald, Ph.D., Keith Nuechterlein, Ph.D., Steven Silverstein, Ph.D., Ian R. H. Falloon, M.D., Christine Vaughn, Ph.D., Isaac Marks, M.D., Robert Drake, M.D., Ph.D., Kim Mueser, Ph.D., Shirley Glynn, Ph.D., Gayla Blackwell, R.N., M.S.W., Sally MacKain, Ph.D., Tania Lecomte, Ph.D., Joseph Ventura, Ph.D., Patrick Corrigan, Psy.D., Will Spaulding, Ph.D., Robert Kern, Ph.D., Paul Satz, Ph.D., Michael Green, Ph.D., Stephen Marder, M.D., Ted Van Putten, M.D., Robert Tauber, M.Ed., and Thomas Backer, Ph.D.

I am particularly indebted to the creative wellspring of Charles "Chuck" Wallace, Ph.D., which has never run dry. We have enjoyed a remarkable 35 years of close, mutually satisfying, and symbiotic collaboration. His original ideas, systematic and scientific pursuit of hypotheses, and ability to clarify the muddled and simplify the complex have nourished me and my work. Because of the quirks of circumstance, I have received the lion's share of recognition for contributions to our field that, in truth, were often created, developed, and evaluated by Chuck.

I also have benefited greatly from the administrative support of Louis Jolyon West, M.D., Fawzy Fawzy, M.D., Frank Turley, Ph.D., Ransom Arthur, M.D., Milton Greenblatt, M.D., Don Flinn, M.D., Rafael Canton, M.D., Fritz Redlich, M.D., and Peter Whybrow, M.D.

Among the redeeming pleasures of academic work are the many collaborations and friendships that are rooted in my international travel to conferences, meetings, consultations, visiting professorships, and workshops for training colleagues in evidence-based practices. These enduring and enriching relationships taught me that the passion and determination to improve the lives of the mentally disabled reside in scientist-practitioners the world round, including Jean Cottraux, M.D., Ph.D., and Bernard Rivière, M.D. (France); Guy Deleu, M.D. (Belgium); Jerome Favrod, R.N., Hans Brenner, M.D., Ph.D., and Volker Roder, Ph.D. (Switzerland); Manfred Fichter, M.D., Iver Hand, M.D., and Annette Schaub, Ph.D. (Germany); César Sotillo Zevallos, M.D. (Peru); Felicitas Kort, Ph.D., and Franzel Delgado Senior, M.D. (Venezuela); Joanna Meder, M.D. (Poland); Jordi Masia (Spain); Toma Tomov, M.D., and Nikolai Butorin, Ph.D. (Bulgaria); Nick Tarrier, Ph.D., and Julian Leff, M.D. (England); Hector Tsang, Ph.D. (Hong Kong); Weng Yongzhen, M.D., and Ying-Qiang Xiang, M.D. (China); Mariano Bassi, M.D., and Gianfranco Goldwurm, M.D. (Italy); Shin-Ichi Niwa, M.D., Emi Ikebuchi, M.D., Nobuo Anzai, M.D., Kei Maeda, Ph.D., and Keiko Kadoya, M.D. (Japan); Chul Kwon Kim, M.D., and Young Hee Choi, M.D. (Korea); Gunnar Gotestam, M.D., Rolf Grawe, Ph.D., Per Borell, Ph.D., and Karl Fagerström, Ph.D. (Norway and Sweden); Louis DeVisser, Ph.D., Mark van der Gaag, Ph.D., Helma Blankman, R.N., Dorien Verhoeven, M.S.W., and Ellen Karman (The Netherlands); and T. Murali, M.D., and R. Thara, M.D. (India).

In addition to my wife Janet's contributions, the book manuscript was substantially improved with the editorial comments and suggestions of Alex Kopelowicz, M.D., and Timothy Kuehnel, Ph.D. Mary Jane Robertson, M.S., my longtime research associate and administrator, was indispensable in preparing graphics that illuminate the principles and practices of psychiatric rehabilitation described in the chapters of the book. I owe a special thanks to John A. Talbott, M.D., for his foreword to this manual as well as to my earlier book, *Psychiatric Rehabilitation of Chronic Mental Patients.* John has been a beacon for the field of psychiatry, ensuring that mental health professionals and systems of care give priority to those patients with psychiatric disabilities. He has made services to the mentally disabled an ethical and moral imperative in his leadership of the American Psychiatric Association, his role as editor-in-chief of the journal *Psychiatric Services,* and his support of research on psychiatric rehabilitation.

Last but not least, the encouragement of Robert Hales, M.D., M.B.A., editor-in-chief of American Psychiatric Publishing Inc., was instrumental in the lengthy gestation for this manual. Bob Hales has extraordinary vision and determination to broaden the field of psychiatric therapeutics beyond traditional psychotherapies and psychopharmacology. His enthusiasm for psychiatric rehabilitation as a mainstay in psychiatry brings the prospects for recovery to all those hampered by disability. It has been a privilege to collaborate with Bob in his capacity as medical director of the Sacramento County Division of Mental Health. Together with the administrative and clinical staff of his division, my team from the UCLA Psych REHAB Program successfully implemented social skills training throughout Sacramento County to the betterment of patients and clinicians alike.

Even now, 40 years after meeting my first patient with schizophrenia, I continue to learn from my patients—not only how to develop partnerships in treatment but also how to accept the disappointments and reversals that inevitably crop up as obstacles to our joint progress toward recovery. My patients are my most admired heroes, struggling to create fulfilling lives for themselves without surrendering to the darkness. Having struggled with the dark beast within myself, I know the importance of persistence and hope born of small stepwise improvements by patient and practitioner alike. A treatment relationship that exudes confidence, competence, cooperation, and compassion is indispensable. Every day, I greet my patients with a gleam in my eye, a smile on my face, and a bounce in my step. And they have rewarded me handsomely.

Introduction

Recovery From Disability offers practical answers to the many questions harbored by mental health practitioners as they face daily challenges in providing effective and compassionate services to persons with psychiatric and developmental disabilities. This manual is not a scholarly text written to sit on a bookshelf, gathering dust while waiting for occasional peeks by academics conducting research or writing articles for publication. However, it is written by a scholar who, in addition to conducting research and developing innovative treatment techniques, has spent his 40-year career as a clinician providing direct services to persons with serious mental and developmental disorders. Thus, the principles and treatment techniques are up-to-date and reflect a consensus of experts in the field regarding evidence-based best practices.

The professional literature for the field of psychiatric rehabilitation and treatment of mental and developmental disabilities is overcrowded with books, chapters in books, articles, and even entire journals devoted to the problems and care of disabled persons. But these publications have little redeeming value for practitioners. They are too technical, written by experts and academics for other experts and academics. Most textbooks or chapters on psychiatric rehabilitation, while full of citations and summaries of the research literature, rarely touch the day-to-day realities faced by practitioners. This manual of psychiatric rehabilitation offers practice-based evidence for helping each unique person work his/her way to recovery wherever he/she receives treatment.

Clinicians wrestle with the unique, individualized needs of each patient. Professionals and paraprofessionals struggle in the clinical trenches to liberate their patients from disabilities. Mental health providers and their consumers can benefit from a road map showing *what services* can be used *how, when,* and *where* in their collaborative efforts to achieve recovery. Disentangling how statistical differences between treatments are revealed by research, this manual offers directions for deciding how evidence-based practices may apply to this or that patient.

Recovery From Disability is written for all disciplines and for clinicians with all levels of experience in working with individuals who welcome practical modes of psychiatric rehabilitation. The purpose of this book is to equip practitioners with a tool kit of rehabilitation techniques. By becoming familiar with the best practices of psychiatric rehabilitation, clinicians will be able to help patients attain their personally relevant goals and a better quality of life.

▶ What Disciplines Can Use the Know-How and Competencies Described in This Book?

This manual of psychiatric rehabilitation is designed for the full spectrum of mental health professionals, paraprofessionals, peer counselors, consumer advocates, and administrators and managers of programs for mentally and developmentally disabled persons. The particular roles, interests, motivation, and previous experience of each individual will determine how the book will benefit them. In particular, the following mental health workers will find the book useful:

- Psychiatrists, psychologists, social workers, and nurses
- Occupational, activity, and recreation therapists; rehabilitation specialists; vocational counselors; employment specialists; and educators
- Case managers, personal support specialists, psychiatric technicians, and nursing aides
- Consumers of services, their families, policy makers, and other stakeholders in public and private services for mentally and developmentally disabled persons

While clinical competencies are rarely obtained by reading a book, I hope that the practical and clinical information in the following chapters is written with sufficient clarity, simplicity, and examples to:

- Enable experienced and self-directed practitioners to use or adapt the methods described in the book.

- Expose a broader range of less experienced practitioners to evidence-based best practices in the hope that their curiosity and desire to expand their therapeutic repertoires will be aroused. Ancillary training and supervision may be required for these workers to achieve competency in the use of the varied rehabilitation techniques.
- Provide administrators, policy makers, and consumers of services—patients, their family members, consumer advocates, and peer support personnel—with lucid and uncomplicated descriptions of contemporary methods of rehabilitation. The aim is to familiarize a broad array of readers with the methods required for optimal services and therapeutic outcomes.

▶ Who Is This Manual Intended For and What Level of Experience Is Needed?

This manual can be used by a wide range of readers with varying experience in psychiatric rehabilitation:

- Novices with little or no experience serving persons with serious mental and developmental disorders—in fact, this book can serve new clinical recruits as a training and orientation manual.
- Mental health professionals with a modest amount of experience and ability in psychiatric rehabilitation—you will find many new principles to light your way as well as useful methods of assessment and treatment to increase your competence.
- Mental health professionals who are knowledgeable and skilled in psychiatric rehabilitation—the 10 chapters of this book will hold many surprises for you: different ways for addressing clinical problems, modalities for removing impairments and disabilities, and pathways for promoting recovery from serious mental disability.
- Mental health teams that want to improve their functioning and clinical impact.
- Teachers and instructors responsible for undergraduate and graduate education, continuing professional education, or consumer education—this book will give you a structure and comprehensiveness that will address almost all of your didactic and seminar needs.
- Researchers—you will find the book useful for generating and testing hypotheses, the first step in designing studies.

● ● ● ● ● ● ● ● ● ● ● ● ● ●

▶ How Did the Subjects or Topics for Each Chapter Get a Place in the Book?

Individuals with mental and developmental disabilities have pervasive problems at the biological, social, psychological, and environmental levels. Therefore, each chapter contributes information, techniques, and treatment methods that address one or more of these problem dimensions:

- Functional assessment for helping patients to select realistic yet personally meaningful goals
- Illness management for teaching patients how to stabilize their symptoms and cognitive deficits
- Training in social and independent living skills for fostering autonomous functioning
- Family education, family support, and behavioral family therapy to help family members and other caregivers to better understand, cope with, and manage their loved one's illness and disability
- Vocational rehabilitation, including supported employment, that can give disabled persons a working life
- Efficient and effective ways to organize and deliver specific treatments to facilitate comprehensiveness, continuity, coordination, and collaboration in services
- Customization of services for individual patients, because "one suit does not fit all"
  - » Persons with more than one disorder (e.g., those with developmental, psychiatric, medical, and/or substance abuse disorders)
  - » Persons whose illness is refractory to customary pharmacological and psychosocial treatments
  - » Persons whose adaptation to community life is marred by aggressive behaviors

▶ How Can You Use This Book?

The book is written as a clinical manual or handbook for everyday use. Pick it up and turn its pages to chapters that give tangible and clear advice and ideas for effective services. You will find rich and graphic information for your practice. Research findings have been translated into practice-based services of immediate utility for those working in mental health centers, clinics and hospitals, day treatment centers, psychosocial clubhouses, community support and self-help programs, and even private offices. Therefore, any rehabilitation practitioner can find and use the book's panoply of basic assumptions and principles, ways to mobilize social supports, and methods of assessment and treatment. There will be no confusion in grasping the concepts and treatment modalities described in this manual. Simple English and a straightforward writing style are used. The author uses a minimum of technical terms and has excised most of the jargon that usually mars books on treatment.

The collective knowledge and abilities described in the book are ready to be plucked off the pages and inserted into treatment planning and services, while monitoring progress and the arduous march toward recovery. It is highly desirable to use this book as the foundation for a training program, course on psychiatric rehabilitation, continuing education workshop, in-service training, and consumer education. A mental health treatment team will find in the book a means of enhancing the clinical impact of the team through use of a common frame of reference. For example, in using flexible levels of intervention, mental health teams may have to offer more support and specific treatment to clinically stable patients attempting to overcome the social and vocational barriers to recovery. Teams and their patients "reading from the same page" enjoy greater consistency, better coordination, tighter collaboration, and superior outcomes.

Recovery From Disability also can be used in its own right with ease by individual practitioners whose patients, clients, or consumers express a desire to improve their social skills to find a friend, learn how to date and have a romance, improve relationships with family members, manage their own medication, develop a relapse prevention plan, or get a job. Effective psychiatric rehabilitation requires an alliance and partnership among disparate disciplines that have all too often been rivals, walled off from one another by tradition and outmoded assumptions about the nature, treatment, and prognosis of disabling mental and developmental disorders.

As physicians, psychiatrists, and all mental health practitioners move farther into the twenty-first century, we must engage our patients in a true collaboration for treatment and rehabilitation. This requires clinicians to educate patients, families, and other caregivers by transferring to them as much of our knowledge and expertise as is feasible and constructive. Then, they can be informed consumers of services with strengthened motivation and persistence in our joint pursuit of a better life. As participatory partners in treatment, our *disabled* patients will be *enabled* to make a successful journey to reach their personally relevant goals and recovery. It is my intention that this book, if its readers apply the principles and practices of psychiatric rehabilitation, can speed our way into a future when recovery is the rule, not the exception.

Terminology

There are certain conventions used in this manual that refer to individuals who provide treatment and those to whom treatment is provided. Other terms that are standardized for the benefit of consistency fall in the realms of type of disorder, illness, or disability. The terms *treatment* and *rehabilitation* are used interchangeably because they are inextricably intertwined. Some readers may associate "treatment" with pharmacotherapy and "rehabilitation" with social skills training. In actuality, patients prescribed medications will be much less likely to use their medications and gain the desired clinical benefits if they do not also receive training in the skills for self-administration and self-monitoring of medication, identifying the therapeutic and prophylactic effects of medication, distinguishing serious from minor side effects and how to react to each type, and negotiating and communicating with prescribing physicians to obtain optimal benefits.

In this volume, the terms *psychiatric rehabilitation* and *psychosocial rehabilitation* have considerable overlap. Both include functional assessment and the full range of psychological and social treatments and services that make up 1) the teaching or training of social and independent living skills and 2) family, vocational, social, peer, professional, and public supports for improved community functioning. Over and above the psychosocial realm, the term *psychiatric rehabilitation* includes assessment procedures related to psychiatric diagnosis, severity and range of symptoms, and cognitive impairments. Unless specific and measurable assessments are integrated into rehabilitative interventions aimed at improving adherence to treatment and remediation of cognitive deficits, progress toward recovery founders at the very start. Also under the rubric of *psychiatric rehabilitation* are psychosocial treatments that focus on reduction or elimination of symptoms and disturbing behaviors of severe mental disorders such as social learning therapy (token economy) and cognitive-behavioral therapy. Thus, *psychiatric rehabilitation* is a more inclusive term than *psychosocial rehabilitation*.

▶ Mental Health Professionals and Other Personnel

We often do not agree about the words describing the work we do, even if we do agree about the principles, values, and outcomes. The terminology that we use is influenced by the country and region where we live; our role and discipline in mental health; the type of patient we provide service to; whether inpatient or outpatient; the type of agency, facility, or program in which we work; and, most importantly, our own personal preferences and experiences.

Providers of treatment comprise the professionals and paraprofessionals who have training and experience in one of the mental health disciplines. Providers include psychiatrists, psychologists, social workers, nurses and nursing assistants, occupational and recreation therapists, psychiatric and rehabilitation technicians, and paraprofessionals of various stripes. Although it is not broadly known, the vast majority of persons who are employed by mental health facilities do not have graduate training in one of the disciplines that are recognized by certifying and licensing bodies. These are paraprofessionals with a college education or less who fill the ranks of clinical case managers and other day-in, day-out providers of services to the mentally ill in public mental health systems.

The term *provider* is avoided as much as possible in referring to those in the healing professions. Instead of a term emanating from an economic model, I have chosen to use terms referring to professionals as having clinical roles. Effective rehabilitation relies on clinicians and patients entering into human relationships that are characterized by genuine concern, nonpossessive warmth, empathy, mutual respect, understanding of cultural differences, and collaboration in setting goals, treatment decision making, and evaluation of progress. Given the indisputable recognition of mental disorders as stress-related biomedical disorders, it is important for helping professionals to enter into relationships in which they have the technical expertise and patients have the best knowledge of how an illness affects them. Treaters and patients need to share their respective perspectives for the sake of progress toward recovery. In the written or spoken word, terms like *provider* and *consumer* convey the view of mental health services as commodities that are exchanged in commercial enterprises. Since "words are eggs" and tend to hatch into concepts and actions that define practices, using terms such as *provider* and *consumer* reduces the humanistic character of the healing arts to a transaction in the marketplace.

By and large, I have used the terms *mental health professional, practitioner, clinician, therapist, trainer,* and *rehabilitation specialist* in making general reference to those who provide services to the seriously and persistently mentally ill—regardless of their discipline, training, or experience. While the professional training and competencies of members of multidisciplinary fields are differentiated, valued, licensed, and necessary for making distinctive contributions to patient care, I have endeavored to avoid the use of terms that identify specific disciplines when the text is referring to the broad class of mental health professionals. Repeating a list of the spectrum of disciplines ad nauseum when referring to generic roles of mental health service workers would be awkward and redundant.

> "The extreme aversion on the part of the caring professions to calling things by their proper names is one of the most vexatious 'issues' I have encountered as a father of a son with schizophrenia. The sick are no longer patients, but clients or service users. And, by implication, considered capable of evaluating their own needs, entering into contractual relations with doctors and other agencies whose function is to deliver the chosen service or care. This seems a surprising way of approaching people who, when ill, are almost by definition 'not in their right minds.'"
>
> TIM SALMON *THE GUARDIAN,*
> NOVEMBER 20, 2006

I have tried to minimize the use of the term *case managers* in describing those personnel who have the responsibility for treatment planning, monitoring, outreach, continuity, advocacy, and direct services for mentally disabled persons. Because it is such a prevalent term, I have not been entirely successful in avoiding its use or its apposite, *case management.* I much prefer the terms *personal support specialist* and *personal support services* because they connote a *personalized relationship* between the worker and the patient and the importance of *support* in the relationship as well as in the *specialist's* advocacy for support services needed by the patient from multiple community agencies.

Specialist is preferred to *manager* also because it conveys the high value inherent in the worker's competence in assessment, treatment planning, direct services, and liaison and consultation with other professionals and agencies. It is clear that the central role of the personal support specialist, when characterized by these competencies, deserves high value and esteem from colleagues as well as the field in general. Our patients with disabilities who are striving for recovery are deserving of specialists with a full spectrum of technical knowledge and skills as well as the ability to form and sustain mutually respectful alliances with their patients.

▶ Patient, Not Consumer

The terms *provider* and *consumer* are used as little as possible in this manual because they connote an impersonal "business relationship" between practitioner and patient. Mental health professionals should not be viewed as commercial entities "selling" their expertise through starchy and detached transactions with patients and families. The terms *consumer* and *provider* emerged in the 1990s when health care dollars became scarce and business people invaded clinical settings to manage health services more efficiently and make profits for their firms. Business jargon became commonplace; *patients* began to disappear, replaced by *consumers,* and *doctors* were supplanted by *providers.* The terms *provider* and *consumer* are perhaps appropriate in the lexicon of administrators and managers of mental health programs, medical economists, and services researchers.

The relationship between practitioner or doctor and patient is characterized by helping, healing, reduction in suffering, commitment, caring, and enduring concern. The "personal contract" that is implicit in this relationship is not unlike those that exist between marriage partners, clergy and parishioners, and teachers and students. If students are not characterized as "consumers" of knowledge and skills and teachers are not referred to as "providers" or "purveyors" of knowledge and skills, why should mental health patients and therapists be commercialized into consumers and providers?

These distinctions may appear trivial, but they are not. You treat patients as if they were members of your family. You talk to them. You comfort them. You take time to explain to them what the future may hold in store. Sometimes that future will be bleak. But you assure them that you will be there to help them face it.

You treat customers quite differently. Customers are in your place of business to purchase health care. You complete the transaction—health care for money. And then they aren't your customers any more. Taken a step further, you can make the case that the less time you spend with your customers, the better your bottom line will be. The doctor–patient relationship is critical to the integrity of the health care system. It is not disposable. Turning doctors into shopkeepers who regard patients as customers is unacceptable.

I know that the term *consumer* is fashionable these days and certainly politically correct. Efforts that empower patients to become more active and decisive in selecting their clinicians and treatment goals are overdue and admirable; however, to use terms like *consumer* and *provider* risks dehumanizing the honorable and venerable patient–doctor or patient–therapist relationship.

At the risk of departing from the zeitgeist and offending those who view the term *patient* as condescending and patronizing, I have used *patient* as consistently as possible throughout the book. In addition, given the scarcity of mental health professionals and the impracticality in almost all public mental health agencies of allowing patients to select their own clinicians, encouraging individuals seeking services that they are *consumers* with choices would only set them up for disappointment and frustration. If mentally disabled persons feel justified in fully participating in the choice of therapists and types of treatment, conflicts could emerge from their interactions with mental health professionals that could harm the therapeutic relationship and diminish the impact of treatment. Patients should be informed about the relative benefits and costs of various treatments as well as the competencies of their treaters in providing these treatments. It is the responsibility of the mental health specialist to educate patients and their families so they become informed, followed by encouragement to participate actively in the choice of treatment.

Patient refers to a person who is in treatment, being cared for, and receiving needed services to reduce symptoms and improve functional capacity. *Patient* is the desired term for individuals seeking treatment from physicians of all medical specialties. Are individuals undergoing surgery or renal dialysis considered consumers of their medical services? Do they wish to be called consumers? Using the term *consumers* for individuals receiving psychiatric services, but not for those receiving other types of medical and surgical services, reflects a troubled and ambiguous role of psychiatry in American health care.

If the point of using the term *consumer* is to enhance the participation and decision-making responsibility of patients in relation to their clinicians, a name change is an ineffective way of accomplishing that goal. Names should be changed to adjust descriptions of disorders or of those giving and receiving services as science reveals more about the conditions that we treat. To reduce stigma and rectify imbalances in the roles of clinician and patient, education and changes in the health care system are the preferred routes. In fact, the main purpose of this book is to provide knowledge, competencies, and attitudes to mental health professionals that will enable them to form collaborative and efficacious therapeutic partnerships with their patients and their patients' family members.

In addition, because the publisher of this book is American Psychiatric Publishing Inc., I have complied with its style requirements by using the term *patient*. Similarly, I have avoided the term *client* because it carries the connotation of being in contractual relationships such as those with lawyers, real estate agents, hairdressers, masseuses, and architects. We should not forget that the term *consumer* reflects a capitalistic way of defining transactions between people (Zealberg 1999). Dentists and surgeons do not refer to themselves as "providers" or their patients as "consumers." To do so in the field of psychiatry and mental health is tantamount to stigmatizing those with psychiatric disorders. Mentally ill individuals who have happily benefited from the type, amount, quality, and impact of the services they have received do not object to referring to themselves as "satisfied patients." Psychiatric disorders are illnesses; hence, the term *patient* is consistent with society's allocating funds for treatment and rehabilitation of persons with illnesses. For millennia, the term *patient* has been associated with an individual who is honorably and ethically in need and deserving of the special status as a recipient of medical treatment. Moreover, payments for medical and psychiatric services are justified by the assumption that the recipient is sick, disabled, and suffering in some way. Using the terms *consumers* and *providers* instead of *patients* and *practitioners* runs the risk of jeopardizing public and private health insurance benefits as well as disability pensions from workers' compensation, the Social Security Administration, and the Department of Veterans Affairs. In an era when health care costs are spiraling out of control, cutbacks in public and private insurance are accelerating, and lack of parity in health insurance continues to bedevil the mentally ill, services may be further constrained and compromised if those providing and using services aver that the individuals they are treating are not patients. Even stigma may be inadvertently increased if the public associates mentally ill persons with the term *consumer* because it may convey the impression that mental disorders are volitional, under a person's control, and not the result of a biomedical abnormality.

Preference is given to the following terms in referring to patients (i.e., clients, consumers) throughout the book: *person (or individual) with a mental disorder (or disability), mentally disabled, mentally ill, psychiatrically disabled, disabled person,* and *participant*. Humanizing those who are in need of psychiatric treatment and rehabilitation by referring to them as *persons* or *individuals* not only sidesteps alternative terms that may stigmatize or diminish the desirability of their taking an active and collaborative role vis-à-vis practitioners, but also highlights the importance of 1) emphasizing the uniqueness of each recipient of service with appropriate emphasis on his/her personal goals, strengths, deficits, and resources; and

2) individualizing treatment and rehabilitation to fit the individual's goals, needs, and phase of illness.

The term *survivor* has been used by a coterie of individuals who view themselves as having "survived" their illness and malevolent psychiatric services. When *survivor* is used to implicate treatment facilities and personnel as harmful, both patients and their treaters are stigmatized. Mental illness and its treatment become a no-win situation. Everyone loses. On the other hand, the term *survivor* can be used suitably to imply that recovery is possible and that mentally ill persons can overcome their disability—similar to survivors of cancer or strokes. The implication is that they are no longer disabled or even mentally ill—similar to survivors of cancer. This may be a felicitous term, since cancer survivors remain vulnerable to relapses, as would persons who may gain remissions and recoveries from their mental disorders. Surviving mental illness also means that individuals live their lives as fully as possible today, tomorrow, and every single day. Maintaining an experience of healthy survival also suggests that the individual has a therapist, psychiatrist, clinician, or treatment team who have been able to convey hope and realistic optimism, even when the patient himself/herself has lost confidence and hope. Surviving means learning about one's psychiatric condition, the therapies that are available, and their likelihood of favorable impact. With this information, survivors participate actively with their clinicians in selecting appropriate and relevant goals and deciding on a treatment plan.

When an individual with a mental disability enters treatment, the important choice of words to identify that individual has nothing to do with terms such as *patient, client, person, participant,* or *consumer.* The diligent and respectful clinician who wishes to engage in a collaborative relationship with the new patient asks the individual, "Would you like me to call you by your first name, your nickname, or your last name?" Giving the patient the choice of his/her preferred way of being addressed infuses esteem and consideration into the developing relationship. Similarly, the clinician should convey to the new patient how he/she prefers to be called: first or second name, prefaced by *Doctor* or not. Surveys have revealed that patients receiving psychiatric services do not harbor strong opinions regarding appellations such as *patient, client,* or *consumer;* in fact, only a tiny minority endorses the term *consumer* (Mueser et al. 1996). When a mental health professional initiates an open and low-key discussion of how a particular patient prefers to be addressed personally or collectively, enhanced feelings of empowerment may contribute to the therapeutic alliance and progress toward recovery. Table 1 lists many of the names used in this book, with their definitions.

● TABLE 1

Terminology for mental health professionals and patients used in this book

Client	An individual who is being treated for mental health or substance abuse problems in a social or rehabilitation setting (e.g., a residential care program) or in the private practice of a psychologist, social worker, marriage and family therapist, or counselor.
Clinician	An individual who uses a recognized scientific knowledge base and has the authority to direct the delivery of personal health services to patients. The term is typically applied in medical settings.
Consumer	An individual who is, has been, or may in the future be receiving care or services.
Mental health professional	An individual with specified training and/or experience in one of the mental health disciplines, such as psychiatry, clinical psychology, social work, psychiatric nursing, recreation therapy, rehabilitation counseling, employment counseling, and marriage and family counseling.
Paraprofessional	An individual who works in the field of mental health but lacks formal training in one of the mental health disciplines. Such individuals tend to learn how to carry out assessment and treatment procedures though observation and direct experience. They almost always have lower levels of responsibility than mental health professionals and are often supervised by the latter.
Patient	An individual who is cared for by a clinician for purposes of diagnosis, treatment, or prevention of illness or for maintaining recovery from illness. The term is usually applied in primary care and specialty medical settings, including psychiatric practice.
Practitioner	An individual who delivers clinical, rehabilitation, or psychosocial treatment to individuals in medical, clinical, or social settings.
Provider	A program, facility, or organization that delivers health care.
Purchaser	A group—such as an employer, unit of government, association, or coalition—that negotiates for and buys health care on behalf of a specified group, generally to cover specific benefits and services at reduced prices.

● **TABLE 1** (cont'd.)

| Stakeholders | Individuals and groups for whom the cost, availability, accessibility, and quality of care hold direct implications. These include individuals who receive care and their families, practitioners, public and private purchasers, managed care companies, accreditation organizations, and policy makers. |

▶ Mental Disabilities Associated With Mental Disorders

As clarified in Chapter 1 ("Rehabilitation as the Road to Recovery") of this book, a large proportion of persons with mental disorders experience disability in their lives for varying periods of time. In severe forms of schizophrenia, bipolar disorder, and treatment-resistant depression, disability can be long-term and even lifelong. Therefore, the term *mental disability* is preferentially used to delineate the disorder afflicting patients who are appropriate recipients of rehabilitation. Other terms are used as well, mostly interchangeably: *mental illness, mental disorder, psychiatric disorder, psychiatric disability*, and *psychiatric illness*. Additional terms used in the text to refer to disabilities affecting individuals for whom psychiatric rehabilitation is helpful are *serious and persistent mental disorders (or disabilities), severe mental illness,* and *chronic mental disorders*. Specific disorders that are associated with disability are also referred to: schizophrenia, bipolar disorder, mood disorders, depression, anxiety disorders, borderline personality disorder, and others. However, to avoid implying that a person with a mental disorder is defined as equivalent to the symptoms of the disorder, I have used terms such as *the person with schizophrenia* or *individuals having a mood disorder.*

▶ Locus of Treatment and the Impact of Treatment

While the book uses terms denoting the locus of treatment as the hospital, mental health center, psychiatric clinic, psychosocial clubhouse, partial hospital, day treatment center, and other facilities, it is the natural environment where the proverbial rehabilitation rubber hits the road to recovery. As much as possible, the modalities of treatment and rehabilitation described in this manual are evaluated in terms of benefits that accrue to patients in their natural environments—homes, work sites, schools, stores, public agencies, recreational facilities, and neighborhoods. Thus, the terms *natural environment, community,* and *everyday lives* are often used to identify the locales where treatment effects are translated into quality of life. Given the importance of mentally ill persons experiencing recovery in nonstigmatizing, normative living environments, segregated communities such as psychosocial clubhouses or day treatment centers are viewed as way stations for those on the road to recovery.

▶ References

Mueser KT, Glynn SM, Corrigan PW, et al: A survey of preferred terms for users of mental health services. Psychiatr Serv 47:760–761, 1996

Zealberg JJ: The depersonalization of health care. Psychiatr Serv 50:327–328, 1999

Rehabilitation as the Road to Recovery

1

Rehabilitation as the
Road to Recovery

Disability is where we start, recovery is our destination, and rehabilitation is the road we travel.

RECOVERY FROM disability is a familiar experience for all people, not just those with mental illness. Disability interferes with our customary abilities to participate in important daily activities, maintain our independence, and pursue our goals in work, family, social, and recreational life. Recovery returns us to our desired quality of life, sometimes with an enhanced appreciation of its value. Each of us has struggled with illnesses or injuries that disabled us in some way. Psychiatric and other types of medical disorders share the same impediments to personal, social, and vocational functioning, albeit in differing extensiveness, intensity, and duration.

An example of a common and universal illness that can disable us is an upper respiratory infection. When we catch a severe cold or flu, our head hurts, our respiratory passages become clogged, our energy dissipates, and our voice softens. We feel fatigue, frustration, and irritability, and we lose our ability to concentrate, to focus, and to plan ahead. These symptoms intrude upon our functional capacities at work, school, and home. Our desire flags for enjoying recreational activities, for communicating with our friends, for attending church, and even for completing basic self-care such as eating, personal grooming, dressing, and exercising. Yet, as the respiratory infection is controlled and eliminated by our natural defense mechanisms and treatment, we recover the functions, energy, enthusiasm, and optimism that were temporarily lost. As the illness is controlled, disability fades and we return to an active, productive, good life.

Enjoying a functional and good life—as good as it can get—is an important milestone for defining recovery. Disability and recovery are universal experiences; our lives are filled with episodes of various ailments that rob us of our previous level of functioning and autonomy for different lengths of time. Shouldn't mental disorders follow the same "laws" as other medical illnesses?

Some might protest that mental disorders are not like medical illnesses. Aren't they lifelong and totally disabling, bringing misery, demoralization, and hopelessness? Don't the seriously mentally ill sit in boardinghouses staring into space year after year? Haven't they lost the ability to communicate, work, make friends, live independently, and remember to take their medication? Isn't it true that mental illness afflicts most of the homeless people who roam our streets? Certainly, there wouldn't be so many mentally ill people in our jails and prisons if their disorders were treatable and reversible.

Yes, it is true that severe mental disorders such as schizophrenia are chronic, not readily reversible, and associated with long-lasting disability. But serious and persisting disability also is associated with illnesses that are viewed as "medical" rather than "psychiatric" or "mental": diabetes, cystic fibrosis, asthma, heart attack with residual angina and exercise intolerance, chronic lung disease, stroke, cancer, multiple sclerosis, HIV/AIDS, arthritis, kidney disease, and epilepsy. There are no cures for these illnesses. They don't go away with treatment—even when heroic treatments, such as heart, liver, and kidney transplants, are used.

The fact that a disease is not reversible or eliminated doesn't necessarily generate pessimism and resignation. Treatment can suppress the symptoms of severe and chronic medical illnesses. Moreover, rehabilitation can help most of those suffering from chronic medical diseases to regain a fairly normal life. After suffering a paralyzing stroke, a person can respond to speech therapy, occupational therapy, and physical therapy, which together can restore independent living. By learning about their illness, taking medication every day, and exercising their civil liberties, individuals with HIV/AIDS can obtain employment and maintain satisfying relationships with friends and family. With anti-inflammatory medication and relentless, customized exercises, persons suffering from rheumatoid arthritis can retain their mobility, work, play, and experience a satisfying quality of life. With effortful monitoring of blood glucose, judicious use of insulin, and regulation of diet, individuals with diabetes can function normally.

Just as persons suffering from severe and chronic medical diseases can recover, given proper treatment and rehabilitation, so too can those with serious and persisting mental disorders. In the past few decades, we have witnessed a sea change in the prospects for a good quality of life for persons with serious mental disorders. Chronic anxiety disorders are now eminently treatable with a combination of antidepressant medications and cognitive-behavioral therapy (CBT). With the advent of antidepressants, CBT, interpersonal therapy, and social skills training, major depressions can be limited to temporary interruptions of a person's life. Bipolar disorder can be controlled with mood stabilizers, adjunctive antidepressants and antipsychotics, family-focused therapy, and social rhythm therapy. Even schizophrenia, the most stigmatized of mental disorders, is rising from defeatism to expectations for recovery. In fact, severe mental disorders now are more effectively treatable and amenable to rehabilitation than most chronic disorders affecting other organs of the body.

> "Invalids should not be fused into a class that sets them apart from the general public, friends or kindred. Invalids should be restored to their original homes, and the communities to which they belong should absorb them, giving them occupations and domestic responsibilities."
>
> SYSTEM FOR THE ECONOMICAL RELIEF OF DISABLED SOLDIERS FROM THE CIVIL WAR (1864)

Of course, there are some notable differences between disorders of the brain and those of other systems of our human physiology. One salient difference is the impairments in cognition, emotion, and insight frequently found in mental disorders—and other brain diseases such as dementia, traumatic brain injuries, tumors, and epilepsy. Persons with serious mental disabilities may not recognize the nature and severity of their symptoms; lack insight, often attributing psychotic symptoms to influences external to themselves; have cognitive impairments that impede learning, memory, judgment, and problem-solving; and lack appreciation of their need for treatment. These problems complicate recovery because diagnosis and treatment are delayed and sometimes completely denied and refused. As for any disease, mental disorders that go untreated for a lengthy period of time grow more chronic and more difficult to treat effectively. The chapters of this manual are dedicated to suggestions for overcoming these unique obstacles to treatment that are inherent in serious mental disorders.

▶ What Is Disability?

People with severe mental disorders also experience disability, with symptoms and cognitive deficits intruding on their functional capacities and a good life. Disability associated with mental disorders is encoded in the *Diagnostic and Statistical Manual of Mental Disorders* criteria for a wide variety of disorders as "symptoms cause impairments in social, occupational, or other important areas of functioning" (American Psychiatric Association 2000). Persons with disabilities stemming from their mental disorders are candidates for psychiatric rehabilitation. Modalities of rehabilitation aim to reverse or compensate for impairments and disabilities, thereby enabling persons saddled with such burdens to function in a more normal

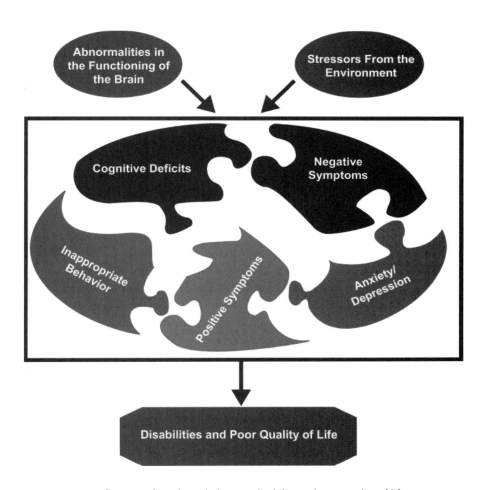

FIGURE 1.1 Influences of psychopathology on disability and poor quality of life.

fashion. Figure 1.1 graphically depicts how psychopathology contributes to disability and a poor quality of life. However, there are many other personal and environmental factors that contribute to disability—factors that are often more decisive than psychopathology and more amenable to treatment and rehabilitation.

HOW IS DISABILITY CONCEPTUALIZED?

Most people would agree that psychiatric disability represents one or more *functional abnormalities that interfere with an individual's autonomy* in work, education, family and social relations, recreation, and independent living. As shown in Figure 1.2, psychiatric disability is one element in a sequence of personal and social consequences of a mental disease. The sequence begins

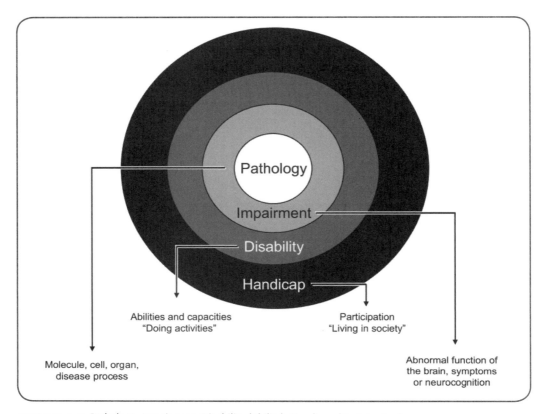

FIGURE 1.2 Pathology–Impairment–Disability (Ability)–Handicap (Participation).

with the presumption that the etiology of mental disorders ultimately will be found to be associated with biological *pathology* in the brain. Abnormalities at the level of genes and molecules, cells, neural networks, neurotransmitter systems, and reverberating connections among brain regions are being investigated for their relevance to psychopathology. Lacking an understanding of the specific etiology of a mental disorder should not deter us from the task of designing effective rehabilitation modalities, because many diseases, such as puerperal fever, scurvy, and cholera, were controlled before the specific pathogen was known.

But the underlying etiology of mental disorders does not only reside in some pathological process in the brain. The genesis of almost all diseases derives from a complex interaction of genetic, environmental, and behavioral influences on the implicated organ. As a result of their genetic endowment, brain functioning, and social development, individuals play an active role in selecting, modifying, and constructing their environments. In turn, their environments affect their behavior and its brain substrates for good or ill (Kendler and Baker 2006). Thus, we can say that it is the balance among genes, brain abnormalities, behavioral and cognitive capacities, and the environment that determines disability.

The adverse effects of the presumptive, pathological abnormalities of the brain on the functions of the central nervous system are termed *impairments*. Pathology of mental disorders, at its molecular and neuronal level, is as yet unknown, but impairments are seen, heard, and felt. Impairments are measurable. They are dysfunctions of learning, concentration, perception, decision making, judgment, and memory, as well as symptoms of mental disorders. In turn, cognitive and symptom impairments lead to *disabilities* in everyday functioning and adjustment. For example, *cognitive impairments* may limit what and how much a person can learn or perform at work or school. If verbal learning and memory are seriously limited, a person is not likely to perform well in school or in a job that requires listening, reading, and remembering. Cognitive impairments, such as poorly sustained attention, inaccurate perception of social and emotional cues, limited verbal memory, and deficits in planning, decision making, and problem solving, have been associated with disabilities in socialization, employment, self-care skills, money management, and treatment adherence. Disabilities also may derive from *symptom impairments* because symptoms can preoccupy a person and interfere with performance of skills and activities of daily living.

When the community or society does not provide supportive services and accommodations to individuals with disabilities that can enable them to function more normally and achieve their personal goals, *handicaps* are said to be present. Handicaps restrict the range of a person's participation in everyday life and citizenship. Some typical handicaps and their accommodations are as follows:

- Inability of paraplegic and other wheelchair-bound individuals to gain access to recreational activities and places of business. *Automated lifts in buses and cars, removal of curbs so wheelchairs can cross streets, and installation of ramps to permit access into buildings are required.*
- Lack of assistance in mobility for blind persons. *Trained Seeing Eye dogs, braille books and books on tape for reading, mobility training with canes, beeps from street crossing lights, and elevators announcing each floor make it possible for visually impaired persons to travel.*
- Insufficient time for mentally ill persons with cognitive deficits to complete school exams in a timely fashion or to learn and memorize concepts and facts. *Disabled student offices provide tutors, assistance in taking notes at lectures, study aides, and longer times to complete exams.*
- Problems that mentally ill or mentally retarded individuals have obtaining and sustaining jobs because of lack of initiative and problem

solving, poor learning, and deficient social skills. *In supported employment, employment specialists and job coaches assist the individual in obtaining a job, teach him/her how to successfully perform in the job, and serve as liaisons among the patient, employer, and responsible mental health treatment team.*

In the most recent revision of the *International Classification of Impairments, Disabilities, and Handicaps,* the terms *impairment, disability,* and *handicap* have been given mirror-image antonyms: *functioning, ability–activity,* and *participation* (World Health Organization 2001). These new appellations highlight the positive attributes of a disabled individual and delineate the goals of rehabilitation. The new terms are also felt to be less stigmatizing to the disabled person, reducing the negative and rejecting attitudes of the public toward the disabled in general and the mentally disabled in particular. The positive concepts used in the new terminology also lend themselves to public education that may further reduce stigma at the level of society.

Disability is not an intrinsic attribute of an individual that is solely determined by the person's *pathology* and *impairments.* The type and extent of disability experienced by a mentally ill person are influenced by a host of stress and protective factors in the 1) person, 2) environment, 3) complexity of the social or vocational roles available in a community or society, and 4) accessibility, comprehensiveness, quality, and efficacy of treatment and rehabilitation services. These manifold factors determining a person's level of disability are shown graphically in Figure 1.3. In this diagram, the degree of disability experienced by a mentally ill person is influenced by the individual's skills, knowledge, problem-solving capacity, medication adherence, family support, role expectations, and community resources. If the environment provides special learning experiences, supportive and compensatory environments, and accessible and high-quality rehabilitation services, the person's disability will be mitigated and his/her abilities will be magnified.

WHO ARE THE DISABLED MENTALLY ILL?

Approximately 14 million Americans live with disabilities resulting from mental disorders that hamper their daily life functioning and impede their quality of life. The number is even greater if the estimated 1.5 million individuals with developmental disabilities are added. Psychiatric rehabilitation can benefit all those whose psychiatric disabilities endure beyond a relatively brief treatment of symptoms. Diagnostic ramifications, as well as

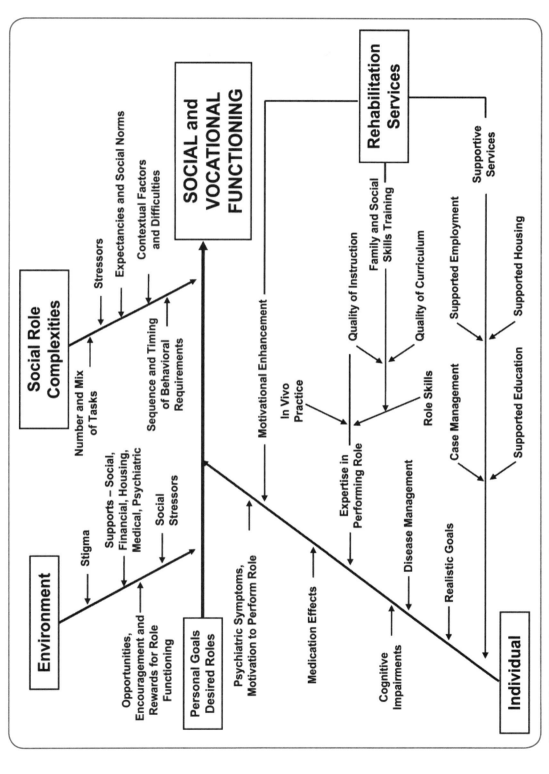

FIGURE 1.3 Factors that influence social and vocational functioning.

legal requirements for determining eligibility for disability benefits from the government, make it essential that the criteria for deciding that someone is disabled be clear and consistent.

Several terms have been used in the literature to delimit the population of the mentally disabled. Most frequent are terms such as *severely mentally ill, chronic mental patients,* and *seriously and persistently mentally ill.* These definitions assume a diagnosis of a major mental disorder, presence of functional incapacities, and receipt of disability benefits from Social Security. The NIMH has specified a three-dimensional definition for demarcating disability among persons with severe mental disorders that is somewhat modified here in accord with recent research. A disabled *mentally ill* patient has a:

- Diagnosis of a schizophrenia spectrum disorder, mood disorder, anxiety disorder, or pervasive developmental disorder.
- Duration of treatment of 2 years or more.
- Extreme psychosocial dysfunction as reflected by a score of 50 or less on the Global Assessment of Functioning Scale on Axis V in the American Psychiatric Association's *Diagnostic and Statistical Manual of Mental Disorders.* This range of scores is consistent with severe difficulty in social, occupational, or school functioning.

Surveys of the mentally ill in several countries have determined that 49% meet the criteria above (Bijl and Ravelli 2000; Ormel et al. 2004). Epidemiologically defined, the prevalence rate for psychiatric disability is 2.32 per 1,000 population. It may be surprising to mental health professionals who work outside the public mental health system to realize that 42% of patients with nonpsychotic disorders meet the criteria for severe dysfunction. That is not so different from the 58% of psychotic patients who are considered severely dysfunctional. Mood disorders, which are so common that approximately 20% of the population will have at least one episode during a lifetime, are the number one cause of work disability among persons in the age group of 15–44. Even when treated with the best, clinically informed, and evidence-based techniques, more than half of persons with major depression are functionally impeded by symptoms and disability.

WHO ARE ADJUDICATED FOR DISABILITY BENEFITS AND CONSERVATORSHIPS?

In many states, some persons with severe mental disorders are considered so severely disabled that they are adjudicated as needing a conservator or guardian. In the best interests of the disabled person, conservators or guardians make judgments, decisions, and actions regarding the individual's treatment, money, and residence. Conservatorships are often granted by courts of law for 1-year, renewable periods. Individuals are candidates for conservatorship if they are unemployed, indolent, friendless, homeless, and dependent on others for daily living needs. If, at the end of a conservatorship period, the person can demonstrate that his/her impairments and disabilities no longer present a danger to self or others or interfere with obtaining appropriate food, clothing, and shelter, the conservatorship can be discontinued.

The federal government, through the medium of the Social Security Administration, has set criteria for determining psychiatric disability. A person must be adjudicated as mentally disabled through a psychiatric and administrative process before disability benefits are made available for life supports. The requirements include such impairments and disabilities as:

- Having the specific symptoms of a bona fide, well-documented mental disorder that meets DSM-IV criteria (American Psychiatric Association 1994, 2000).
- Failure to carry out activities of daily living—self-care, personal hygiene, home maintenance, care of personal possessions, use of public transportation, and buying, preparing, and eating appropriate foods.
- Lack of communication skills, resulting in poor social relations with marked social isolation or withdrawal.
- Inability to maintain a reasonable pace and persistence in work or worklike tasks.
- Likelihood of relapsing when exposed to stressors inherent in entry-level jobs.

Eligibility for Social Security disability benefits is reevaluated on an annual basis, since it is recognized that treatment, rehabilitation, and time could all make a difference in the individual's level of functioning.

A large number of individuals with disparate mental disorders, listed here, are often deemed disabled as defined by the various criteria delineated above.

- Schizophrenia
- Bipolar disorder
- Major depression and dysthymia
- Obsessive-compulsive disorder
- Social phobia
- Panic and agoraphobia

> "The psychosocial impairment associated with mania and major depression extends to all areas of functioning and persists for years, even among individuals who experience sustained resolution of clinical symptoms."
>
> CORYELL ET AL. (1993)

> "Among 2839 patients with bipolar disorder who were in continuing treatment and self-help groups, 64% were unemployed and few were symptom-free for six months."
>
> KUPFER ET AL. (2002)

> "In a cohort of 117 persons with bipolar disorder, 51% were unemployed, 21% worked part-time or as volunteers and only 27% had full-time, competitive employment."
>
> DICKERSON ET AL. (2004)

> "When studies of psychosocial outcome in bipolar disorder are examined in aggregate, upwards of 60% [of individuals] fail to regain full functioning in occupational and social domains, suggesting that comprehensive rehabilitation may be essential to reduce the morbidity of this disorder."
>
> MACQUEEN ET AL. (2001)

- Posttraumatic stress disorder
- Some personality disorders such as borderline, schizotypal, and schizoid
- Developmental disorders such as pervasive developmental disorders, and Down's syndrome

The challenge of rehabilitation is to power the movement of disabled persons toward recovery by helping them develop abilities and skills and creating supports in vocational, educational, recreational, and social realms that enable them to participate fully as citizens. While this book will focus on the reversal of disabilities associated with mental disorders, the same principles and techniques of rehabilitation can be adapted for application to those with developmental disorders. Because the functioning of developmentally disabled persons has been hampered from the very start of their lives, the term *habilitation* may be more appropriate than *rehabilitation*.

How Is Recovery Related to Disability?

As indicated in Figure 1.2, abilities are still present in the face of disabilities. People with serious mental disorders are individuals who have many interests, goals, and strengths, debunking the view that mental illness must be a defining attribute for a person. Disabled individuals are not disabled or mentally ill 24 hours a day, 7 days a week. Even patients with severe mental disorders, such as schizophrenia, continue to participate in their daily lives, with their families, and in their communities, despite the burden of cognitive, behavioral, and social dysfunction, as well as the handicaps of stigma, neglect, and atrocious housing foisted on them by an aloof society. Recovery demands that we and our patients identify positive qualities that can be tapped for the arduous march toward a more functional life. We need only to look and listen for the personal assets held by the mentally ill. This important task does not require digging a mine into the unconscious or peering into the brain. Strengths are on the surface for all to see if we focus on them for creating a treatment plan.

Even in persons with the greatest disability, positive attributes can be found. The glass is always half full *and* half empty. Rehabilitation challenges practitioners to recognize and build on each person's abilities, attractiveness, endearing qualities, uniqueness, and heroic persistence in the face of adversity. Catch people doing and saying normal and adaptive things and let them know that it made you feel good, gave you a boost, made your day, put a smile on your face, and gave you respect for them. A responsive social environment is the cement that builds strengths needed for the long journey to recovery. Rehabilitation provides positive, responsive environments. It has a dual function: to reduce impairments and disabilities while strengthening cognitive, social, family, vocational, recreational, self-care, money management, and other independent living skills.

What interventions derive from therapeutic environments? Since medications come from pharmaceutical companies and prescribing psychiatrists, they are important elements from the environment. While medications exert their effects on the brain, they do so as agents of the environment. Similarly, cognitive-behavioral therapies, social skills training, supported employment, and assertive community treatment are also elements available from a therapeutic environment. When we talk about "wellness" and a "healthy society," we are in actuality pinpointing all of the salutary, environmental influences that can affect skills, relationships, cognitions, imagery, physiology, emotions, and relationships.

A mutually valued human relationship is the bedrock of effective rehabilitation. Whether involving a professional practitioner, paraprofessional, peer advocate, outreach worker, clergyperson, family member, or other natural support person, a therapeutic relationship is marked by:

- Development of a helping and confiding connection that conveys confidence that the unique attributes and strengths of the disabled person will permit a life with satisfaction and self-acceptance.
- Personal qualities of the helping person that engender positive expectations for the future, even in the face of periodic reversals, frustrations, and failures.
- A therapeutic process that provides opportunities for success experiences with shared enthusiasm and celebration.
- Understanding that meaningful changes in the quality of life can occur

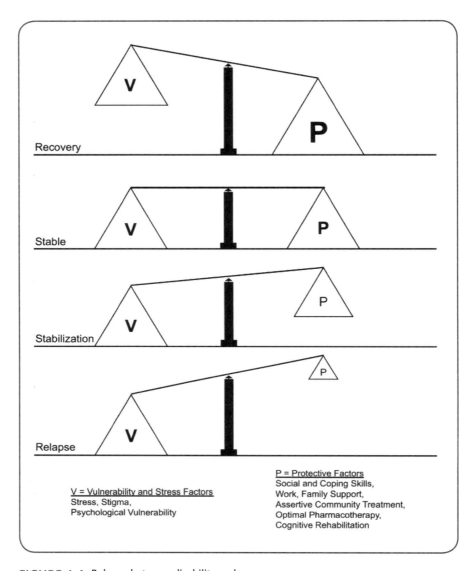

FIGURE 1.4 Balance between disability and recovery.

along with gradual insight into the nature of the illness and disability linked to the importance of treatment.

Resourcefulness and strengths at the level of the person and community are counterweights to impairments and disabilities of serious mental disorders. The dynamic balance between factors promoting wellness and those associated with disability is shown in Figure 1.4. By adding rehabilitation to the teeter-totter, using available evidence-based interventions, we can shift the balance from impairments, disability, and handicap to recovery and integration into the community. A mental health practitioner who does not grasp the capabilities of a patient is like the captain of a ship without a rudder.

EXAMPLE

"Recovery can mean many things. It can be a process as well as an endpoint. It is not necessarily the disappearance of symptoms, but the attainment of meaningful goals for one's life. Recovery means finding hope and the belief that one may have a better future. It is achieving social re-integration, finding a purpose in life and work. In addition, religious and spiritual faith plays a positive role in facilitating recovery." (Murphy 2007)

What Is Recovery?

Trying to define recovery is akin to the proverbial blind men who try to describe an elephant by feeling its various body parts. Just as an elephant is not solely its trunk, eyes, ears, legs, feet, abdomen, or tail, recovery comprises many interconnected definitions within an overarching concept. The facets or dimensions of the concept of recovery derive from:

- The vantage points of those who are offering their definitions.
- Objective versus subjective criteria identified by professionals and consumers for the definition.
- A focus on clinical and functional outcome versus personal experience and values.

Practitioners and researchers tend to emphasize objective, measurable criteria for defining recovery—for example, holding a job or attending school, living independently, and self-managing medication. Thus, clinical definitions of recovery center on operational descriptions of outcome at some point in time. Consumers emphasize subjective indications of recovery such as meeting the challenge of disability throughout the course of a disorder with hope for the future and aspirations to gain a sense of self-value and purpose in the present. Through their own perspective of what is important, psychiatrists tend to emphasize symptomatic remission and adherence to medication regimens. Psychologists emphasize cognitive functioning, self-efficacy, and social, family, and work functioning. Sociologists focus on economic well-being, reduced use of mental health services, social networks, and coping with stigma.

In fact, recovery encompasses all of these meanings. We can conceive of definitions and terms related to the subjective experiences of persons as they recover from a mental disorder. This includes experiences from the very beginning of a disorder, since struggling with the symptoms, hospitalizations, medication side effects, and attempting to return to a functional and self-respecting life begin almost immediately following the onset of any illness. We might define this phase as "recovering from mental illness," as it involves making efforts to gain control over the illness, to develop a collaborative relationship with one's treaters and caregivers, and to achieve progress in reaching one's personal goals and reclaiming selfhood. We can also define recovery from a clinical point of view—as an outcome of treatment, rehabilitation, community support, and personal striving that results in a level of functioning that is tantamount to normal.

EXAMPLE

Several programs have been initiated to promote recovery by changing the irrational fears and trepidation that constitute stigma among all segments of the population. *Stamp Out Stigma,* or SOS, combats the negative myths and stereotypes associated with mental illness through the efforts of recovered patients who give presentations to audiences in schools, colleges, commercial enterprises, and voluntary associations. They discuss their experiences with mental illness, treatment, and recovery, as well as answer questions about mental health issues. A similar antistigma effort, *In Our Own Voice,* is sponsored by the National Alliance on Mental Illness (NAMI). NAMI also seeks to change public opinions through *StigmaBusters,* a group of family members that scrutinizes the media—especially television and the movies—exerting pressure to change or remove stigmatizing terms like "crazy" and programs that reinforce misconceptions of mental illness.

HOW IS RECOVERY DEFINED WHEN VIEWED THROUGH AN OBJECTIVE, CLINICAL LENS?

Most people would agree that recovery from any illness is consistent with a life within the broad, widely accepted range of normalcy. For those with symptoms, cognitive impairments, and disabilities of a major mental disorder, normal functioning is elusive. Symptoms such as depression, mania, hallucinations, delusions, obsessions and compulsions, severe anxiety, and thought disorder intrude on the everyday life activities of persons with mental disorders. Cognitive impairments such as deficits in memory, social perception, and learning impede satisfactory involvement in social and vocational roles. For disabled persons, functioning is laborious, accompanied by restrictions, loss of pleasure, and loss of spontaneity.

The definition of recovery encompasses functioning within normal limits in those very same dimensions of life that are abnormal for disabled persons. Thus, to be considered *recovered* from a serious mental disorder, a person should have:

- A sustained remission of symptoms that constitute the diagnosis at a subclinical level of frequency and severity.
- Full- or part-time engagement in an instrumental role activity, such as work or school, that is constructive, productive, and age-appropriate.
- A life independent of supervision by family or other caregivers such that the individual is responsible for day-to-day needs in managing money, medication, appointments, shopping, food preparation, and personal possessions.
- Cordial family relations.
- Recreational activities in normative places and settings.
- Satisfying peer relationships characterized by participation in an active friendship, with companions or a social network.

While other medical diseases use various durations of the criteria above for determining recovery (e.g., in cancer, 5-year survivals), my colleagues and I consider 2 years of continuously fulfilling the criteria as meeting the definition of the state of *recovered*. It should be noted that significant alleviation or reasonable remission of symptoms is not, by itself, sufficient for a person to have reached a state of recovery. There are many patients who have received effective pharmacological and psychosocial treatments, with excellent reductions or remissions of their symptoms, but continue to experience functional difficulties. Some readers may find this operational definition too restrictive, too optimistic, or not sufficiently inclusive; for example, some would argue that having a satisfying quality of life and self-esteem should be included as criteria. I have elected not to include these as required elements because they are often highly correlated with the other criteria; also, they are not always present in persons who meet the other criteria for normality and have no mental disorder.

The objective criteria for recovery, especially independent living, are almost impossible to attain if appropriate housing is not available. Housing is not only a basic need and foundation for stability in pursuing the goals linked to recovery; it also enables individuals to participate in community life (O'Hara 2007). Because of stigma, lack of federal and local funding, and the disconnect between agencies responsible for mental health services and housing, enormous numbers of persons with mental disabilities do not have decent, safe, affordable, and secure housing that meets their needs and preferences. One can view the humanistic ethos of a society by how its mentally ill are treated and housed. By that reckoning, the United States falls far behind many western European countries that provide more generous financial entitlements for the mentally disabled. With more disability income, mentally ill individuals in Sweden, Norway, Denmark, and Holland can choose to live in apartments that are indistinguishable from those of the general population.

The mentally ill prefer to live in less restrictive, supported housing that is integrated into ordinary neighborhoods—not segregated in homeless encampments, group homes, or other facilities earmarked for psychiatric patients. Substantial barriers are posed by segregated housing to developing friendships, enjoying family life, participating in normative social and recreational activities, working or attending school, taking responsibility for independent functioning, and gaining access to evidence-based services (Fakhoury et al. 2002; Tanzman 1993). In the United States, family members are the primary spark plugs in creating and advocating for better housing.

EXAMPLE

Homes for Life is a nonprofit organization in Los Angeles formed by family members of the mentally ill. Fund-raising and grants have enabled their mentally ill residents to live in newly constructed or renovated apartments and homes that offer assured, lifelong residences with supportive services that are available to meet each person's needs throughout the various phases and levels of disability stemming from a mental disorder.

HOW IS RECOVERY DEFINED WHEN VIEWED THROUGH A SUBJECTIVE, PERSONAL LENS?

The process of *recovering* from a serious mental disorder takes place on a continuum, with progress over time marked by many challenges and the development of resilience. By the time a person reaches the specific operational criteria that define recovery, there has been an accumulation of social and independent living skills, personal strengths, and more positive self-

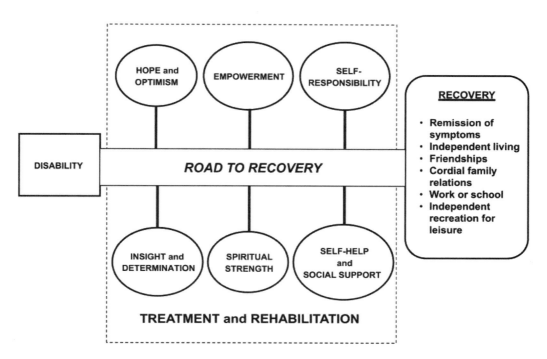

FIGURE 1.5 Positive factors propelling progress toward recovery.

appraisals. The process can be seen as the growth of the individual toward a normal and satisfying life.

As shown in Figure 1.5, moving on the pathway to a state of being recovered involves efforts to persist in coping with the symptoms and functional restrictions of a mental illness while carving out a meaningful life and valued sense of integrity. Many subjective experiences, as well as objective features, are often present as an individual moves along the continuum from illness and disability to recovery. These include:

- *Hope* or realistic optimism for a better future that comes from active coping with symptoms and disability as well as reclaiming a positive sense of self.
- *Empowerment* that comes from success in reaching one's goals, participating in treatment, and finding new roles that are satisfying and valued by society.
- *Spiritual strength* that can overcome adversity and connect people with faith and hope.
- *Self-help and social support from peers* that are eroding the harmful legacy of patronizing and authoritarian treaters.
- *Destigmatization* of mental illness and of those who suffer from it.

The close connections between factors related to positive movement on the road to recovery on the one hand and to the state of recovery on the other are shown in Figure 1.5. For example, while hope, realistic optimism for the future, and greater acceptance of oneself all help to propel patients along the road to recovery, these positive attitudes remain operative even after a person meets the criteria for having recovered. In fact, sustaining the state of recovery is almost always dependent upon maintaining an optimistic mind-set together with the kind of empowerment that comes from treatment relationships infused with informed choice, shared goals, and active collaboration by the patient. In short, subjective and objective experiences of recovery are interdependent and reciprocal.

The process of *recovering* is a journey that features liberation from symptoms by "getting a life" despite an illness with persisting symptoms. The process of recovery is quickened by exchanging alienation for meaningful relationships, responsibility for oneself rather than dependence on others, and integration into the community. The acronym REFRESH sums up elements that contribute to a normal life in the community. *Refresh* is an apt term for the concept of recovery because it signifies renewal, restoration of spirit, endurance, and reinvigoration. To refresh is to enliven a disabled person for *growth and development*. In addition, the process of recovering from a serious mental disorder is refreshing.

Relationships	people with whom to share experiences, feelings, and dreams
Empowerment	self-respect that comes from participation, success, and achievement
Family	cordial relations with reciprocity of affection and consideration
Recreation	enjoying community activities in normal places
Education	learning the knowledge and skills required for independent living
Spiritual	strength for the struggle for personal meaning, belief that one is not alone
Hope	having goals with positive expectations for self-improvement

HOW OFTEN DO SERIOUSLY MENTALLY ILL PERSONS RECOVER?

There have been efforts to define recovery from substance dependence disorders, major depression, and bipolar disorder as well as schizophrenia. However, both the concept and the definition of recovery from addictions have been restricted to abstinence from alcohol or illicit drugs. Recovery from mood disorders has focused exclusively on remission of symptoms of depression and mania and prevention of relapses. Recovery from schizophrenia has been defined more broadly and has received much more empirical investigation. Using various operational definitions that include sustained symptom remission and reasonably normal social and personal functioning, investigators in Europe, the United States, Canada, and Japan have reported recovery rates for schizophrenia patients at all stages of the illness—from young persons with recent onset of illness to more chronic patients with illnesses lasting as long as 30–40 years.

WHAT DOES LONG-TERM FOLLOW-UP OF RECOVERY IN PATIENTS WITH CHRONIC SCHIZOPHRENIA TELL US?

Long-term follow-up studies of patients who had schizophrenia for 20–40 years have consistently found recovery rates from 45% to 68% (Harding et al. 1992; Liberman and Kopelowicz 2005). These results, graphically depicted in Figure 1.6, were unexpected because they challenged conventional wisdom on schizophrenia as a disorder entailing lifelong disability. The field of psychiatry was not prepared to accept such an optimistic picture of persons with schizophrenia. As a result, the research was buried in journals collecting dust in libraries and was exhumed only recently by interest in the concept of recovery.

The extent of normalization in patients with long-standing schizophrenia in what is arguably the best of these studies, as highlighted in Table 1.1, makes clear the good quality of life of persons who had gradually recovered from their illnesses over many years of treatment and rehabilitation. Contrary to popular misconceptions, the recovery of persons who have had schizophrenia for most of their lives is not a result of the illness "burning out" because of aging. When a control group of patients matched for age, duration of illness, social class, and geographic locale were evaluated later in life, only half as many met criteria for recovery. The main difference in rates of recovery between sites is the comprehensiveness, continuity, consistency, and consumer-responsiveness of the treatment and rehabilitation available over many years.

The recent publication of an extraordinary, prospective study of more than 1,000 persons with schizophrenia from 14 countries in the developed and developing world shines new light on our understanding of recovery from schizophrenia (Hopper et al. 2007). Careful follow-up assessments were conducted over a 2-year period 12–26 years after the cohort was first diagnosed and evaluated. Structured and reliable instruments were used in the assessments. An amazing 60% of the individuals were rated as recovered as judged by clinical ratings and overall symptom and disability status at the

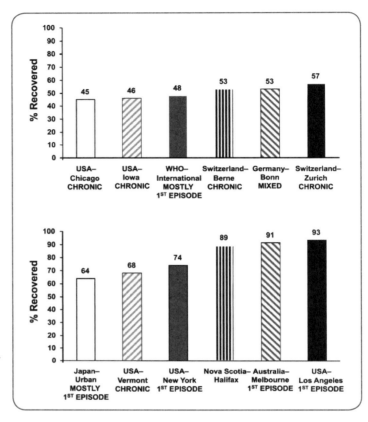

FIGURE 1.6 Rates of recovery in long-term follow-up studies of schizophrenia.

● **TABLE 1.1**

Outcomes of patients with long-standing schizophrenia who recovered

Global Assessment Scale above 61 points (in normal range)	66%
Not hospitalized in past year	82%
Two or fewer hospitalizations in past 20–25 years	64%
No current psychotic symptoms	68%
Taking antipsychotic medication regularly	25%
Have close friends	68%
Currently employed or involved in worklike activity	60%
Living independently and meeting self-care needs	81%
Leading a "full life" (self-reported)	~66%

Source. Harding et al. 1987.

time of follow-up, and 74% of the schizophrenia patients were employed to some extent. The best predictor of recovery was the proportion of time that the individual was psychotic during the 2 years after onset of illness. This finding is consistent with other research suggesting that duration of untreated psychosis is a salient prognostic indicator and may even serve as an index of enduring damage to certain structures in the brain. Fortunately, this obstacle to recovery is modifiable through early detection and case-finding, followed by rapid treatment intervention.

The "clinician's illusion" also yields an underestimation of the extent to which persons with schizophrenia and other serious mental disorders function normally, thereby meeting the objective and subjective criteria for recovery. For example, practitioners tend to disproportionately see and treat patients with schizophrenia who have disorders of longer duration, greater chronicity and severity, and more comorbidity. Approximately half of persons with schizophrenia are not in treatment at any one time, as determined by epidemiological studies (Mezzich and Ustun 2005). Many of these individuals would meet our definitions of recovery. Thus, the selection bias inherent in determining patienthood places another large group of individuals who have recovered from schizophrenia below treaters' radar screens.

HOW RAPID IS RECOVERY IN RECENT-ONSET SCHIZOPHRENIA?

Young people with schizophrenia bounce back from their illness with particular resilience. Studies of individuals within the first few years of their onset of schizophrenia have shown substantial remissions of positive and negative symptoms in over two-thirds of cases. Results from two reports (Figure 1.7) illustrate the rapid recovery of young patients with schizophrenia who are given the benefit of comprehensive treatment and rehabilitation. At the UCLA Schizophrenia Aftercare Clinic, over 80% of patients achieved good remission of positive symptoms, and over 90% were able to return at least half-time to work or school (Nuechterlein et al. 2006) (Figure 1.7, bottom). Similar good results have been reported from the Nova Scotia Early Psychosis Program (Whitehorn et al. 2002). In the latter program, over 60% of the patients achieved normal community functioning, and over 50% returned to their pre-illness life trajectory (Figure 1.7, top). At both sites, multidisciplinary teams offered optimal antipsychotic medication; flexible, need-based case management; individualized goal-oriented therapies; family and patient education; and state-of-the-art vocational rehabilitation.

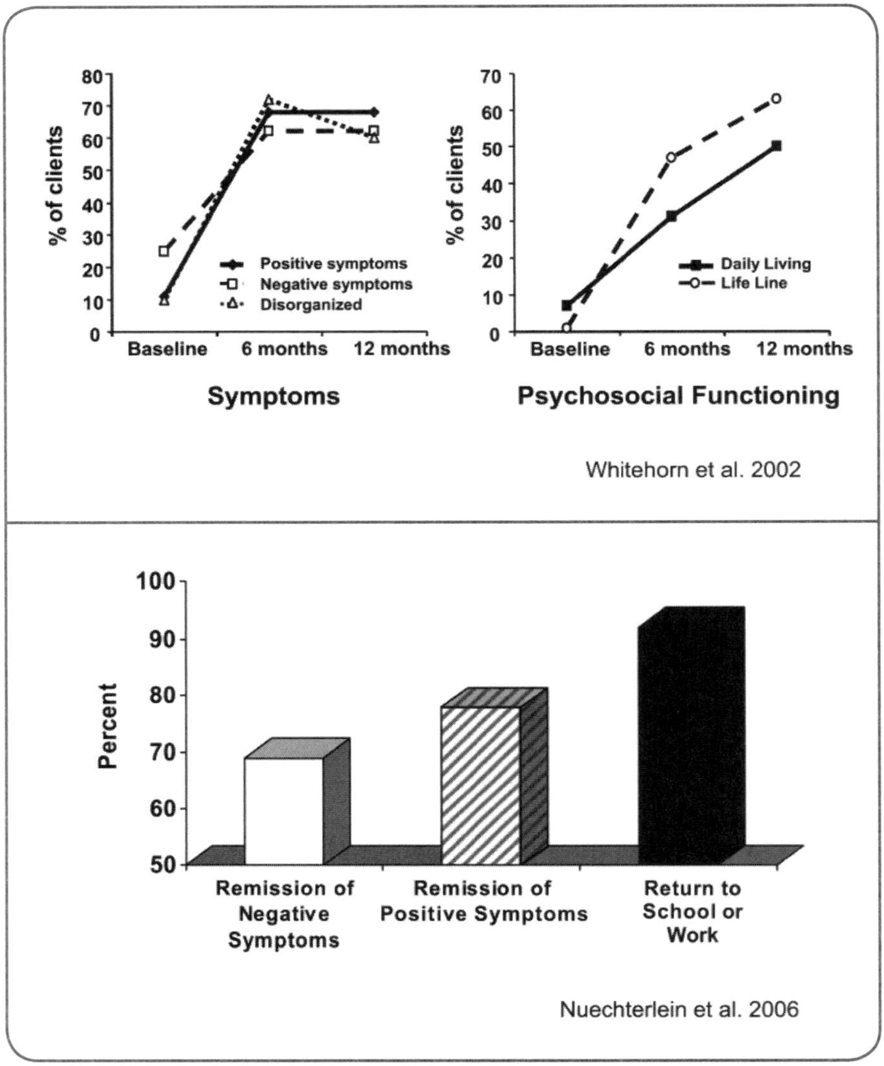

FIGURE 1.7 Recovery of young persons with recent onset of schizophrenia. (Top) Rate of recovery after 12 months of treatment for young persons with schizophrenia following their first psychotic episode. Definition of recovery includes symptom remission, unsupervised daily living, and resumption of their lifeline in appropriate social and occupational roles. (Bottom) Rate of recovery after 12 months of treatment for young persons within 2 years of their first psychotic episode. Recovery defined by symptom remission and resumption of employment or school in normal settings. *Source.* Data from (Top) Whitehorn D, Brown J, Richard J, et al.: "Multiple Dimensions of Recovery in Early Psychosis." *International Review of Psychiatry* 14:273–283, 2002. (Bottom) Nuechterlein K, Ventura J, Gitlin M, et al.: "Determinants of One Year Outcomes in Recent Onset Schizophrenia." Paper presented at the International Conference on Schizophrenia, St. Moritz, Switzerland, April 22, 2006.

WHAT ACCOUNTS FOR THE NEWLY FOUND POPULARITY OF RECOVERY?

The confluence of many developments, listed in Table 1.2, has created the current interest in recovery. It has taken decades of improvement in treatment, advocacy, and destigmatization for an optimistic outlook for serious mental disorders to develop. Recovery as a benchmark for all stakeholders in treatment of serious mental disorders has crystallized because of a crescendo of interest and validation from such varied sources as research, clinical service, and consumerism. The appearance of recovery on the collective radar screen has been powered by the consumer movement; families and patients have become strong advocates for improved services and better outcomes.

● **TABLE 1.2**

Sources propelling stakeholder interest in recovery from mental disorders

- Evidence that symptomatic and social recovery occur in patients with chronic illness
- Accelerated recovery in young patients with recent onset of schizophrenia
- Relapse prevention techniques for disease management that reduce relapse rates by one-half
- Destigmatization of mental illness, which encourages greater access and receptivity to treatment
- New and increasing forms of evidence-based treatments that are more effective than previous treatments
- Consumer-driven emphasis on recovery as hope, empowerment, and achieving a full life regardless of symptoms and disability
- Self-help and peer support organizations of consumers (patients)
- Powerful impact of advocacy groups for improved research, treatment, and rehabilitation: National Alliance on Mental Illness, NARSAD, Depression and Bipolar Support Alliance, Mental Health Association, Academic Consortium, American Psychiatric Association
- Growing prominence and influence of psychiatric rehabilitation, with recognition that chronicity of serious and persisting mental illness is a result of insufficiency of comprehensive, continuous, coordinated, collaborative, consumer-oriented, competency-based, and compassionate care

Other influences arose from clinical experience, such as the development of evidence-based, psychosocial therapies. Research has lent its thrust to the recovery movement through awareness of the plasticity and malleability of the brain, suggesting that even a diseased brain can repair itself with the help of a facilitating environment. The arrival of novel medications, resulting from research on neurotransmitter systems, has enabled psychiatrists to customize treatment to each patient, making it more likely that individuals with mood and psychotic disorders will find a drug that produces therapeutic benefits. As an example, the advent of clozapine has enabled many patients with schizophrenia to recover whose illness had been previously refractory to all other antipsychotic drugs.

RECOVERY IS MORE THAN COPING WITH A DISABLING MENTAL DISORDER

The emphasis on recovery is a salubrious development in psychiatry, expanding our view of mental disorders from biologically determined diseases catalogued by symptom-dominated diagnoses. Recovery denotes having a normal life that is incompatible with the stigma fomented by a mental disease. Normality emphasizes the positive attributes of a person who has overcome symptoms and social and vocational limitations with a quality of life unhampered by dependency and functional segregation. The conceptualization of "normality" is broad, congruent with the capacious standards of society. Thus, a person would be considered normal who is working or volunteering part-time, who has only one friend with whom he socializes, and who may have phone or face-to-face contact with his family only at Christmas. Similarly, an individual would be considered living within the normal range who experiences frequent auditory hallucinations but is able to carry on with social, recreational, and employment activities without disabling intrusions from her symptoms.

Individuals with spinal cord injuries, strokes, or renal failure can recover from their symptoms and disabilities if they are able to work, have friends, live independently, and initiate and enjoy normal recreational activities. Accommodations, physical therapy, compensatory supportive services, and dialysis enable them to overcome obstacles to their normal functioning. Dignity, self-esteem, and participation in the full range of normal community activities and privileges are now available to persons with physical disabilities, thanks to motorized wheelchairs, modified driving controls in automobiles and other conveyances, accommodations in public transport, accessibility to shops and public buildings, and availability of personal support specialists who facilitate independent living in normal residences.

For certain, each person in our democracy, whether mentally ill or not, should be able to define for himself/herself the meaning of enjoying a full and dignified life, having hope and optimism for the future, feeling empowered to make his/her own choices, and experiencing growth through relationships and a supportive environment. But idiosyncratic and highly personalized definitions of a "full, meaningful, and dignified life," "hope and optimism for the future," "feeling empowered to make choices," and "experiencing growth" could easily broaden the concept of recovery beyond all social norms. Would "recovery from a mental disorder" be a useful term to describe an individual whose:

- "full life" was delimited to a regimented board-and-care home with rare forays into the community,
- "dignity" derived from being able to smoke two packs of cigarettes each day,
- "hope and optimism for the future" referred to looking forward to the annual Thanksgiving dinner or weekly visits from a recreational therapist for games of Monopoly,
- "feeling empowered" meant being able to intimidate his roommate so the latter would share his money and possessions,
- "making choices" meant being able to stay in his room and nap all day long, and
- "experiencing growth" referred to eating as much as desired despite morbid obesity?

There are logical deficiencies in relying solely on subjective criteria for defining recovery. Personal satisfaction with life and one's treatment and living arrangements has been shown to be unrelated to improvement in symptoms and functioning (Garland et al. 2003). Is a homeless and impoverished person with bipolar disorder to be considered "in recovery" if he is enjoying his life, feeling empowered to choose the street or doorway for sleeping, making the choice to refuse medication and other mental health services, and experiencing growth because his panhandling has resulted in increased income? Is such a person experiencing recovery if he unequivocally states that he has learned to live better with his illness and accept himself with dignity (Dickerson 2006)? Vague, confusing, and highly individualistic definitions of recovery that are not anchored in reliable measures or empirical validity can endanger the funding of mental health services, undermine the status of psychiatry in the eyes of the medical and health services establishment, and have unintended effects on worsening stigma toward the mentally ill (Brekke et al. 2001).

Certainly there is an enormous difference between definitions of recovery when individuals share personal meaning, contentment, and satisfaction, but the definitions diverge on the following functional criteria:

- Making autonomous decisions about daily routines, solving problems independently, working in normal employment, using recreational facilities in common with other community citizens, and managing one's own money and medications
- Following scheduled activities planned and led by paid staff, being accompanied by a case manager to deal with social agencies and shopping, having money and medications managed by others, and participating in sheltered or transitional employment within a mental health club

A definition of recovery that is left to the idiosyncratic, personalized, and subjective view of each person risks circular reasoning whereby anyone can be said to have recovered who feels good about himself/herself by "living a satisfying, hopeful, and contributing life even with the limitations caused by illness" and developing "new meaning and purpose in one's life as one grows beyond the catastrophic effects of mental illness" (Anthony 1993). The term *recovery* can be turned into a catchword or slogan that can be applied to almost any mentally ill person who, while making no discernible change in level of functioning, is persuaded by beneficent professionals and peer advocates that he/she is dignified, hopeful, empowered, responsible, and satisfied with life. To emphasize a rhetoric of recovery without building skills and supports to overcome disability is to court disaster for our patients.

A "feel good" definition of recovery is so loose that it can encompass anyone who may be coping with a debilitating medical or mental illness *but who is still disabled and lacking the capacity to live and participate in normal ways and places in society.* We may admire persons who have dignity, love of life, and determination to make each day count while dealing with their catastrophic illnesses: individuals who are living in hospice with terminal cancer, bedridden with disabling heart failure, hospitalized with schizophrenia, or homebound with amyotrophic lateral sclerosis. But unless they are living and working in ways compatible with what would be considered within the normal range, considering them as "recovered" would be a misnomer. There is no question that practitioners should strive to help their patients find self-affirmation, hope, courage, satisfaction, and value in their daily lives within the constraints of disability. But without bolting the meaning of recovery to a foundation of a normal life, as defined by society, ideological exuberance runs the risk of promising too much and delivering too little.

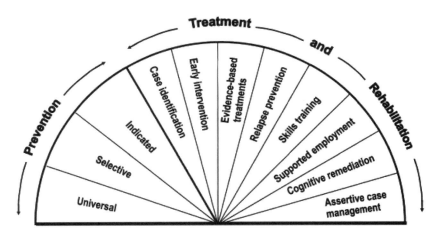

FIGURE 1.8 The continuum from prevention to treatment and rehabilitation prohibits artificial distinctions between treatment and rehabilitation.

▶ What Is Psychiatric Rehabilitation?

If rehabilitation is the road to recovery, how can the mentally disabled make the journey successful? The overall goal of psychiatric rehabilitation is to ensure that persons with a psychiatric disability have maximum opportunity to recover as normal a life as possible. This means ensuring access to the social, vocational, and recreational responsibilities and privileges of citizens participating in their communities. Rehabilitation connects the personally relevant goals of the mentally ill to services that reduce disability and promote recovery.

From the outset, let's understand that there is no qualitative boundary between *treatment* and *rehabilitation*. As shown in Figure 1.8, treatment and rehabilitation are used interchangeably in this book because they have no fundamental differences. Some academics and practitioners make the distinction between these terms by viewing treatment as pharmacological interventions for the acute phase of a mental disorder versus rehabilitation as psychosocial services for mentally disabled persons who have been stabilized through treatment. As the forthcoming chapters clearly articulate, this distinction is fatuous, since psychosocial services such as education about the nature of mental illness and promotion of adherence and teaching coping skills must be delivered together with medications during the acute phase of the disorder. Treatment and rehabilitation are two sides of the same coin.

Rehabilitation varies in form, intensity, and duration depending upon the type of mental disorder and the amount of disability. There are many disorders in which patients have never learned the abilities to function effectively in society and still others in which patients' abilities have eroded

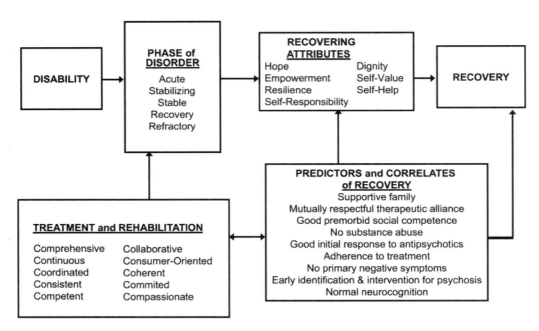

FIGURE 1.9 Determinants of movement from disability to recovery.

or atrophied through long periods of disuse. Examples of the former are schizophrenia and developmental disorders and of the latter, major depression, bipolar disorder, and panic with agoraphobia. For patients with substantial cognitive deficits and poor premorbid functioning, rehabilitation may require lengthy teaching of skills and carefully organized supports and resources in the community to improve quality of life.

The major determinants of recovery from serious mental disorders are displayed in Figure 1.9. At any one time in their lives, patients' locations on the road to recovery depend upon the interactions among the type of disorder, quality of treatment and rehabilitation, and prognostic features of the individuals. Fortunately, most of the factors that influence disability are malleable and hence can be modified to promote recovery. As they move from their starting point of disability toward their destination of recovery, patients experience increasing amounts of hope, empowerment, self-responsibility, dignity, and self-esteem. These attributes promote further progress on the continuum from disability to recovery. Rehabilitation comprises the practices that affect and are affected by the personal and social outcomes of individuals as they advance

> Recovery from serious mental disorders is possible if treatment and rehabilitation are comprehensive, continuous, coordinated, collaborative, consistent with patient's personal goals, competent, connected flexibly with phase of illness, compatible with patient's culture and individualized needs, cooperative with community agencies, consumer-oriented, and compassionate.

toward recovery. A basic assumption of rehabilitation is that all patients with psychiatric disabilities can benefit from its services to varying degrees regardless of their initial level of functioning, rate of progress, and prospects for recovery.

Psychiatric rehabilitation provides a spectrum of services that enable disabled individuals to perform those cognitive, emotional, social, intellectual, and physical skills needed to live, learn, work, and function as normally and independently as possible in the community with the least interference by symptoms. Each of the chapters of this manual describe current, evidence-based services that practitioners can use to help their patients reach this overarching aim of psychiatric rehabilitation. The methods by which this aim is achieved, delineated in Chapters 3 through 10, involve the following:

- Medications, cognitive remediation, and disease management procedures to remove or ameliorate intrusive symptoms and cognitive deficits that interfere with social functioning and a good quality of life.
- Functional assessment of all dimensions of an individual's experiences that are linked to recovery and personally relevant goals: social competence and social problem-solving, personal hygiene, money management, independent living, work or school, spiritual life, family relations, and care of personal possessions.
- Teaching persons specific skills that are way stations toward achieving personally relevant goals.
- Arranging and designing supportive environments and programs that compensate for deficits in education, work, and independent living.
- Involving families in services for the seriously mentally ill.
- Vocational rehabilitation.
- Delivering treatments and services so they are maximally accessible to those with mental disabilities living in the community.
- Special services for special people, such as treatments for persons whose illness is refractory to all therapeutic endeavors or individuals with concurrent substance abuse and mental illness.
- Providing professional and natural supports consistent with a satisfying and full life.

Considerable differences in impairments and disabilities with consequent type and amount of rehabilitation needed are found even among persons with similar mental disorders. Differences exist in the severity, chronicity, and comorbidity of their disorders and their responsiveness to medications. The form and extensiveness of rehabilitation also are determined by diversity of intelligence, capacity for learning, social competence, cognitive functioning, developmental history, education, cultural and ethnic backgrounds, social class and income, family support, and satisfaction with their current quality of life. In addition, variations in availability of mental health services and community resources determine how far and fast along the road to recovery each person will go. Given each person's values and choice of personal goals, patients will differ in their progression on the continuum from disability to recovery.

Rehabilitation is a clinical science, guided by theory-driven principles and empirically based interventions and services. The principles and practices of psychiatric rehabilitation are described in the next chapter. Each of the chapters in this book describes the rationale, methods of assessment, evidence-based treatments, benefits, and outcomes that compose the modes of rehabilitation. As new methods of rehabilitation become available and are linked to the varied and specific needs and goals of disabled persons, progress will be steadily made in extending the benefits of recovery to a greater number of patients. With the translation of basic behavioral and biological sciences into clinical applications, the future will brighten for the mentally disabled. The pessimism and stigma so long associated with psychiatric disorders will recede into musty obscurity. A paradigm shift from disability to recovery will reveal to all that "under white ashes embers will glow."

▶ Summary

Embarking on the road to recovery, patients and their mental health professionals need a key to open the gate of disability. The key to effective rehabilitation is a process that starts with engaging the patient in a collaboration for identifying goals that can enrich the person's life. Proceeding along the road of rehabilitation involves overcoming symptoms and cognitive impairments; building on the person's coping, social, and independent living skills; strengthening the person's social support system; and finding resources in the community for enhancing participation in society. The work of rehabilitation is always in the present but with eyes on the future.

In planning and evaluating rehabilitation, it is important for patients, family members, and practitioners to be viewed as doing the very best they can within the context of their personal attributes and competencies and the scope and quality of rehabilitative services. With a realistic optimism and respect for individual differences, practitioners will be able to find and emphasize each person's positive characteristics. As one patient stated, "My recovery was about gaining other people's confidence in my abilities and potential and in their expectations of what I could achieve." The purpose and value of psychiatric rehabilitation depend upon practitioners adding impetus to the desire that each person has for a better life. When professionals hold positive attitudes, communicate hope, and use evidence-based practices, disabled individuals are able to experience improved psychosocial functioning, community participation, and personal fulfillment.

▶ Key Points

- Disabilities arise when the symptoms and cognitive dysfunctions of mental and developmental disorders, combined with stressors, interfere with a person's functioning in work, school, family, friendships, recreation, spiritual life, and independent living.
- Psychiatric symptoms and cognitive disturbances are neurodevelopmental impairments that can be treated by medications and environments that reduce the stress impinging on an individual with a mental disorder.
- Abilities, the converse of disabilities, can be promoted through learning skills and supportive, remedial social interventions.
- The more than 15 million Americans with psychiatric disabilities have a wide spectrum of diagnoses requiring treatment beyond 2 years and, in addition to medication, psychosocial rehabilitation to restore personal, vocational, and social functioning.
- Recovery from mental disorders is achieved when symptoms and cognitive dysfunctions are in abeyance, vocational and social functioning have improved to permit active participation in community life, and individuals gain a sense of empowerment and self-direction, self-respect, personal responsibility and value, hope for the future, and satisfaction in their everyday lives.
- With treatment and rehabilitation that is continuing, comprehensive, coordinated, collaborative, consumer-oriented, competently connected to evidence-based practices, consistent with the phase and type of a person's disorder, and compassionate, recovery can be achieved by 50% or more of persons with psychiatric disabilities.
- Psychiatric rehabilitation encompasses coordinated and comprehensive biobehavioral services that enable disabled persons to perform those cognitive, emotional, social, intellectual, and physical skills needed to live, learn, work, and function in the community as normally and independently as possible.

▶ Selected Readings

Anderson J: Empowering patients: issues and strategies. Soc Sci Med 43:697–705, 1996

Davidson L, O'Connell M, Tondora J, et al: The top ten concerns about recovery encountered in mental health system transformation. Psychiatr Serv 57:640–645, 2006

Davidson L, O'Connell M, Tondora J, et al: Recovery in serious mental illness: a new wine or just a new bottle? Prof Psychol: Res Pr 36:480–487, 2005

Deegan PE: Recovery: the lived experience of rehabilitation. Psychosocial Rehabilitation Journal 11:11–19, 1996

DeSisto MJ, Harding CM, McCormick RV, et al: The Maine and Vermont three-decade studies of serious mental illness. Br J Psychiatry 167:338–342, 1995

Drake RE, Green AI, Mueser KT, et al: The history of community mental health treatment and rehabilitation for persons with severe mental illness. Community Ment Health J 39:427–440, 2003

Engel GL: From biomedical to biopsychosocial: being scientific in the human domain. Psychosomatics 38:521–528, 1997

Harding CM, Brooks GW, Ashikaga T, et al: The Vermont Longitudinal Study of Persons With Severe Mental Illness, II: long-term outcome of subjects who retrospectively met DSM-III criteria for schizophrenia. Am J Psychiatry 144:727–735, 1987

Jacobson N (ed): In Recovery: The Making of Mental Health Policy. Nashville, TN, Vanderbilt University Press, 2004

Kessler RC, Berglund P, Demler O, et al: The epidemiology of major depressive disorder. JAMA 289:3095–3105, 2003

Kopelowicz A, Liberman RP: Integrating treatment with rehabilitation for persons with major mental disorders. Psychiatr Serv 54:1491–1498, 2003

Kopelowicz A, Liberman RP, Zarate R: Psychosocial treatments for schizophrenia, in A Guide to Treatments That Work, 3rd Edition. Edited by Nathan PE, Gorman JM. New York, Oxford University Press, 2006, pp 243–269

Kopelowicz A, Wallace CJ, Liberman RP: Psychiatric rehabilitation, in Gabbard's Treatments of Psychiatric Disorders, 4th Edition. Edited by Gabbard GO. Washington, DC, American Psychiatric Publishing, 2007, pp 361–379

Liberman RP: Psychiatric Rehabilitation of the Chronic Mental Patient. Washington, DC, American Psychiatric Press, 1988

Liberman RP: Handbook of Psychiatric Rehabilitation. New York, Macmillan, 1992

Liberman RP: Recovery from schizophrenia. Int Rev Psychiatry 14:1–103, 2002 (special issue)

Liberman RP, Kopelowicz A: Recovery from schizophrenia: a concept in search of research. Psychiatr Serv 56:735–742, 2005

Liberman RP, Kopelowicz A, Silverstein S: Psychiatric rehabilitation, in Comprehensive Textbook of Psychiatry/VIII, 8th Edition. Edited by Sadock BJ, Sadock VA. Baltimore, MD, Lippincott Williams & Wilkins, 2004, pp 3884–3930

Mintz J, Mintz L, Arruda MJ, et al: Treatments of depression and the functional capacity to work. Arch Gen Psychiatry 49:761–768, 1992

President's New Freedom Commission on Mental Health: Achieving the Promise: Transforming Mental Health Care in America. Rockville, MD, U.S. Department of Health and Human Services, 2006. Available at: http://www.mentalhealth-commission.gov. Accessed 2007.

Ralph O, Corrigan PW (eds): Recovery in Mental Illness. Washington, DC, American Psychological Association, 2005

Resnick SG, Rosenheck RA, Lehman AF: An exploratory analysis of correlates of recovery. Psychiatr Serv 55:540–547, 2004

Skodol AE, Gunderson JG, McGlashan TH, et al: Functional impairments in patients with schizotypal, borderline, avoidant or obsessive personality disorder. Am J Psychiatry 159:276–283, 2002

Warner R: Recovery From Schizophrenia: Psychiatry and Political Economy, 3rd Edition. New York, Brunner/Routledge, 2004

Watts FN, Bennett DH: Theory and Practice of Psychiatric Rehabilitation. New York, Wiley, 1983

▶ References

American Psychiatric Association: Diagnostic and Statistical Manual of Mental Disorders, 4th Edition. Washington, DC, American Psychiatric Publishing, 1994

American Psychiatric Association: Diagnostic and Statistical Manual of Mental Disorders, 4th Edition, Text Revision. Washington, DC, American Psychiatric Publishing, 2000

Anthony WA: Recovery from mental illness: the guiding vision of the mental health service system in the 1990s. Psychosocial Rehabilitation Journal 16:11–24, 1993

Bijl RV, Ravelli A: Current and residual functional disability associated with psychopathology. Psychol Med 30:657–668, 2000

Brekke JS, Kohrt B, Green MF: Neuropsychological functioning as a moderator of the relationship between psychosocial functioning and the subjective experience of self and life in schizophrenia. Schizophr Bull 27:697–708, 2001

Coryell W, Scheffner W, Keller M, et al: The enduring psychosocial consequences of mania and depression. Am J Psychiatry 150:720–727, 1993

Dickerson FB: Commentary: disquieting aspects of the recovery paradigm. Psychiatr Serv 57:647, 2006

Dickerson FB, Boronow JJ, Stallings CR, et al: Cognitive functioning and employment status of persons with bipolar disorder. Psychiatr Serv 55:54–58, 2004

Fakhoury WK, Murray A, Shepherd G, et al: Research in supported housing. Soc Psychiatry Epidemiol 37:301–315, 2002

Garland AF, Aarons GA, Hawley KM, et al: Relationship of youth satisfaction with mental health services and changes in symptoms and functioning. Psychiatr Serv 54:1544–1546, 2003

Harding CM, Brooks GW, Ashikaga T, et al: Vermont Longitudinal Study of Persons

With Severe Mental Illness. Am J Psychiatry 144:727–735, 1987

Harding CM, Zubin J, Strauss JS: Chronicity in schizophrenia: revisited. Br J Psychiatry Suppl October (18):27–37, 1992

Hopper K, Harrison G, Janca A, et al: Recovery From Schizophrenia: An International Perspective. New York, Oxford University Press, 2007

Kendler KS, Baker JH: Genetic influences on measures of the environment: a systematic review. Psychol Med 36:1–12, 2006

Kupfer DJ, Frank E, Grochocinski VJ, et al: Clinical characteristics of individuals in a bipolar case registry. J Clin Psychiatry 63:120–125, 2002

Liberman RP, Kopelowicz A: Recovery from schizophrenia: a concept in search of research. Psychiatr Serv 56:735–742, 2005

MacQueen GM, Young LT, Joffe RT: A review of psychosocial outcome in bipolar disorder. Acta Psychiatr Scand 103:163–170, 2001

Mezzich JE, Ustun TB: Epidemiology, in Comprehensive Textbook of Psychiatry/VIII, 8th Edition. Edited by Sadock BJ, Sadock VA. Baltimore, MD, Lippincott Williams & Wilkins, 2005, pp 656–672

Murphy MA: Grand rounds: recovery from schizophrenia. Schizophr Bull 33:657–660, 2007

Nuechterlein K, Ventura J, Gitlin M, et al: Determinants of one year outcomes in recent onset schizophrenia. Paper presented at the International Conference on Schizophrenia, St. Moritz, Switzerland, April 22, 2006

O'Hara A: Housing for people with mental illness. Psychiatr Serv 58:907–913, 2007

Ormel J, Oldehinkel AJ, Nolen WA, et al: Psychosocial disability before, during, and after a major depressive episode. Arch Gen Psychiatry 61:387–392, 2004

Tanzman B: An overview of surveys of mental health consumers' preferences for housing and support services. Hosp Community Psychiatry 44:450–455, 1993

Whitehorn D, Brown J, Richard J, et al: Multiple dimensions of recovery in early psychosis. Int Rev Psychiatry 14:273–283, 2002

World Health Organization: International Classification of Functioning, Disability and Health (ICF). Geneva, Switzerland, World Health Organization, 2001

Principles and Practice of Psychiatric Rehabilitation

Principles and Practice of Psychiatric Rehabilitation

If I were to wish for anything, I should not wish for wealth or power, but for the passionate sense of the potential and for the eye which sees the possible. What wine is so sparkling, so fragrant, so intoxicating, as possibility?

SØREN KIERKEGAARD (1813–1855)

PRINCIPLES OF psychiatric rehabilitation guide practitioners' efforts to promote recovery in persons with mental disabilities. Reflecting the values and standards held by society and the rehabilitation and recovery communities, principles are the overarching values and aims that govern the delivery of rehabilitation services. They form the basic assumptions, core beliefs, and professional ethos of practitioners who serve individuals with psychiatric disorders. Drawn from conceptual foundations as well as from practical and empirical needs for services, principles are fundamental to the design, development, and implementation of treatment practices. Inspired by the humanistic principles of rehabilitation, its practices enable individuals

- to learn skills and gain supports
- for living as independently as possible
- with integration into normal community life
- at the highest level of functioning that is feasible
- as free of symptoms as possible, and
- with a meaningful life that offers personal satisfaction and self-efficacy.

The seven principles of psychiatric rehabilitation are presented in Table 2.1 with examples of specific practices that each principle subsumes.

The vision and mission of psychiatric rehabilitation are imbued by its principles. The vision of psychiatric rehabilitation is to *enable individuals with mental disabilities to recover and to live as normally as possible in the community.* The mission of the field is to *engage patients and their families or caregivers in a collaborative treatment process that teaches skills and provides*

● TABLE 2.1

Principles of psychiatric rehabilitation, with exemplary practices

● **Recovery of a normal life** in the community is possible for many persons with mental disabilities if **best practices** of rehabilitation are provided.

» Our part of the bargain is to mobilize as many of the evidence-based treatments as are available and relevant for helping our patients achieve their personal goals en route to recovery. Giving value and credence to recovery as an uncompromising goal and vision for rehabilitation can also motivate practitioners, patients, family members, managers, policy makers, and other stakeholders to reform our current systems of care by bringing evidence-based services into everyday practice.

● **Impairments, disabilities, and handicaps can be reduced or overcome by integrating pharmacological and psychosocial services with advocacy for improved clinical, educational, vocational, and governmental policies and practices.**

» Governmental policies such as those covering disability benefits, the Americans with Disabilities Act, and nondiscriminatory employment and housing make it possible for mentally disabled persons to have funds for subsistence, employment with reasonable accommodations, and residences in normal community neighborhoods.

● **Individualization of treatment** is a fundamental pillar of rehabilitation.

» Rehabilitation rests on respect for the uniqueness of each individual, including an understanding of how family, cultural, and ethnic diversity inform diagnosis, functional assessment, and treatment response.

● **Rehabilitation** is more effective and recovery more rapid when patients and families are **actively involved** in planning and participating in treatment.

» Formation, maintenance, and continuity of a collaborative, positive partnership among practitioner, patient, and family are achieved through interpersonal competencies of the practitioner.

● **Integration and coordination** of services are essential to enhance progress toward recovery.

» Multidisciplinary collaboration and communication are necessary among practitioners and agencies responsible for optimal blending, coordination, and consistency of pharmacological and psychosocial services.

● **Building on patients' strengths, interests, and capabilities** is a cornerstone of rehabilitation.

» Practitioners utilize educational and behavioral techniques to enhance learning of skills. Empowerment, responsibility, and self-esteem are acquired through success in obtaining skills, using one's abilities, and attaining one's personal goals.

● **Rehabilitation takes time, proceeds incrementally, and requires perseverance, patience, and resilience** by patients, families, and practitioners.

» Practitioners solicit and set functional, attainable, and specific short-term goals that are stepping stones toward patients' longer-term, personally relevant life goals.

supports for fostering illness management, psychosocial functioning, and personal satisfaction. Principles of psychiatric rehabilitation give purpose and direction to the vision and mission. For example, the vision of recovery is more likely to become a reality when *patients and families are actively involved in treatment* and when *best practices of rehabilitation are employed.* The mission of *teaching skills and providing supports* is accomplished when *treatments are individualized* and *services are integrated.*

Specific treatments or practices are guided by principles and used in the service of the vision and mission. Thus, *social skills training* and *supported employment* are specific practices that fall under the *principle of building skills and supports for improving social and vocational functioning.* Practices of psychiatric rehabilitation empower patients to achieve their personal goals and move toward recovery, while principles provide the framework within which practices are delivered. Values-based principles are the strategies of psychiatric rehabilitation, while practices give "marching orders" to practitioners in their daily work. If we view principles as being the rules of the road to recovery, then practices are the engines that keep the patient and practitioner moving in the direction of recovery. Principles and practices turn possibilities into realities.

When treatments and community resources are delivered and mobilized competently by practitioners, desirable outcomes are more likely to ensue. Practices fall into the following categories:

- Functional assessment
- Engagement and maintenance in treatment
- Therapeutic relationships
- Illness management
- Training skills
- Developing and maintaining family involvement in treatment
- Personal support services (i.e., case management)
- Supported employment and related vocational rehabilitation
- Cognitive-behavioral therapy
- Psychosocial clubs
- Peer support and self-help
- Community supports
- Organizing new resources for meeting patients' personal goals

The boundaries among the various principles are sometimes porous. It is neither possible nor desirable to erect walls between principles that collectively influence the direction of the field of rehabilitation. Therefore, some of the practices described under one principle may also be relevant to others. For example, therapeutic relationships that enlist the participation of patients in the planning and choice of treatment convey hope and empowerment to those patients, as does rehabilitation that builds skills and supports. Principles overlap, intersect, and reverberate with one another. This interaction is valuable, as it reinforces the collective salience of principles for practitioners, permitting rehabilitation to become more strongly embedded in the mental health field.

Conceptual Foundations of Psychiatric Rehabilitation

Principles and practices of psychiatric rehabilitation have been influenced by two primary sources: *practical needs for services* and *conceptual foundations*. Concepts relevant to rehabilitation have given focus to principles and stimulated the development of practices. Some of the most important innovations in psychiatric rehabilitation were spawned by philosophical ideals of humanism, civil liberties, individualism, freedom of choice, and personal responsibility. Psychosocial rehabilitation had its birth in the mid-nineteenth-century era of moral therapy. Reformists such as Samuel Tuke of the Quaker York Retreat in England and Dorothea Dix in the United States believed that moving the mentally ill from overcrowded, unsanitary, and crime-ridden cities into spacious, airy hospitals located in the rural countryside would improve their mental faculties and morale. Rehabilitative principles were inspired by a combination of liberal democracy, the pursuit of happiness, the spread of public health measures, and a revolt against the atrocious warehousing and torpor of the mentally ill in almshouses and jails. Leaders of moral therapy grasped the importance of compassion, cleanliness, work, and scheduled activities for improving thoughts, feelings, and behavior. The founders of state hospitals believed that patients could recover if the institutions gave them opportunities to behave normally. In this early period of rehabilitation, as well as more recently, necessity was the mother of invention.

Unfortunately, as the country's population soared with immigration in the second half of the nineteenth century, hospitals became crowded and custodial and therapeutic nihilism became ascendant. When the large state hospitals began to discharge thousands of chronic patients 50 years ago, there were no places or programs for them to spend their time, socialize, or enjoy recreation. The community mental health centers and their professional staff were not prepared to offer appropriate services to the seriously mentally ill. Other than family members, there was no one to take responsibility to ensure that patients would adhere to their medication or attend outpatient treatment. After living in regimented hospitals, ex-patients experienced a vacuum in their lives that led to resurgence of symptoms and frequent rehospitalizations. Their residual symptoms, cognitive impairments, bizarre behavior, psychosocial disabilities, and stigma were enormous barriers to community reintegration.

With little more than donated space and furniture, the first psychosocial clubs were established 50 years ago by determined and humanistic social workers and charitable citizen-volunteers and through the self-help efforts of formerly hospitalized patients. As was the case in moral therapy, healthy behaviors of patients were elicited and reinforced through normal social and work activities. In the face of urgent personal and social needs of psychiatric patients, pioneers in social psychiatry assumed correctly that treatments for the mentally ill would be most helpful if the treatment environment and professional staff encouraged and expected normal functioning. In addition, individuals were granted freedom of choice in how they would participate in the club and even whether or not they would attend. Psychiatric treatment was not offered by the clubs, participants were called "members," and the roles of staff and members were purposely blurred.

While psychoanalytic therapy was ineffective for mentally disabled persons, its optimism that psychiatric disorders could be cured and social problems alleviated through insight and awareness inspired the Community Mental Health Centers Act in the early 1960s. Leaders of American psychiatry laid the groundwork for community reintegration of the mentally ill and for the more recent emergence of the "recovery model" in public mental health. The belief that recovery is an individually defined journey for a meaningful life requiring self-awareness and responsibility has its philosophical roots in the psychoanalytic movement as well as in egalitarianism.

More recently, the model of service delivery called *assertive community treatment* has demonstrated that patients, even those who are homeless, can be treated effectively wherever they might live. Endorsing freedom of choice for individuals with serious mental illness, assertive community treatment teams accept full responsibility for persuading patients to voluntarily accept services. This model was developed to blunt the high rates of rehospitalization among the seriously mentally ill. As described in Chapter 8 ("Vehicles for Delivering Rehabilitation Services"), these interdisciplinary treatment teams assertively reach out to patients wherever they may be in the community, thereby overcoming denial of illness, reluctance for treatment, and social isolation.

❱ Scientific Foundations of Psychiatric Rehabilitation

Insemination of rehabilitation by scientific concepts has more recent origins. As psychiatric rehabilitation becomes more academically respectable with a proliferation of books and journals as well as an expansion of research funds, translation of basic biobehavioral sciences to rehabilitation will accelerate in the coming years. Increasingly, theoretical concepts will generate new treatments that will be submitted to hypothesis testing in research. In a reciprocal manner, empirical findings and experiences that emerge from theory-driven clinical practice will shape and refine the theories. Theory must always be the servant of rehabilitation, not its master. To be of value, concepts and theories beg to be challenged by clinical realities, to be modified, and even to be discarded.

The constructive interactions among *principles,* their *conceptual foundations,* the *practices* used in rehabilitation, and the resulting clinical, social, and personal *outcomes* accruing to patients are shown in Figure 2.1. In this part of the chapter, I provide an overview of each of the scientific concepts that have contributed to the principles and practices of psychiatric rehabilitation: the vulnerability-stress-protective factors model of mental disorders, cognitive science, social learning theory, and life span developmental psychology.

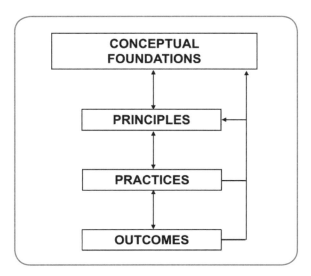

FIGURE 2.1 Reciprocal relationships among conceptual foundations, principles, practices, and outcomes of psychiatric rehabilitation.

▶ Vulnerability-Stress-Protective Factors Model of Mental Disorders

Principles of psychiatric rehabilitation and their associated therapeutic practices are elucidated by the vulnerability-stress-protective factors model. As shown in Figure 2.2, this conceptual model posits that *socioenvironmental stressors,* when experienced by individuals who have enduring *psychobiological vulnerability,* can adversely affect the course and outcome of serious mental disorders. The course and outcome of a disorder can be described in terms of continua from disability to recovery in symptoms, cognitive impairments, social functioning, and quality of life. The brain's vulnerability to stressors is thought to stem from genetic and neurodevelopmental roots. Stressors from the environment, which cause perturbations in a vulnerable brain, include alcohol and drugs of abuse; an overheated emotional climate within the family; mismatch between practitioners and services and the personal goals and needs of the individual patient; social isolation and its obverse, overstimulating social situations; losses and personal rejection; traumatic experiences; and an accumulation of daily hassles.

The negative impact of stressors on a vulnerable individual leads to symptom exacerbation and relapse, increased cognitive impairments, greater personal and social disabilities, and degradation of the person's quality of life. As depicted in Figure 2.2, when this occurs, the course and outcome on the four domains shift toward the right, or dark, end of the continua. When stressors subside and/or protective factors are strengthened, the direction of course and outcome on the domains shifts toward the left, or the brighter, end of the continua. We do not have treatments to directly affect the enduring vulnerability of the brain nor can we insulate our patients from stressors, since the latter are ever-present in daily life and are unpredictable hazards of living in modern society. Even the anachronistic notion of the psychiatric hospital as a stress-free asylum is belied by the personal experience of anyone who has had to endure hospital stays. Hospitals are very stressful places. Patients lose their privacy, choices, autonomy, and freedom of movement.

Protective factors constitute the conceptual domain that offers opportunities to creatively and effectively shield mentally ill individuals from the combined noxious effects of vulnerability and stress. Protective factors include personal attributes such as resilience, social competence, and normal cognitive functioning, as well as supportive factors in the environment such as family support, reliable housing, and a trusting relationship with one's therapist and psychiatrist. Each person carries his/her own vulnerability, stress, and protective factors when seeking psychiatric assistance. In

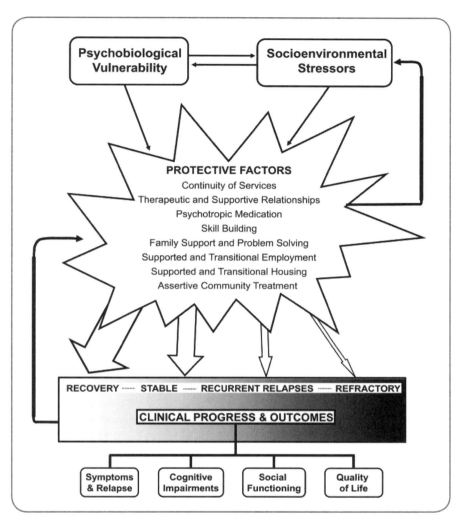

FIGURE 2.2 Vulnerability-stress-protective factors model of mental illness. Evidence-based protective factors can reduce relapse and improve cognitive functioning, social functioning, and quality of life.

developing a treatment plan, this concept requires practitioners to identify a distinct profile of protective factors from among personal, family, social, vocational, educational, and community attributes. Strengthening protective factors can shift the balance from disability to recovery.

Evidence-based practices also confer protection against stress and vulnerability. Best practices embody protective factors, including optimal pharmacotherapy, strategies of disease management, social skills training, judicious family support, supported employment, normalized residential options, and assertive community treatment. Each of these evidence-based practices is the subject of a separate chapter in this book. Rehabilitation practices are protective and facilitate recovery when they are organized and delivered in a manner that is comprehensive, continuous, competent, coordinated, collaborative, consumer-oriented, and compassionate. Under these circumstances, impairments, disabilities, and handicaps dissolve and individuals move in the direction of normal participation in their communities.

The teeter-totters pictured in Figure 2.3 show the precarious balance between stressors and vulnerability on one side and protective factors on the other. When stress and vulnerability are weighty, the individual is pushed "up in the air"; when protective factors such as social support and social skills increase, their combined weight brings the individual down to earth with his/her "feet on the ground." This therapeutic shift can occur even if vulnerability and stressors remain relatively constant. Among the most "weighty" protective and supportive factors are the continuous, collaborative therapeutic alliance and evidence-based treatments. Thus, progress toward recovery ensues when noxious stress, superimposed on vulnerability, is outweighed by protective factors.

The development of structured and behavioral forms of family intervention has been one of the most important evidence-based practices advanced by research on vulnerability, stress, and protective factors. During the past 40 years, researchers have noted that many families with a mentally ill relative experience stress and tension, unrealistic expectations, emotional overinvolvement, criticism, and hostility—collectively termed *high expressed emotion.* In these high-stress families, the relapse rates are two to three times greater than in families that are able to protect themselves from stress and its adverse consequences on the mentally ill relative. Conversely, supportive families who are educated about the illness and have realistic performance expectations for a mentally disabled family member are powerfully protective against the hazards of stress and vulnerability. This relationship between attributes of the family and relapse has been shown to hold for many stress-related mental and physical disorders: schizophrenia, bipolar disorder, depression, obsessive-compulsive disorder, eating disorders, asthma, and ulcerative colitis.

When families are engaged in rehabilitative programs that offer them education about the nature of their sick relative's illness, training in communication skills, and practice in problem solving, relapse rates tumble by one-half or more. Thus, when the needs of families are neglected by mental health professionals, the buildup of stress will often have harmful effects and block the pathway to recovery. On the other hand, families that are equipped with knowledge, coping, communication, and problem-solving skills can confer protective benefits on patients' course and outcome.

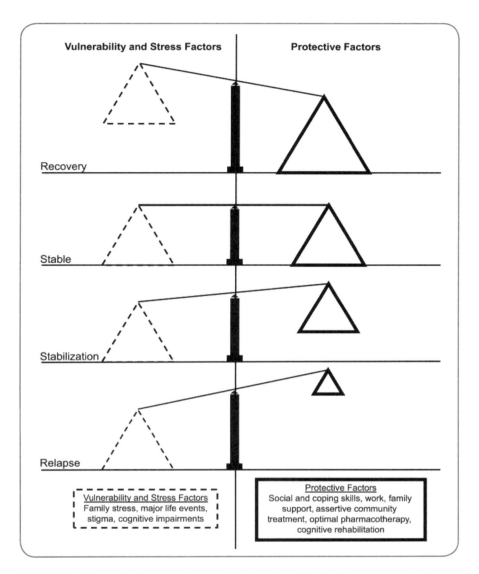

FIGURE 2.3 Protective factors such as social and coping skills, family support, optimal pharmacotherapy, and evidence-based psychosocial services can accumulate with treatment, thereby counterbalancing and outweighing the noxious effects of vulnerability plus stress.

▶ Cognitive Science

Cognitive functions refers to those basic brain mechanisms responsible for accurate perception of people and events, social contacts and personal relationships, sustained and selective attention to tasks, learning, memory, concept formation, organization and execution of behavioral responses, language and speech, decision making, problem solving, abstract reasoning, formation and stability of beliefs and attitudes, and interactions among emotions, thoughts, and actions. In short, cognitive capacities are the interface between ongoing experiences of individuals and their responses to and coping with their everyday world. One way to grasp the significance of these disparate cognitive functions is through the concept of *information processing.*

Information is received by our sense organs as signals, stimuli, words, and conversation. The incoming information often presents us with a problem to solve or an expectation of others to meet. Next, our cognitive capacities enable us to process that information, make sense of it, prioritize it, and process it so that appropriate responses to the situation can be made. The processing phase also involves using our stored memories of similar experiences for sorting out prospective, alternative responses to the situation. If we have effective cognitive functions, we are more likely to choose one or more responses that will have a desired impact on the external world.

The final step of information processing involves using verbal and nonverbal communication to send our chosen responses to the persons with whom we are interacting. Obtaining constructive, intended effects in the social situation not only provides protection against stressful events but also further strengthens our cognitive capacities and social skills for successful responses to future situations. The interactions among the brain, behavior, and the environment are illustratively presented in Figure 2.4. When information processing in the brain functions well, social competence, with its verbal and nonverbal behavior, has a favorable effect on the social environment. Often this means getting one's request fulfilled by others or getting an interpersonal problem solved. Obtaining positive feedback from others strengthens both the individual's social skills and his/her cognitive functions. Normal cognitive functions and information processing enable individuals to function satisfactorily in everyday life, reach their personal goals, obtain their needs, and have a good quality of life.

Unfortunately, most individuals with serious and persisting mental disorders have abnormalities in cognitive functions. In fact, there is evidence that some of these abnormalities are present even prior to the onset of the mental illness. Lacking the cognitive functioning for understanding, organizing, and responding effectively to the world around them, seriously mentally ill persons are impaired in meeting the challenges and requirements of everyday life. Considerable research has documented the relationship between cognitive and social functioning in the severely mentally ill. Thus, if impairments in cognition impede patients' social and vocational functioning, can rehabilitation remedy or prevent resulting disability?

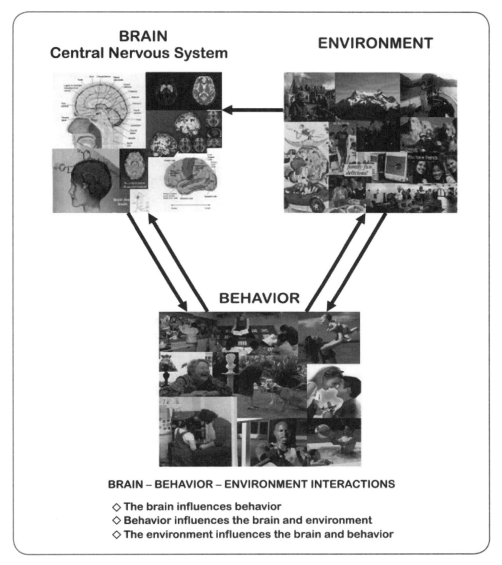

BRAIN
Central Nervous System

ENVIRONMENT

BEHAVIOR

BRAIN – BEHAVIOR – ENVIRONMENT INTERACTIONS

◇ The brain influences behavior
◇ Behavior influences the brain and environment
◇ The environment influences the brain and behavior

FIGURE 2.4 Interactions among brain, behavior, and environment. Influenced by normal neuro-cognition, adaptive behavior has a favorable impact on the environment that generates positive reinforcement. Positive reinforcement has a strengthening effect on both neurocognition and social competence.

Three therapeutic strategies are available to protect the individual from disability:

1. Improve cognitive functioning, thereby reducing impairments.
2. Teach skills and abilities that can compensate for cognitive impairments.

Provide supportive services and environments that offer accommodations for the disabilities and handicaps that are consequences of symptoms and cognitive impairments.

Because of the approximately one trillion neurons in the brain and their enormous, weblike interconnections, this organ has the potential for flexibility in its functions and compensatory actions. Termed *brain plasticity,* the functioning of the central nervous system is flexible and can be influenced for good or bad by events that take place at the biological, behavioral, and environment levels of the individual person. New medications offer promise by having salutary, biological effects directly on those brain functions responsible for regulating cognition. *Cognitive remediation techniques,* described in Chapter 10 ("New Developments for Rehabilitation and Recovery"), can improve cognitive functions such as attention, learning, and memory by *training the brain.*

Social skills training is an effective rehabilitation modality because it utilizes methods that depend upon implicit or procedural learning. Procedural learning occurs without burdening the verbal or explicit learning mechanisms that are impaired in schizophrenia and other disorders. Impairments in verbal learning, verbal memory, and symbolic and abstract associations account for patients' limited insight into their illness and the fatuity of using "talk therapy" or discussion groups in rehabilitation. In contrast, implicit or procedural learning takes place when individuals acquire skills through active learning. They learn by:

- Watching others, on video or in vivo, as role models perform the skills.
- Practicing the skills repeatedly until proficiency develops.
- Obtaining positive reinforcement and coaching for successful use of the skills in real-life situations.
- Experiencing natural, positive consequences and mastery in achieving personal goals.

A third strategy for overcoming cognitive deficits is through *supportive interventions.* Professionals with requisite expertise can organize supportive social and environmental mechanisms that provide a bridge over the cognitive dysfunctions. This is done by modifications of the social, residential, educational, or vocational situation to accommodate the person's cognitive problems. Two examples come from supported education. A disabled person with deficiencies in memory, learning, sustained attention, decision making, and problem solving is eligible to obtain 1) a tutor who can take notes during lectures and provide the repetition needed to learn the academic material in a one-to-one, quiet setting, and 2) more time to complete tests, which compensates for deficits in sustained attention, decision making, and problem solving. These specially designed social supports effectively compensate for the cognitive deficits, enabling a person to succeed in school.

CLINICAL EXAMPLE

A patient with schizophrenia completed his bachelor's and master's degrees by taking assiduous notes, tape-recording the class lectures, and then typing his notes, with editing, using a word processor after class. The repetition in his study habits enabled him to learn the required information and concepts despite his memory and concentration problems. He studied the edited notes repeatedly and was able to learn the course material and receive good grades through a combination of compensatory and cognitive remediation procedures. Research has shown that the hippocampus, the brain region responsible for storage of memories, shows adaptive changes in neural patterning during exposure to repeated learning that don't occur during rapid presentation of information. Years later, switching him from haloperidol, a first-generation antipsychotic drug, to risperidone, an atypical antipsychotic, led to improvements in his cognitive functioning, which were, in part, a result of his being able to discontinue Cogentin (benztropine), an antiparkinsonian agent that further compromises cognitive functioning beyond that caused by the illness itself.

▶ Social Learning Theory

Our development as functional and unique human beings throughout life is shaped to a large extent by our cumulative learning experiences. Our genetic endowment, cognitive capacities, personality traits, and intelligence limit what and how fast we can learn, but within those boundaries we have considerable latitude in achieving our personal goals through the processes of learning. Principles derived from learning theory give us important therapeutic techniques for leveraging desired changes in our patients' behavioral and social functioning. Therefore, our competent use of learning principles is of great therapeutic importance. Considering the widespread functional deficits of the seriously mentally ill, if we hope to use principles of learning to shift their trajectory from disability to recovery, then practitioners must view themselves as teachers, educators, and trainers.

Rehabilitation specialists serve as educators either by teaching skills directly or by providing supports and accommodations in the community for whatever skills the person may already have. For persons with cognitive or symptom impairments, establishing accommodating environments and ensuring their provision facilitate learning in those settings. Given the significance of educational approaches for rehabilitation, how can clinicians become effective teachers? Familiarity with learning theory and the ability to adapt learning principles to the special needs of the mentally ill are prerequisites. Because most seriously mentally ill persons have cognitive deficits that interfere with conventional modes of learning, psychiatric rehabilitation must offer *special education,* not unlike that used with persons who have learning and developmental disabilities.

BEHAVIORAL PRINCIPLES

From the basic laboratories of learning theorists, a scientific study of behavior emerged over the past century. As a result, changes in the frequency and form of human behavior, including symptoms and functional abnormalities, are now understandable and often predictable. The cardinal principle of human learning is the temporal relationship of behavior to the environment in which it occurs. As shown graphically in Figure 2.5, *behavior* is a generic, multimodal term encompassing signs and symptoms, cognitive

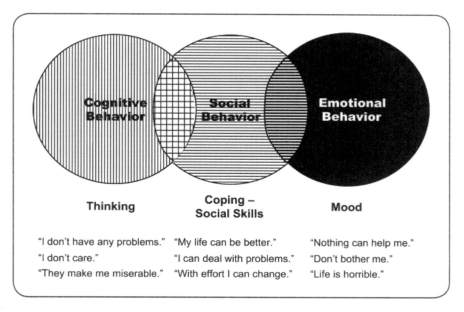

FIGURE 2.5 Overlapping and interacting domains within the construct of behavior: thoughts, social interaction, and emotions.

> ● TABLE 2.2
>
> **Operationalization of behaviors for measuring change brought about by the multimodal scope of rehabilitation in all domains of functioning**
>
> ● The patient talked to himself three times during the 20-minute treatment session.
> ● Complaints of feeling slowed down and stressed did not interfere with his working full-time.
> ● He succeeded in socializing with friends three times during the past week.
> ● She reported having two job interviews since the last treatment session.
> ● A moderate level of depression was rated with a Beck Depression Scale score of 19.
> ● He engaged in seven "healthy pleasures" during the month, including bicycling and a movie.

functions, emotions, beliefs, attitudes, actions and reactions, conversations, imagery, affect-laden communications, verbal and nonverbal social skills, work, aggression, and cognitions. If it's observable and measurable, even indirectly, it's behavior.

Describing the occurrence, frequency, and intensity of behavior in measurable terms conveys a broad spectrum of functioning that is the focus of psychiatric rehabilitation. Examples that illustrate the specificity and breadth of behavioral measurement are shown in Table 2.2.

Rehabilitation is more likely to be effective when the patient and practitioner are able to identify personal goals in behaviorally specific and operational terms and then monitor goal attainment so that progress can be evaluated. Measuring symptoms, skills, and stepwise progression toward patients' personal goals is essential if the rehabilitation enterprise is to be efficiently guided by each step's success or failure. The clinical utility of monitoring the behavior of interest is shown in Figure 2.6 (p. 54). The feedback loops depicted in the figure provide vital information for joint decision making about treatments by the clinician and the patient.

Two learning principles are critical for social rehabilitation of persons with severe mental disorders. One of these principles is *repeated practice of verbal and physical behaviors that are novel or previously learned but in need of strengthening*. William James, a pioneer in empirical psychology, highlighted this principle when he stated, "Repetition is the soul of learning" (James 1890). The other principle that is highly relevant to learning is

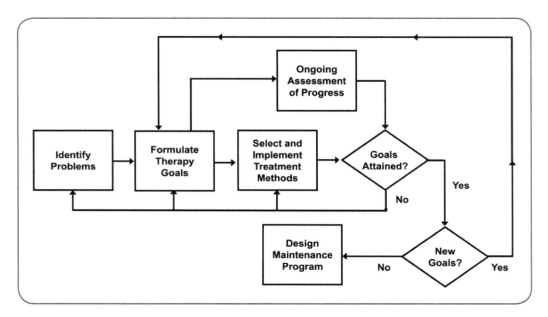

FIGURE 2.6 Clinical decision-making process informed by ongoing assessment of progress toward goals.

direct instruction, also termed *precision teaching*. Precision teaching leads to mastery through continuous engagement of students in practicing tasks that shape a fluent performance. This process is accomplished through instructional routines such as presentation, practice, feedback, review, and homework.

Teachers who are effective in direct instruction start each session with a statement of the session's goals and objectives, followed by a review of the skills taught in the previous sessions, and then present new skills in small steps with explicit directions for practicing them. Precision teaching requires ongoing monitoring of students' performance with frequent feedback and other remedial actions until the learner performs fluently. These principles have been validated by decades of basic and applied research in the fields of psychology and education.

CONSEQUENCES AND CONTINGENCIES: REINFORCERS

Learning theory focuses on the A–B–C's of changing behavior, both abnormal behavior that needs to be weakened and adaptive behavior that needs to be strengthened. The "A" stands for *antecedents of the target behavior*, the "B" for the *target behavior* itself, and the "C" for the *consequences of the behavior*. Depending upon how the antecedents and consequences are arranged and coordinated with the behavior of interest, learning and change will or will not take place.

Consequences given contingent upon desired behavior are called *positive reinforcers* when they have the effect of increasing the probability that the desired behavior will occur in the future. Positive reinforcement is illustrated by a therapist giving verbal and nonverbal acknowledgment and encouragement when a patient is participating actively in a supported employment program. Receiving positive feedback in a genuine and spontaneous manner will strengthen the patient's subsequent participation in the program.

Turning off attention toward counterproductive and undesirable behavior is a consequence that reduces that behavior. In learning theory, this is called *extinction*. An example of extinction is when the therapist strategically ignores a patient's hypochondriacal complaints and shifts the focus of therapeutic interaction to the patient's activities at work or enjoying time with a friend. *Negative reinforcement* occurs when some specific behavior increases by virtue of its enabling the individual to avoid or escape from some aversive or unpleasant consequence. Thus, when we drive within the speed limit to avoid getting a citation from the police, safe driving is negatively reinforced. Rehabilitation programs aim to accentuate or reinforce socially appropriate and adaptive behaviors while ignoring or providing constructive and corrective feedback for symptomatic and counterproductive behaviors.

What constitutes a positive reinforcer varies considerably from person to person. Cultural and religious values can determine reinforcers. For most Americans, alcoholic beverages are reinforcers, but for observant Muslims, Mormons, and Seventh Day Adventists, such beverages are not. In addition to consumables, sex, and material goods, reinforcers may be identified from among the everyday behaviors or activities that individuals prefer to do. Hence, watching TV, sitting in a favorite easy chair, playing computer or video games, and interacting with a pet can be powerful reinforcers that can strengthen personal goals that are new, unfamiliar, and occur too infrequently.

Shaping Behavior

Giving positive reinforcement for very small approximations to the desired goal leads to gradual acquisition of the behavioral goal. This is sometimes referred to as the *law of successive approximations*. It is familiar to all of us, since teaching patients with cognitive impairments requires breaking down any functional goal into its constituents or elements and then giving contingent reinforcement for those small elements. An example of shaping is the positive feedback given by group members in a social skills training class when a participant demonstrates an effective conversational opener with an acquaintance as a starting point for learning how to establish a friendship.

Antecedents and Discriminative Stimuli

Practitioners tend to identify stressful or noxious events or experiences that occurred in the recent past to explain the cause for symptom exacerbation or a dysfunctional emotional response. Triggers or precipitants of a maladaptive behavioral response—for example, aggression that follows an insult—do play a role in learning theory. Triggering events, stressors, life events, and other precipitants are called *discriminative stimuli.* Discriminative stimuli are empowered to become predictable cues for a behavioral response by virtue of frequently occurring temporal relationships among the discriminative stimulus, some behavior, and a reinforcing consequence of that behavior.

A discriminative stimulus can be illustrated by a pleasant greeting that a practitioner offers to a patient at the start of a treatment session. Over many repeated sessions, the pleasant greeting has been associated with an affirming response by the patient and continued positive, empathic, and supportive interest by the therapist in the patient's self-disclosure of recent events, feelings, and problems. Thus, the initial pleasant greeting of the practitioner becomes a discriminative stimulus for getting a treatment session under way in a cooperative and optimistic manner. Discriminative stimuli may also be antecedents to terminating some behavior. Thus, patients can be taught to recognize nonverbal expressions of disinterest or boredom as "no go" signals for ending a conversation.

From a learning theory perspective, many of the events that are considered precipitating factors for relapse or exacerbation of symptoms are not sufficient causal explanations by themselves, but rather are embedded in a repeated cycle of antecedents–behaviors–consequences. A notorious example of this comes from family interactions that lead to exacerbation of symptoms of various mental disorders. If a family member criticizes a relative with depression or schizophrenia, the individual is very likely to respond with a defensive remark, pouting, hostility, or a self-deprecating comment. A frequent consequence of that type of behavioral response is the family member responding in like fashion with a somewhat higher emotional pitch. This cycle has been found to continue in a self-perpetuating, escalating fashion until the patient begins to exhibit subsyndromal or prodromal signs and symptoms of the mental disorder.

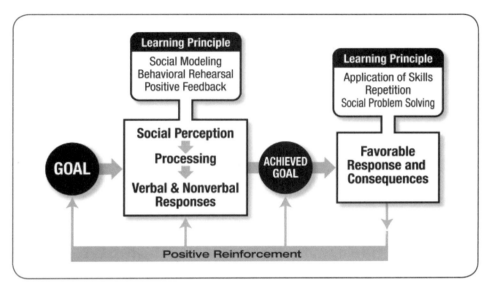

FIGURE 2.7 Role of behavioral learning principles in social skills training. **In** social skills training, behavioral learning principles provide sources of motivation for the acquisition of skills at the levels of social perception, processing incoming information, and making judgments and decisions about how to respond and to implement those decisions using socially appropriate verbal and nonverbal responses.

Social Modeling

Social modeling, another important principle derived from learning theory, is sometimes referred to as imitative learning, observational learning, or vicarious learning. It takes place when an individual acquires some behavior or behavioral skill by observing another person perform that behavior or skill. Most complex social, occupational, and athletic skills are learned in this manner. Social modeling conforms to the aphorism "A picture is worth a thousand words." When a student is in training to become a mental health professional, social modeling is of critical importance in learning interviewing, diagnostic, and treatment skills. The model is usually a faculty member or mentor, but classmates also serve as models for each other. In social skills training, modeling makes a major contribution to the learning process as patients observe the trainer or other patients demonstrating effective communications such as making positive requests of others, making assertive statements, or asking open-ended questions to maintain a conversation.

The role of learning principles in social skills training is displayed in Figure 2.7. A patient has a personally relevant goal that involves interacting and relating with others. During the role-play segment of social skills training, social modeling and behavioral rehearsal are used to teach appropriate interpersonal skills in the dimensions of social perception, processing of incoming information from the other person in the role-play, and then making decisions regarding how best to send verbal and nonverbal behavior back to the other person. Immediate positive reinforcement is given as feedback during the skills training session to strengthen the patient's social behaviors. When the patient succeeds in his/her goal in real life, the natural reinforcement that comes from the benefits accruing from the interpersonal situation further strengthens the person's social skills for the future. Reporting that the goal was achieved during the subsequent social skills training session is the occasion for further social reinforcement from the clinician and other members of the group.

▶ Life Span Developmental Psychology

The overarching goal of psychiatric rehabilitation is to assist persons with mental disabilities to achieve relatively normal, meaningful, valued, and satisfying lifestyles. Conceptions of *abnormal* and *deviant behavior* are derived from psychiatry. In contrast, rehabilitation emphasizes *normalization of behavior congruent with community expectations and integration.* This field requires definitions of normality in the context of community acceptance. The field of life span developmental psychology places normality within a frame of reference of age-appropriate behavior.

The development of normal, age-congruent social behavior has been mapped from childhood to adulthood. In the developmental sequence through adolescence, children's social behavior changes in the direction of cooperation, problem solving, independence from adult supervision, control of anger, negotiation, and compromise. Higher levels of complex, reciprocal social relatedness and perspective taking develop as the prefrontal cortex matures along with its interconnections to other brain regions. Social competence also develops as children and adolescents identify with both peer and adult role models and learn from social norms and rule-governed behavior and through the positive and negative consequences of their behavior.

Considerable research has shown that children and adolescents who later develop schizophrenia achieve their developmental milestones later, with many of them displaying significant deficits in premorbid social adjustment even as early as childhood. In monozygotic and dizygotic twin studies, delays in social competence have been noted in the twin who later developed schizophrenia. One seminal study using home movies and videos taken by parents during early childhood demonstrated that trained observers could differentiate siblings who subsequently developed schizophrenia from the brothers and sisters. The children who later developed schizophrenia we more passive, reacted and deferred to others rather than initiating activities, stayed closer to their parents, engaged in less independent and cooperative play, and took fewer risks. These early, premorbid abnormalities in social behavior are believed to be genetic and neurodevelopmental indicators of the vulnerability to schizophrenia.

Because candidates for rehabilitation are most often adults, adequate milestones used for framing their personally relevant goals within the normal range derive from research on adult development. These milestones are shown in Table 2.3. Especially in schizophrenia, the onset of the disorder during late adolescence or early adulthood has two major, adverse impacts on the individual's social development: 1) the illness interrupts further maturation of social functioning, and 2) symptoms of the illness—especially negative symptoms—interfere with the use of already acquired social skills.

In defining what is normal or mentally healthy, it is important to recognize that mental health is not incompatible with the presence of

● TABLE 2.3

Tasks for the stages of adult development

Early adult stage (ages 17–45)
- Undergoing individuation and realignment of relationships with parents
- Forming and pursuing life goals and aspirations
- Establishing and raising a family
- Pursuing a career or occupation, with financial independence

Middle adult stage (ages 46–65)
- Sharing one's experience, knowledge, and skills with others
- Developing a more compassionate, judicious, and reflective view of life
- Experiencing fewer external demands for accomplishments and less stress and adopting a more balanced lifestyle
- Confronting risk of midlife crisis

Late-life transition
- Anticipating and accommodating losses of roles, work, and relationships
- Experiencing decline in physical health and awareness of mortality
- Taking on new roles: retirement careers and activities, grandparenting, more leisure time
- Experiencing, paradoxically, increased satisfaction with life than at earlier stages

some amount of psychopathology—as long as symptoms do not intrude excessively on one's positive functioning. Definitions of normality incorporate variations associated with culture, geography, age, and family and personal values. Nonetheless, a consensus has been reached among scholars who have identified characteristics consistent with adult maturity and wellness. These characteristics, listed in Table 2.3, can be used as benchmarks for assisting patients in setting their overall personal goals for rehabilitation.

The fact that most serious mental disorders have their onset in the adolescent and early adult periods is partly explained by the stressors impinging on young people at a time in their lives when they are expected to make a transition toward self-definition, independence, and achievement. In particular, the adolescent or young adult with schizophrenia or disabling mood and anxiety disorders experiences years of restricted progress, aborted life goals, and regression at the same time that peers are continuing their trajectory into adult roles. Failure to establish independence and withdrawal from interpersonal relationships, school, and work are devastating to his/her self-esteem and personal identity. At a time when peers are forming friendships and intimacy and achieving self-support, the seriously mentally ill young person lapses into the role of patient, with constricted social contacts revolving around family, mental health professionals, and other mentally ill patients.

This conceptualization of stunted transition into adulthood has many consequences for treatment and rehabilitation. The painful discrepancy between aspirations and reality evokes denial of illness, rejection of treatment, demoralization and depression, irritability, and hostility; moreover, these emotions, combined with impaired functioning, interfere with the patient setting and working toward realistic, incremental goals. When best practices of psychiatric rehabilitation are used from the very beginning of the engagement process, hope can be implanted by educating patients and families experiencing these traumas about the following:

- The nature of the illness
- The ways in which treatments can stem symptoms and cognitive impairments and stabilize the illness
- The malleability of many of the functional problems that interfere with recovery

Using a Socratic approach, the practitioner can bring the patient and family to see for themselves how stepwise progress toward meaningful life goals can be accomplished through participating in evidence-based services. These initial interventions, plus enthusiastically inviting the family and patient to become intrinsic members of the treatment team, can shift the gears of treatment so that the patient and family are empowered to move forward with a more hopeful, realistic optimism toward the future.

Two normative elements in the transition to adulthood offer hope to mentally disabled persons for achieving satisfying roles in the years to come: 1) because there is considerable fluidity in the timing and progression of adult tasks and socialization, these are not strictly bound by age, and 2) modern society recognizes great variations in the pathways taken within the normal range. The capacity to realign, transform, or make up lags in social development through setting personally relevant goals, learning social and occupational skills, and creating individually meaningful life roles gives hope to mentally ill persons who wish to undertake the journey to recovery. Rehabilitation can be useful at any age and for any pace of improvement however deliberate and slow.

▶ Principles and Practices of Psychiatric Rehabilitation

The seven principles of psychiatric rehabilitation are presented in this section with illustrations of intervention practices that illuminate them. Examples of practitioner competencies are given for some of the practices because fidelity to evidence-based services promotes favorable therapeutic outcomes.

....

1. **Recovery of a normal life in the community is possible for many persons with mental disabilities if best practices of rehabilitation are provided.**

....

Psychiatric disorders do not yield easily to medication alone or to singular psychosocial practices such as case management or social skills training. Especially when the aim is to facilitate a return to relatively normal functioning, a comprehensive array of competently delivered, evidence-based services needs to be provided continuously and flexibly with coordination among treatment providers. As a cautionary note, we must understand that at this point in our fragmented systems of service, only a minority of the seriously mentally ill—especially those with conditions within the schizophrenia spectrum—will be able to gain a level of recovery within the normal range of community participation. However, achieving as full and normal a life as possible can be a reasonable and hope-inspiring goal for most of our patients.

> ... at social re-
> ...ry is not a recovery in the real
> sense of the word. But it seems
> beyond argument that there is an
> improvement in personality if one
> changes from obvious and dis-
> abling psychosis to a considerable
> measure of ability to live in one's
> own environment. The fact that
> the patient can be helped to the
> point where he knows how to keep
> out of trouble is at least economi-
> cally and pragmatically useful. It
> seems a century or two too early
> for expecting perfection in this one
> field of human welfare."
>
> HARRY STACK SULLIVAN, M.D.
> (1892–1949)

Our part of the bargain is to mobilize as many of the evidence-based treatments as are available and relevant for helping our patients achieve their personal goals en route to recovery. Giving value and credence to recovery as an uncompromising goal and vision for rehabilitation can also motivate practitioners, patients, family members, managers, policy makers, and other stakeholders to reform our current systems of care by bringing evidence-based services into everyday practice.

Best practices and evidence-based treatments can speed recovery. These include:

- Involving patients and their families in functional assessment helps identify personally relevant goals to enrich and bring meaning, self-respect, and optimal independence and satisfaction into one's life.

- Evidence-based pharmacological and psychosocial treatments remove or attenuate symptoms and cognitive and emotional impairments that interfere with the quest to reach one's goals.

- Motivational enhancement instills hope for a better future, thereby sustaining the persistence required for years of learning social and independent living skills.

- Structured and supportive programs for work, school, and housing enable patients to achieve higher levels of independent functioning.

- Teaching families and patients to improve their coping, communication, and problem-solving skills helps to build realistic expectations and generate positive reinforcement for progress.

- Proactive, long-term, intensive, flexible, and indefinite case management by personal support specialists assists patients in using survival skills for community integration.

- Enlightened and recovery-oriented administrators and managers in mental health agencies give priority to incorporating best practices into the competencies and performance standards of clinicians and multidisciplinary teams.

2. **Impairments, disabilities, and handicaps can be reduced or overcome by integrating pharmacological and psychosocial services**

with advocacy for improved clinical, educational, vocational, and governmental policies and practices.

In promoting recovery from serious mental disorders, rehabilitation specialists face a daunting task. Dislodging impairments, disabilities, and handicaps that are obstacles on the road to recovery requires energy, activism, realistic optimism, tolerance for frustration, and always seeing the glass as half full. Fortunately, there is aid and comfort for the beleaguered practitioner. The past several decades have seen the emergence of a coherent set of rehabilitation strategies for controlling or reversing impairments, remediating disabilities, and removing barriers in the community that are responsible for handicaps in the mentally ill. Medications and cognitive rehabilitation can remove or ameliorate impairments such as symptoms and deficits in sustained attention, memory, learning, and problem solving. Reducing symptom and cognitive impairments improves the chances of success for learning abilities and skills that can pave the way to recovery.

The two most important approaches for enhancing the functional capacities of the mentally disabled are 1) inculcating social and independent living skills through educational and training techniques and 2) supportive services that compensate for the specific behavioral deficits that interfere with functioning. Personal support specialists (i.e., case managers) can provide assistance to mentally disabled persons, enabling them to work, attend school, deal with social agencies, become informed consumers, make friends, improve family relations, or live successfully in a community home. A pictorial representation of the role of the personal support specialist is shown in Figure 2.8, and the various levels of intervention for reducing disabilities and handicaps are shown in Figure 2.9.

Advocacy and Stigma-Busting

Dealing with handicaps that interfere with patients' full participation in society requires major efforts that often reside in social advocacy rather than in clinical interactions. Remedies for society's stigma toward the mentally ill have been introduced in the past 15 years. One notable example is the Americans with Disabilities Act, which prohibits employers from discriminating against persons with disabilities. Applicants for jobs need not disclose their disabilities unless these are directly related to the requirements of the job. Employers are expected to offer accommodations to workers with disabilities so the latter can be productive.

Other examples of changes in the social system that have improved the prospects of the mentally disabled to participate more fully and normally in society are:

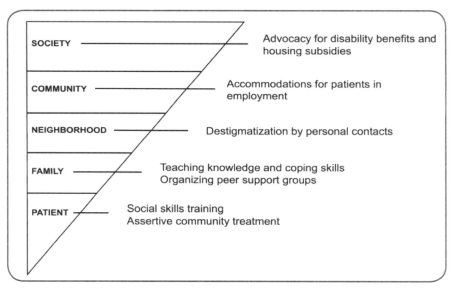

FIGURE 2.8 Role of personal support specialists (i.e., case managers) in psychiatric rehabilitation. Personal support specialists can provide opportunities, encouragement, and reinforcement of social and independent living skills in the community.

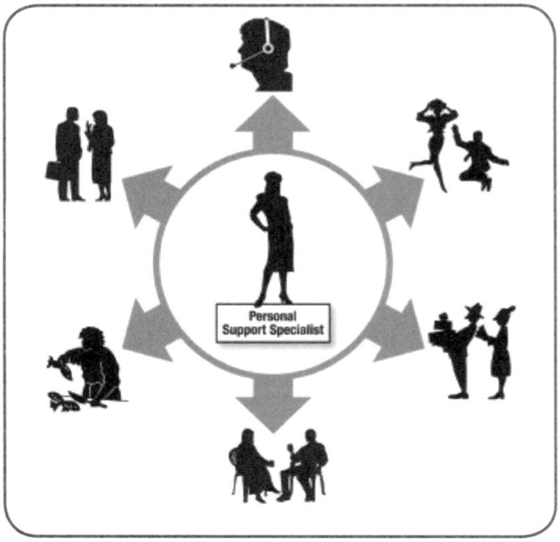

SOCIETY —————————— Advocacy for disability benefits and housing subsidies

COMMUNITY —————————— Accommodations for patients in employment

NEIGHBORHOOD ——————— Destigmatization by personal contacts

FAMILY ————— Teaching knowledge and coping skills Organizing peer support groups

PATIENT Social skills training Assertive community treatment

FIGURE 2.9 Multiple levels of intervention to reduce disability and handicap in mentally disabled patients.

- Tax credits extended to employers for hiring disabled persons.
- Supported education that encourages mainstreaming of mentally ill students in all levels of the education system. Offices for disabled students provide individualized supports such as tutoring, more time for test taking, and in-school psychiatric consultation.
- Work incentive programs to encourage the disabled to gradually shift from Social Security benefits to being self-supporting workers.

- Affirmative action aimed at encouraging the employment of disabled persons by the federal government and companies that have contracts with the federal government.
- Assertive community treatment teams that are mobile and reach out to persons with mental illness who may find conventional mental health services inaccessible or threatening.

Recovery from mental illness is sabotaged by stigma. Stigma discourages mentally ill individuals and their families from seeking treatment, makes them second-class citizens, excludes them from neighborhoods, and feeds the misapprehension that they are always dangerous, bizarre, unpredictable, and untreatable. Mentally ill persons, harmed by stigma at the family, community, cultural, and economic levels, experience shame, devaluation, rejection, and bruised self-esteem. Family members also experience stigma when they disclose their relative's illness and attempt to advocate for better services.

When stigma declines, another barrier to recovery is removed. Fortunately, in recent years, stigma as a handicap has been on the defensive, under attack from a variety of directions, which are identified in Table 2.4.

- **TABLE 2.4**
Salutary developments in reducing stigma of mental illness

- Celebrities are "coming out of the closet" and very publicly speaking and writing about their mental illnesses and, more importantly, how their treatments enabled them to recover.
- Rehabilitation and self-help programs are winning publicity for their success in restoring the capacity for work, citizenship, responsibility, and independence of the mentally ill.
- Advocacy organizations like the National Alliance on Mental Illness pressure the media to curtail stigmatizing productions.
- Numerous Web sites offer factual information about mental illness and the effectiveness of current treatments.
- Media campaigns highlight the importance of early identification and treatment of mental illness with attendant prevention of chronicity.
- Education and training of key personnel who have direct contact with the mentally ill have enlightened police, judges, physicians, teachers, and employers.
- Testimonies of mentally ill individuals have allowed them to articulate how treatment has been instrumental in their recoveries.
- Opportunities for face-to-face contact by the seriously mentally ill with neighbors, friends, and community businesspeople have increased.

3. Individualization of treatment is a fundamental pillar of rehabilitation.

"One size does not fit all."

"Only penguins look alike."

"Always remember that you are absolutely unique, just like everyone else."

Tailoring treatment planning and implementation for each person is based on the simple but pervasive reality of individual differences. Diversity is reflected by lives that change over time, never to repeat the past in exactly the same way. Disorders may reflect common abnormalities in neurotransmitter systems, but patients are unique in how their learning histories, coping, resilience, and social supports protect them from those abnormalities. The importance of recognizing each person's special features is pictorially shown in Figure 2.10.

Matching treatments to individuals' levels of cognitive, behavioral, and social functioning is one of the most important principles of psychiatric rehabilitation. Differences between patients affect the choice of appropriate treatment, as do differences from one time to another within the same individual. What will be helpful to a patient at the time of acute exacerbation of psychosis will not be helpful when the same patient has reached the stable phase of his/her illness.

"Sometimes we think that we won't find another human being inside a person who is different from us and who seems strange, unpredictable and hard to understand. Maybe we are reluctant to make the effort to communicate or expect the other person to avoid us, so we give up without even trying. How sad it is that we would give up on any other person who's more like us than we think."

FRED ROGERS (1928–2003)
Mr. Rogers' Neighborhood

Regrettably, rehabilitation practitioners all too often lose sight of this basic principle because it is much more convenient to assemble everyone in a program in the same activities. Even in group activities considerable individualization is possible. For example, a patient who is functioning at a high level will proceed more rapidly in a social skills training group. That person could remain in the group as an esteemed member by serving as a "teaching assistant" or tutor for individuals who are at lower levels of functioning. Effective rehabilitation requires us to guard against grouping, stereotyping, and homogenizing patients, whose individuality then disappears behind diagnostic labels. Reifying disorders imprints a lifeless uniformity on our patients' experience and on our treatment efforts.

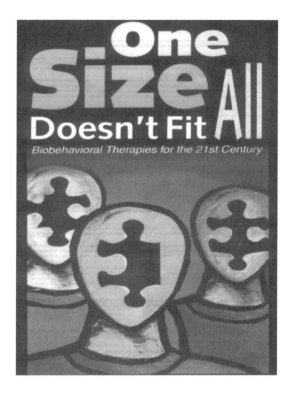

FIGURE 2.10
Importance of recognizing each person's special qualities in treatment planning. Treatment outcomes are improved when practitioners recognize the unique attributes of each patient and conform services to the person, not to the disorder.

Evidence-Based Treatment Is Never Provided to the "Average" Patient

Practitioners should not adopt a particular evidence-based treatment or program without using clinical judgment in shaping the intervention to fit the individual patient. Treatments are documented as "evidence-based" in large-scale, controlled clinical trials, in which the *average outcome* for subjects is found to be significantly better than the *average outcome* for those assigned to the standard treatment. The fact that a treatment, on average, is statistically more effective than a comparison treatment has very little significance in choosing an appropriate treatment for a single *specific individual*.

Practitioners provide treatment not to "average individuals" but rather to real patients whose attributes may, in fact, contraindicate the use of a particular evidence-based service. It may be inappropriate to apply an evidence-based treatment to an individual whose type, severity, or duration of disorder, personal goals, language and cultural barriers, and strengths and weaknesses make him/her different from those who responded to the treatment in the large-scale, published research. One example of this comes from supported employment, an evidence-based treatment for vocational rehabilitation. While approximately 50% of patients who participate in supported employment have been able to get jobs, only individuals who assertively express a strong interest in working are selected for this program. Thus, by referring a patient to supported employment, a practitioner could be setting a patient up for failure if the individual is not inclined to work or is ambivalent about working.

Cultural and Ethnic Differences

Rehabilitation assessments and interventions must be adapted for congruence with the family and cultural context of the individual. Approximately one-fourth of individuals receiving services from the public mental health system in the United States identify themselves with one of the many ethnic groups that have recently emigrated to this country. Without rehabilitation programs that are sensitive and compatible with individuals representing the diverse ethnic and language groups prevalent in our society, obstacles to accessibility, effectiveness, and satisfaction with services will be discriminatory. Failing to use a "cultural lens" to make accurate diagnoses, select appropriate goals, and offer treatments that are modified for their familiarity and acceptability to the individual patient will result in the disproportionate use of emergency, inpatient, and involuntary interventions for minority patients. Cultural competence, described in greater depth in Chapter 9 ("Special Services for Special People"), is essential for helping individuals affiliated with various ethnic groups recover from their mental disabilities.

Recognizing and Promoting Spirituality

Because of the secular origins of mental health disciplines and their practitioners, religion and spirituality are often neglected rather than being harnessed to rehabilitation. Ignoring a domain that distinguishes individuals and pervades their personal identity handicaps both patients and their clinicians. Most patients express the wish that their health and mental health providers would address religious and spiritual issues in their clinical care. Empathy in the therapeutic alliance requires an understanding of each individual's spiritual beliefs, customs, values, and affiliations. Awareness of our patients' religious and spiritual qualities helps us to select the most appropriate tools for relieving distress and motivating adherence to treatment.

Religious beliefs are associated with well-being, personal adjustment, and coping with medical and psychiatric disorders. Belief in a higher power, religion, prayer, and faith in God are repeatedly cited in first-person accounts as important in the process of recovering from a serious mental disorder. Given the frightening experience of being out of control of one's thinking, emotions, and volitional behavior, persons with psychiatric disabilities search for ways of dealing with their limitations, helplessness, and loss of direction in life. As shown in Table 2.5, practitioners can encourage patients to use spiritual and religious beliefs to make sense of complex events, accept distress and disappointment, and cope with frustration.

4. **Rehabilitation is more effective and recovery more rapid when patients and families are actively involved in planning and participating in treatment.**

The key that opens the door to effective rehabilitation is *engaging* the patient and family members in a collaboration for identifying and achieving goals that can lead to a more functional and satisfying life. Through active participation in treatment, patients become more invested and motivated in treatment. It is the responsibility of clinicians and mental health organizations to design and implement their treatment programs so that active participation becomes a norm. Very few patients with serious mental disorders initially

---

● **TABLE 2.5**

Sensitivity to a patient's spiritual and religious needs and beliefs is a practitioner competence

- Providing a nonjudgmental, accepting, and empathic approach toward eliciting information about the patient's religious and spiritual beliefs
- Taking time to understand the patient's spirituality as it may relate to symptoms and functioning
- Asking, "What religious or spiritual resources in your life might help you cope with your problems?"
- Encouraging individuals with religious beliefs to gain strength and support from knowing that God is a loving and supportive life force
- Seeking consultation and information from appropriate sources concerning the patient's spiritual beliefs and traditions, including referral to relevant clergy and mental health practitioners

come to treatment in an active mode. Passivity is instilled by the sick role and its accompaniments: hopelessness, dependency, stigma, negative symptoms, and demoralization. How then can practitioners and clinical administrators mobilize active involvement and participation by patients and their families? Each of the subsequent chapters in this book elucidates methods for gaining the vigorous involvement of patients in rehabilitative services, a principle of rehabilitation that animates practices of the entire field.

> "Life is short, opportunity fugitive, experience deceptive, judgment difficult. It is the duty of the physician, not only to do that which immediately belongs to him, but likewise to secure the cooperation of the sick."
>
> HIPPOCRATES (CA. 460–377 B.C.)

Only recently have practitioners in the mental health disciplines, as well as medicine in general, recognized the importance and therapeutic value of gaining the involvement of their patients, families, and other caregivers as full partners in the treatment enterprise. This recognition represents a major shift from the traditional authoritarian, patronizing, and "doctor knows best" roles. In point of fact, the patient and family are "experts" in the mental illness under treatment because they experience the symptoms, impairments, and disabilities 24 hours a day, 7 days per week. Their experiences complement the technical and professional expertise of the practitioner. Valuing their experiential expertise is a building block for erecting a therapeutic relationship infused with mutual respect.

The partnership among the patient, family, and practitioner begins with the initial evaluation, when patient and relatives provide information about their experiences with past treatments—what was helpful and what was harmful or indifferent. Who knows better than the patient and family about side effects, tolerability, and efficacy of past medications and psychosocial treatments? Involving the family should not violate the patient's confidentiality in any way if all concerned understand that treatment becomes more effective when the family is actively participating. It's a rare patient who refuses open sharing of all relevant clinical information with responsible family members when he/she grasps the therapeutic significance of having his/her relatives as full members of the treatment team.

A consumer-oriented approach to treatment and rehabilitation engenders collaboration, empowerment, mutual respect, a stronger therapeutic alliance, and better adherence to treatment. By presenting reasonable treatment alternatives for patients to choose from, accompanied by information on the positive and negative trade-offs involved, therapeutic outcomes improve, regardless of which option the patients actually choose. Once treatment goals and interventions are selected, involving the patient in regularly scheduled re-evaluations of the progress being made informs jointly made judgments about maintaining, tweaking, or changing the treatment program. (The cycle of goal setting, treatment, and evaluation was shown in Figure 2.6 earlier in this chapter.)

The experience of being an active participant in the treatment process lends confidence to patients and their families and raises their optimism and hope for a better future. Hope is strengthened when patients know that they can express their deepest fears, worries, concerns, and suffering to receptive treaters who are empathic, encouraging, realistically optimistic, and persistent in the face of reversals and uncertainty. As shown in Figure 2.11, working together as a collaborative team enables patients, with the support of families, practitioners, and peers, to persevere with hope through arduous and lengthy treatment in the pursuit of recovery.

Hope for improvement and recovery is supported by relationships with

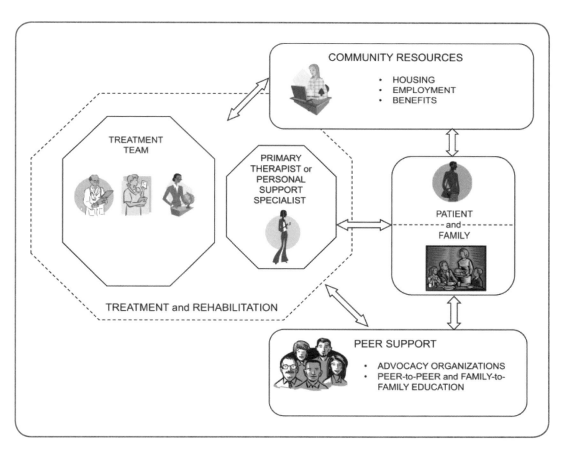

FIGURE 2.11 Facilitation of recovery by teamwork among treatment team, patient, family, peers, and community resources.

practitioners and family members who never give up on the patient and whose decision making aligns with the patient's strengths and interests. Practitioners and family members in such relationships have the ability to accept mentally ill persons in whatever phase of illness they happen to be in and find positive attributes to acknowledge and reinforce. Neither hope nor empowerment materializes from thin air or rhetoric. Empowerment and hope derive from making a difference in one's life, whether as patient, family member, or practitioner. These important forms of self-efficacy are inculcated by achieving incremental treatment goals that enable all parties to see light at the end of the tunnel. Realistic optimism aerates the practitioner–patient relationship when both realize that goals can change to become more attainable and that it's always possible to try another way to reach one's goals. Without confidence in the resourcefulness for improving one's life, futility is the predator of hope.

5. Integration and coordination of services are essential to enhance progress toward recovery.

No single treatment or quick fix is sufficient for restoring functional and satisfying lifestyles to persons with serious and persistent mental disorders. Because an array of treatments is required for the multifaceted problems that are associated with disability, integration and coordination are key elements in achieving recovery. Psychosocial and pharmacological treatments need to be integrated at three levels—the 1) patient, 2) practitioners or team treating the patient, and 3) agencies contributing varied services in the system of care.

At the simplest level, integration supports the efficacy of pharmacological and psychosocial treatments. Patients require education to understand how medications and psychosocial treatments can be mutually beneficial or in conflict. Side effects of medication, such as sedation, tremor, or akathisia, may interfere with psychosocial treatment. This situation calls for accommodations, with changes in type or dose of medication with or without concomitant changes in psychosocial treatment. On the other hand, an overstimulating psychosocial treatment may trigger an exacerbation of psychotic or depressive symptoms that calls for changing the psychosocial treatment and/or augmenting the medication regimen.

Integration at the Level of Treatment Teams

At the level of the treatment staff, integration of multiple treatments is essential for assessment, treatment planning, and treatment. A proper assessment is almost always an interdisciplinary effort. The responsible clinician or treatment team has to integrate the information obtained by various members of the multidisciplinary team regarding the patient's history, symptoms, diagnosis, psychosocial functioning, cognitive status, family relationships, and educational or vocational functioning. Without a well-integrated, comprehensive, and thoughtful assessment, any treatment plan is bound to be suboptimal.

Once a plan of treatment is embarked on, the patient's progress must be monitored and communicated among the responsible clinicians. For example, communication between an employment specialist providing supported employment and the rest of the multidisciplinary treatment team is critical for solving a problem that surfaces on the job. Perhaps intervention is needed when, for example, there is an emotional eruption between the patient and a family member or roommate, there is a change in medication for insomnia that results in the patient being sleepy on the job, or the patient is trying to cope with anxiety provoked by a letter from Social Security cutting off benefits.

Integrating treatment at the patient and staff level becomes an enormous challenge when a patient is receiving services from more than one agency. Who takes what specific responsibility for coordinating and communicating information on assessment, treatment, and progress for each agency when a patient is involved with separate organizations providing services for substance abuse, mental health, money management, probation, residential housing, conservatorship, vocational rehabilitation, and medical problems? Given the fact that comorbidity is often the rule rather than the exception, this scenario is not uncommon. In such situations, competencies for diplomacy, negotiation, administration, and information processing are required if the multiplicity of services are to be cumulative in their effects.

Clinical collaboration can work reasonably well among agencies if representatives from each entity become acquainted, learn to respect and rely on one another, and maintain regular communication regarding the respective services they are providing to the patient. Little can be expected from a solo practitioner who is constrained in the range of services that he/she can provide. In a survey of 615 psychiatrists who were treating schizophrenia patients in clinical practice, medications were used freely but psychosocial services were rarities. Only 38% of the patients had case management, 13%

were participating in social activities, and just 3% were receiving vocational rehabilitation—despite the fact that 73% were unemployed (West et al. 2005).

Integration at the Organizational Level

Systems of care, whether in urban or rural areas, face considerable challenges in organizing the diverse services that are needed by persons with serious mental disabilities. Obtaining housing; Social Security benefits; vocational, educational, and family supports; and substance abuse services falls within the role of the personal support specialist or case manager. There is no particular discipline assigned to this coordinating role, although it is often a social worker because of his/her training in community organization and supports. Models of case management arose in response to the need to orchestrate a host of services in the community that are not offered under the same roof.

Successful integration of disparate services provided by different agencies ultimately depends not on individual patients, families, and practitioners but rather on organizational actions. Unless top and middle managers and program administrators of services—within a given catchment area or system of care—provide supports and mandates for high-fidelity use of an integrated approach, even the best-designed programs will have little impact on patients over the sustained period required for incremental improvement and recovery. Support for integrated treatment and rehabilitation at the management and organizational levels is partly dependent upon adequate funding by policy makers. The constraints facing public and private funding of mental care have perilous consequences for improved services and long-term recovery. But even when agencies and clinicians are motivated to implement better-quality services, they will not be able to do this alone—they will need training and consultation from experts or "knowledge transfer brokers" to learn new, evidence-based approaches and gain competence and confidence in their everyday use.

6. **Building on patients' strengths, interests, and capabilities is a cornerstone of rehabilitation.**

Through the patient's eye, rehabilitation aims to help the individual to "get a life" that is meaningful and rewarding, despite the imprint of symptoms, cognitive and emotional impairments, and disability. In contrast with the traditional focus of psychiatry on the treatment of symptoms, rehabilitation shifts the focus to the day-in, day-out functioning of disabled individuals. In particular, the focus is on what the patient is able to do, how the patient can solve problems, with whom the patient has developed relationships, and when the patient has accomplished a task and achieved a goal. Patients and their families, in league with their practitioners, can be challenged to live in the present and plan for the future. Helping patients to answer the question "How will you act today to change your situation tomorrow?" keeps the focus on positive, short-term goals that lead to hope, empowerment, self-responsibility, and, eventually, a better quality of life. Progress by patients toward attaining their personal goals is facilitated by our using social skills training and other evidence-based treatments to *build on existing strengths*.

If we look for strengths to build on, we will find them, as in the following examples.

- Henry had artistic skills and enthusiasm about his creativity but needed social skills training to negotiate the pathways for obtaining a vendor's permit so he could exhibit his work in the public park. Then he learned some sales skills to win customers—the first time he earned money for his artistic skills.

- Jill placed her name on a waiting list for independent housing and learned through skills training how to advocate for obtaining priority— she used the phone and in-person visits to ask about her place on the waiting list. When she informed the officials in the housing authority that she would volunteer her experience and ability in gardening to improve the grounds of an apartment building, she was put at the top of the waiting list.

- Struggling with his lifelong disability caused by social anxiety, depression, and paranoid personality traits, Simon continued to cherish his dream of becoming a physician. His persistence and determination were the strengths that enabled him to proceed through a series of therapists until he found one who used cognitive-behavioral therapy that overcame his chronic anxiety and depression. His grades and Medical School Admission Test scores were acceptable, but social skills training provided him with the ability and sustained effort through many medical school interviews until he was finally accepted.

- When Janice asked her psychiatrist about returning to college, he cautioned her to give up that goal and to think instead about a volunteer job. "He told me that, given my schizophrenia, I should consider myself retired and needing a long rest." Despite her illness, she was a bright young woman with the ability to concentrate and

> ● **TABLE 2.6**
> **Guidelines for practitioners in building skills and supports and encouraging their use**
>
> ● Provide assistance and choices for patients in identifying short-term goals that are stepping-stones toward their long-term personal goals, imbuing patients with decision-making opportunities.
> ● Persuade patients to select goals that are attainable and functional for them.
> ● Ensure that skills for which training is provided have meaning for everyday situations and longer-term life goals.
> ● Use existing skills as a base for adding new ones.
> ● Employ social learning principles with an active, directive style.

learn. Her engaging personality warmed a helping relationship with a counselor in the disabled students office of a local community college. Aided by supported education services, she was able to complete course work over 3 years that made her eligible for admission to a 4-year college.

Rehabilitation that builds upon patients' preexisting abilities, interests, and endearing personal qualities is empowering only if patients are able to put their skills into everyday use. Transferring their skills to the natural environment depends upon practitioners, families, and friends who can create opportunities and encourage and reinforce the patients' modest, stepwise efforts to use their skills and supports in their natural environment. As shown in Table 2.6, accentuating the positive fosters rehabilitation by concentrating on what can be improved, not on what cannot.

7. **Rehabilitation takes time, proceeds incrementally, and requires perseverance, patience, and resilience by patients, families, and practitioners.**

Given the serious impairments and disabilities that characterize most mentally disabled individuals embarking on the road to recovery, realistic expectations for improvement must be governed by patience and persistence. Rehabilitation enables mentally disabled persons to gradually reach their long-term goals as symptoms become quiescent, skills are acquired, supportive services are organized, and community resources are mobilized. Improvement comes slowly because treatment and rehabilitation must be tailored to the changing phases of a person's illness. Only after a period of sustained stability can evidence-based treatments such as supported employment be most effectively deployed to accelerate movement toward recovery. Even when a patient has had long periods of stability, intensive rehabilitation may require a deliberate pace. Potholes and detours make the road to recovery treacherous, bumpy, and grueling. Going slow is sometimes faster.

As evidenced by the following example of successful rehabilitation, recovery-oriented treatment requires a considerable amount of "tincture of time."

Patients and practitioners should be cautioned to avoid excessive zeal in pursuing overly ambitious goals. A vigilant clinician is sensitive to subtle indicators that a patient may be surpassing his/her threshold of vulnerability. Anxiety, irritability, problems concentrating, and other warning signs of relapse are often the best guide for pacing rehabilitation, as each individual tends to have his/her own degree of vulnerability to environmental stimulation and challenge. To endure is more important than to race.

CLINICAL EXAMPLE

Debbie was 25 years old when she joined the weekly group for social skills training. She had been discharged from the hospital 3 months before but was still troubled by frequent and unpleasant delusions and hallucinations. Even more of a handicap for her participation in the group were her negative symptoms and overwhelming social anxiety. She had spent almost all of her time since age 19, when her schizophrenia began, secluded in her family home. For the first 2 months of attending the group, her anxiety disrupted her participation. She was encouraged to take a break, step outside, and return when she felt more comfortable. The other group members were friendly and accepting of her limited involvement. During the next 6 months, the flexibility of the group leader and cohesion of the group members enabled Debbie to gradually increase her tolerance for the group process. By the sixth month she was able to remain in the group for the entire 90-minute session. Her growing comfort in the group was aided by a combination of exposure in vivo and vicarious desensitization from watching her peers actively participating, planning goals, achieving them, and enjoying the process. The shaping of her increasing involvement was accomplished by positive social reinforcement for successive increments of participation offered by fellow patients and the group leader.

She was now ready to set long-term, personal goals as the first step in becoming actively involved in the specific procedures of social skills training: modeling, role-playing, coaching, positive reinforcement, and homework assignments. She said she wanted to become more socially active, to do things outside the home, and to get married. While her goal of marrying seemed elusive given the severity and chronicity of her illness, the group leader realized that her "dream" of marriage could serve as a motivator for pursuing less ambitious goals. He encouraged tiny improvements that were in accord with her desire to have more social contact:

- Giving positive feedback to other members of the group as they role-play their goals
- Participating in role-plays herself
- Completing homework assignments such as doing shopping for her family and attending church services
- Expressing appreciation to her parents and other relatives for their helpfulness to her and sticking with her throughout the many years of her illness and disability
- Asking questions of clerks and store managers
- Greeting fellow parishioners at church
- Attending Bible study class and introducing herself to others in the class
- Registering for an art class and, later, a jewelry-making class

After 18 months in the group, she asked to join a second group, the *Basic Conversation Skills Module.* This modality also emphasized incremental learning steps, from recognizing when people would be responsive to her starting a conversation to conversational openers, maintaining a conversation, and appropriate turn-taking and self-disclosure. The skills that she gained in conversation were the raw material for her further steps into the real world. She became more active in church groups, took driving lessons and obtained her license, invited peers to join her for coffee and meals, asked open-ended questions in her art class, and obtained a part-time volunteer job in a church-affiliated preschool.

By this time she was fully participating in the group and orienting new members as well. Her psychotic symptoms were in full remission—probably a result of the long-term, gradually increasing efficacy of her antipsychotic medication plus the salutary experiences she was having in the group and in her everyday life.

Throughout this period, she had only monthly appointments for medication reviews with her psychiatrist and no other treatments aside from social skills training. She was learning in the group to serve as her own case manager—setting and achieving goals herself.

She spent a year consolidating her progress in interacting with varied people and places and practicing her newly learned social skills. She began to make better eye contact and speak with more expressiveness, including gestures and body language. Then, in response to the dating goals and achievements of another female group member, Debbie asked to join a special *Friendship and Intimacy Module,* which included training on safe and satisfying sex, as well as development of sustained friendships and dating skills. She completed this module in 3 months and began a slow, steady ascent toward her dream of marriage. Over the next 3 years, she set and accomplished weekly goals that included:

- Calling the local recreation district to sign up for tennis lessons.
- Inviting one of her tennis partners out to dinner.
- Signing up for a wellness seminar where she could get information on nutritious meals and exercise.
- Persuading a friend from church to walk with her three times a week.
- Posting her personal profile on a computer dating service that specialized in her religious denomination.
- Engaging in practice dates with male members of her social skills training group who were eager to help her.
- Participating (with a female peer from the group) in speed dating sessions.
- Going on more than a dozen dates, which were primarily meetings in coffee shops for conversations.
- Pairing off with a man whom she met through a computer dating service.
- Using her friendship and dating skills to get acquainted and build a companionable relationship.
- Going on dates and engaging in kissing and necking, first tentatively and then enthusiastically.
- Agreeing to go steady with this boyfriend.

Almost to the day of her sixth anniversary of joining the social skills training group, Debbie entered the session with a big smile on her face. When asked by peers why she seemed so happy, she recounted that her boyfriend had surprised her with flowers and a musical evening at the Walt

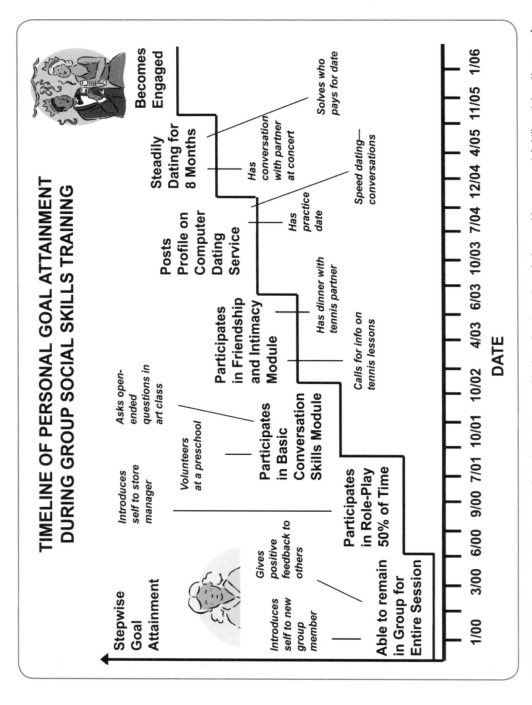

FIGURE 2.12 Personal goal attainment for Debbie, a 25-year-old schizophrenia patient, during weekly group social skills training. Six years of gradual, slow but steady improvement in this patient's social skills enabled her to reach her long-term, personally relevant goal of marriage.

Disney Concert Hall in Los Angeles. Then she said, with happiness pouring out of her face and words, "I'm engaged to be married." Her boyfriend had proposed to her after the concert. Six months later, Debbie was busy preparing for her wedding; however, she continued to attend the weekly group, where she practiced interpersonal situations with her fiancé, family members, and people who were to be in the wedding party. The unhurried, measured accomplishments that Debbie earned over 6 years are shown in Figure 2.12. Two big accomplishments that took more than 4 weeks of persistent communication were persuading her fiancé to accompany her to the city hall to obtain their marriage license and coming to an agreement with her mother on various differences they had about the wedding arrangements. On August 20, 2006, Debbie was married.

▶ Summary

The 10 "C's" listed in Table 2.7 are guidelines for "best practices" in rehabilitation. They interrelate reciprocally with the basic principles of our field. These 10 guidelines for psychiatric rehabilitation are incorporated by evidence-based services and are beacons for practitioners and patients on their voyage toward recovery.

Comprehensive services are necessary for most seriously mentally ill persons because their disorders are characterized by diverse personal, social, and occupational disabilities. If recovery is the goal, each patient needs a humanistic, longitudinal relationship with a mental health professional who makes possible access to appropriate psychosocial and pharmacological services. Psychotropic medications must be combined and coordinated with psychosocial services to render essential comprehensiveness for the journey toward recovery. Comprehensiveness of services alone is not sufficient as they must be delivered by practitioners who have requisite competencies for delivering evidence-based practices.

Coordination of pharmacological and psychosocial services is the key to efficacious treatment by integrated, multidisciplinary teams. Mechanisms for frequent, as-needed intercommunication among team members regarding individual patients are easier said than actually implemented. Obstacles to communication among practitioners sharing patients can be overcome to a large extent by phone, email, and fax as well as by team meetings. Practitioners who contribute their respective expertise to drug and psychosocial treatments need to communicate about the therapeutic and adverse effects that are being produced. Practitioners, their treatment teams, and agencies need to maintain cooperative and coordinated relationships with an array of

> ● **TABLE 2.7**
>
> **The 10 "C's" of psychiatric rehabilitation: guidelines informed by principles and used in the design of best practices**
>
> - Comprehensive
> - Continuous
> - Coordinated
> - Collaborative
> - Consumer-oriented
> - Consistent with phase of disorder
> - Competence in using evidence-based services
> - Connected with patient's strengths, skills, and deficits
> - Compassionate
> - Cooperative with community agencies and resources and commitment by program managers and policy makers

community resources and agencies. This ensures that those services needed by the seriously mentally ill person are consumer-oriented, made available, and delivered with compassion and competence through evidence-based practices.

Consumer-oriented services require a shift in the traditional roles of practitioner and patient. The new egalitarianism recognizes that each has his/her own knowledge and experience to contribute to planning and implementing treatment. Collaboration and compassion are energized by empathy, mutual respect, and shared perseverance and courage in pursuing recovery through a veritable minefield of treacherous pitfalls. These guidelines, more than any others, carry with them the responsibility for informed value judgments by practitioners. Collaborative relationships with patients help to ensure that goals, treatment plans, and evaluation of services are consumer-oriented. It is not a simple matter for a practitioner to accept the patient's personal goals, especially when they appear to be unrealistic and influenced by psychopathology. But there is no alternative to adhering to values that are in accord with a "customer approach" to treatment. Value-free rehabilitation is not an option.

Patients with serious and disabling mental disorders retain their vulnerability to relapses and persistent symptoms for a lifetime; therefore, treatment that is flexibly and consistently attuned to the phase of a person's

CLINICAL EXAMPLE

A psychiatrist was understandably skeptical of accepting his patient's personal goal of becoming a writer. The patient, who had a history of schizoaffective disorder and grandiose delusions, had spent many years reading voraciously, taking courses in the humanities at a community college, and writing a memoir of his illness and its lengthy course. Once the psychiatrist read the memoirs, he was impressed with the high quality of his patient's writing acumen. The two of them worked together on finding outlets for writing as an avocation if not a remunerative career. Over the following years, the patient wrote columns for the newsletter of a self-help consumers' organization, essays on mental illness for a national magazine, articles for an environmental magazine, and letters to the editors of local newspapers on various topics.

disorder must be available continuously. Intensive and comprehensive treatment will be needed only at certain times, but compassionate, consumer-oriented treatment enlivened by a collaborative therapeutic relationship should be accessible indefinitely. This has been well accepted for the lifelong provision of maintenance medications for schizophrenia, mood disorders, and disabling anxiety disorders. Availability of lifelong services is even more relevant for psychosocial treatments, since patients' readiness for vocational and social rehabilitation, as well as independent living, changes over time. The gradual accretion of skills, judgment, insight, and self-directed functioning occurs opportunistically and unpredictably, thereby demanding long-term availability of psychosocial services.

Because providers of services come and go, collaborative involvement of educated family members assumes great importance since they serve as the unbroken thread of knowledge, support, and advocacy for the patient. We must not forget that family members also are consumers and deserve a host of educational and support services from mental health agencies. In particular, practitioners, along with the National Alliance on Mental Illness and local mental health agencies, have the responsibility of coaching family members to be assertive proponents for seeking and obtaining services consistent with their mentally ill relative's changing needs. Failing to prepare family members for this critical responsibility is tantamount to preparing to fail. Families as well as practitioners need to establish cooperative relationships with various community agencies and resources so their relatives can access them. These include Social Security, housing authorities, Medicaid and Medicare, substance abuse services, medical and dental services, emergency mental health outreach, and hospitalization. Importantly, family members should be schooled by practitioners and patients themselves to remain connected with the patients' strengths rather than focusing solely on symptoms and disabilities.

Integration of comprehensive, coordinated, continuous, collaborative, and consumer-oriented rehabilitation requires a strong commitment by agency managers and policy makers for provision of resources, administrative support, and mandated services. Unless the top managers and program administrators—locally and systemwide—lend credence to the requirements for high-fidelity use of integrated, evidence-based practices, the likelihood of practitioners using them is nil. Improvements in the quality of care are dependent upon administrators who manage by walking around to observe services in action and dispense positive reinforcement to practitioners who are doing exemplary work. Evidence-based practices, guidelines, and principles of rehabilitation should be integrated into job descriptions and performance standards and evaluations of clinicians. Why else would practitioners change their traditional ways of working?

As the field matures, more effective treatment practices may bring different principles into view. In this chapter, I have outlined the principles that are currently marking the territory of psychiatric rehabilitation and briefly described some of the practices that add clinical substance to the principles. The next seven chapters of this manual describe in greater depth and detail those practices that have been spawned by overarching principles and, in turn, give clarity and significance to the principles.

While progress is extending the benefits of psychiatric rehabilitation to greater numbers of the mentally disabled, it is slow. Reforms of mental health systems of care have resulted in little improvement for the vast majority of patients; however, building in regular, empirically based reviews of program and system performance may accelerate the delivery of high-quality services. Regular, repeated assessment of progress toward goals—whether at the level of the patient, program, or system of care—has the potential to guide decisions about treatment of the individual as well as to improve the accomplishments of programs and systems. The principles and practices of psychiatric rehabilitation can stimulate change through introducing evidence-based practices and new approaches to treatment. Satisfaction with the status quo will only breed futility, which is "continuing to do the same thing over and over again while expecting a better result in solving a problem" (Albert Einstein).

▶ Key Points

- Modalities of rehabilitation have emerged from practical exigencies as well as from the vulnerability-stress-protective factors concept of mental disorders. Protective factors counterbalance the noxious effects of stress and psychobiological vulnerability to confer functional capacities on disabled individuals.

- There are myriad protective factors. Some derive from the individual's attributes, such as premorbid social competence, intactness of cognitive functioning, and adherence to treatment; others are found in the person's environment, including a supportive family, skills training, assertive community treatment, structured remedial services for deficits in vocational, educational, and self-care responsibilities, and evidence-based pharmacotherapy.

- Cognitive science, social learning principles, and life span developmental psychology contribute to the design, development, and validation of new rehabilitative modalities.

- Evidence-based treatments, such as behavioral family therapy and social skills training, have emerged from social learning theory and cognitive remediation from cognitive science.

- Individualization of treatment is a pillar of psychiatric rehabilitation. Treatment must be linked to the person's phase of illness as well as to his/her strengths and deficits. "One size does not fit all" dictates a comprehensive assessment of specific attributes of each individual as well as the person's spiritual needs, community supports, and resources for rehabilitation.

- Building on the strengths of the individual is a keystone of rehabilitation. Treatment starts "where the patient is at" and beefs up the individual's resilience and coping capacities by providing training for skill development and offering supportive services that compensate for behavioral and cognitive deficits.

- Psychosocial and pharmacological treatments need to be integrated for the patient, for the multidisciplinary team working with the patient, and for all those agencies contributing services to the patient.

- Rehabilitation fosters recovery through incremental goal attainment. On the road to recovery, mentally disabled persons and their professional helpers "go faster by going slower." The recovery race is won not by the fleet of foot but by the persistent.

▌ Selected Readings

Agras WS, Wilson GT: Learning theory, in Comprehensive Textbook of Psychiatry/VIII, 8th Edition. Edited by Sadock BJ, Sadock VA. Baltimore, MD, Lippincott Williams & Wilkins, 2004, pp 541–553

Anthony WA, Liberman RP: Principles and practice of psychiatric rehabilitation, in Handbook of Psychiatric Rehabilitation. Edited by Liberman RP. Needham Heights, MA, Allyn & Bacon, 1992, pp 1–30

Cloninger CR: Fostering spirituality and well-being in clinical practice. Psychiatr Ann 36:157–162, 2006

Colby A: Competence and Character Through Life. Chicago, IL, University of Chicago Press, 1998

Damasio AR: The Feeling of What Happens: Body and Emotion in the Making of Consciousness. New York, Harcourt Brace, 1999

Hermann H, Harvey C: Community care for people with psychosis: outcomes and needs for care. Int Rev Psychiatry 17:89–95, 2005

Isohanni Murray EK, Joikelainen J, et al: The persistence of developmental markers in childhood and adolescence and risk for schizophrenia psychoses in adult life. Schizophr Res 71:213–225, 2004

Griffith J, Griffith M: Encountering the Sacred in Psychotherapy: How to Talk With People About Their Spiritual Lives. New York, Guilford, 2001

Group for the Advancement of Psychiatry: Beyond Symptom Suppression: Improving Long-Term Outcomes of Schizophrenia (Report No 134). Washington, DC, American Psychiatric Press, 1992

Kopelowicz A, Liberman RP: Recovery from schizophrenia. Directions in Psychiatry 21:287–305, 2001

Kopelowicz A, Liberman RP: Integrating treatment with rehabilitation for persons with major mental illness. Psychiatr Serv 54:1491–1495, 2003

Liberman RP, Kopelowicz A, Silverstein S: Psychiatric rehabilitation, in Comprehensive Textbook of Psychiatry/VIII, 8th Edition. Edited by Sadock BJ, Sadock VA. Baltimore, MD, Lippincott Williams & Wilkins, 2004, pp 3884–3930

Miller WR (ed): Integrating Spirituality Into Treatment: Resources for Practitioners. Washington, DC, American Psychological Association, 1999

Nuechterlein KH, Dawson ME: A heuristic vulnerability-stress model of schizophrenia. Schizophr Bull 10:300–312, 1984

Nuechterlein KH, Dawson ME, Gitlin M, et al: Developmental processes in schizophrenic disorders: longitudinal studies of vulnerability and stress. Schizophr Bull 18:378–425, 1992

Nuechterlein KH, Dawson ME, Ventura J, et al: The vulnerability/stress model of schizophrenia relapse. Acta Psychiatr Scand Suppl 382:58–64, 1994

Perlick DA, Sirey J, Link BG, et al: Stigma as a barrier to recovery. Psychiatr Serv 52:1613–1638, 2001

Vaillant GEH, Vaillant CO: Normality and mental health, in Comprehensive Textbook of Psychiatry/VIII, 8th Edition. Edited by Sadock BJ, Sadock VA. Baltimore, MD, Lippincott Williams & Wilkins, 2004, pp 583–597

Warner R: Local projects of the World Psychiatric Association programme to reduce stigma and discrimination. Psychiatr Serv 56:570–575, 2005

Yank GR, Bentley KJ, Hargrove DS: The vulnerability-stress model of schizophrenia: advances in psychosocial treatment. Am J Orthopsychiatry 63:55–69, 1993

▶ References

James W: Principles of Psychology. New York, Collier Books, 1890

West JC, Wilk JE, Olfson MR, et al: Patterns and quality of treatment for patients with schizophrenia in routine psychiatric practice. Psychiatr Serv 56:283–291, 2005

Illness Management

3

Illness Management

It is more important to know the patient who has the disease than the disease afflicting the patient.

SIR WILLIAM OSLER (1849–1919)

THE SYMPTOMS of a disease are not the primary reason that people seek medical or psychiatric care. Patients are keen to eliminate symptoms and suffering, but they also want to regain their functional capacities for work, family life, friendships, and recreation. The patient being treated for severe depression wants the tormenting symptoms to remit so he can again welcome the morning light, resume his job, interact spontaneously with his family, and enjoy food, sex, and social and recreational activities. The aim of *illness management* is to equip disabled patients with the skills and supports to control their illness and move toward a more functional life and recovery. Relapses, rehospitalizations, and recurrent episodes of intrusive and disabling symptoms inevitably disrupt one's life, produce stress, and undermine one's hope, personal success, well-being, and self-control. Learning how to work closely with one's physician, personal support specialist, or therapist to minimize symptomatic disturbances is a critical step for moving toward one's personal goals and an active, meaningful, and satisfying life.

As a core element of psychiatric rehabilitation, illness management provides clinicians with tools to engage patients and their families in a practical collaboration to reach seven goals:

- Reduce signs, symptoms, and relapses of their illness by employing optimal pharmacological and psychosocial treatments.
- Overcome demoralization, passivity, and stigma by gaining self-efficacy through success in coping with their illness.
- Learn skills for self-management of their illness that is translated into

empowerment for achieving their personal goals as they move toward recovery.

- Become informed about the cognitive impairments, signs, and symptoms of their illness together with recommendations for evidence-based treatment with medications.
- Share in decision making regarding medications as informed consumers of psychotropic drugs, and use medications reliably.
- Actively participate in developing and pursuing their personal goals.
- Gain realistic optimism and hope for recovering valued, daily life activities and a normal lifestyle in the community.

While self-help and peer support are to be encouraged, these extremely helpful approaches for education of patients should not be viewed as releasing mental health professionals from their responsibilities for illness management. As a starting point for rehabilitation, illness management builds a collaborative, consumer-oriented bridge between the psychiatrist and other mental health professionals on one side and the patient, family members, and other caregivers on the other. The collaboration is forged by equals in expertise; the practitioner has expertise regarding diagnosis, clinical assessment, and treatments, while the patient and family are the experiential experts, knowing first-hand what symptoms and disability are like to live with.

▶ Diagnosis: The Beginning of Illness Management

Little progress can be made in illness management unless a practitioner can make an accurate diagnosis. Having the correct diagnosis enables practitioners to:

- Prescribe the appropriate medication for a patient.
- Understand how to tailor the patient's psychosocial services in terms of intensity, duration, and frequency.
- Make predictions regarding the patient's likely response to treatment.
- Orchestrate the appropriate education of the patient and family regarding the illness, its treatment, prognosis, and ways of coping with symptoms and disability.

Psychiatric diagnosis and *functional assessment* drive treatment and rehabilitation. Functional assessment is the focus of the next chapter. Psychiatric diagnosis rests on the quality and sources of information available to the diagnostician. Important sources, often overlooked, are the family and others who are familiar with the patient, particularly those who have had long-term relationships with the individual. Some family members keep diaries and records of the illness and treatments that are highly specific, including lists of medications and their doses over time, as well as the side effects and efficacy of each drug. Welcoming such information from patients, relatives, and others serves as an invitation by the practitioner for consumers of services to become active partners in the assessment and treatment process, thereby facilitating the development of therapeutic relationships.

An unstructured and unsystematic approach to interviewing will not yield reliable and accurate diagnoses. Simply asking patients about the experience of symptoms for particular disorders listed in the *Diagnostic and Statistical Manual of Mental Disorders* will result in underestimating or overestimating the presence of disorders. Interviewing guidelines that can improve the accuracy of diagnosis are provided in Table 3.1. Structured diagnostic interviews that yield better-quality information for making diagnoses are available from American Psychiatric Publishing Inc. (www.appi.org).

Making a diagnosis of schizophrenia, bipolar disorder, or even recurrent major depression consigns most individuals to a lifetime of medication and treatment by a psychiatrist and other practitioners. There are other serious consequences, such as medication side effects, stigma, and adverse effects on personal identity, relationships with others, and career goals. A diagnosis follows patients for the rest of their days, since subsequent practitioners tend to rely on past chart diagnoses, without conducting fresh, systematic diagnostic evaluations. Thus, the diagnosis of a major mental disorder should be made carefully. Sufficient descriptive information and specific examples of symptoms must convince the diagnostician that the criteria for the symptoms are indeed present.

▶ Managing an Illness: Reciprocity and Collaboration in a Therapeutic Relationship

Practitioners cannot teach patients to gain control over their mental illnesses without first establishing a helping relationship. Establishing yourself as a knowledgeable, credible, and caring clinician is the first step. Strengthening your relationship with your patients throughout the course of their illnesses will make the difference between success and failure in the therapeutic endeavor. Being authoritative in the practice of evidence-based psychiatry

● **TABLE 3.1**

Guidelines for diagnostic interviews: reliable eliciting and rating of symptoms of mental disorders

Make questions specific to the symptom of concern, and ask them in the vernacular of the patient.

● "Have you ever thought that people on the street, in restaurants, or in places that you frequent are looking at you, taking special notice of you, talking about you, or having critical attitudes toward you?" This question helps the patient to understand that the subjective experience of ideas or delusions of reference is being queried.

   If the patient gives an affirmative response to any question aimed at eliciting a criterion symptom of a disorder, always ask for a specific, graphic description of a personal example. "When I was in a restaurant yesterday, I noticed that some people at another table across the room were staring at me and talking to each other about me in a derogatory manner." This response is specific enough to confirm the presence of referential thinking; however, it is not clear whether the symptom is an idea or delusion of reference.

Determine the degree of personal conviction that the patient has regarding the actual reality of his/her belief.

● "Do you believe for sure that they were saying negative things about you or that this may or may not have been happening?" Any doubt in the strength of conviction of the personalized interpretation of the perception would put into question the delusional nature of the experience and shift the clinician's judgment toward an idea of reference. "When I was in the restaurant, I was sure that they were talking about me. I could see their lips move, and they occasionally looked around toward my table." In contrast to delusions, ideas of reference, persecution, grandiosity, or control are not rated as a psychotic symptom. In this example, the patient had full conviction that the experience was actually true, and the belief therefore meets the criteria for a delusion of reference.

is not to be confused with a detached, authoritarian persona. The prevailing medical wisdom assumes that important decisions regarding treatment are made from a position of detached concern or what might be viewed from the patient's perspective as "detachment with a veneer of tenderness" (Halpern 2001). While few psychiatrists and other mental health professionals have a natural ability for empathic listening for emotional tones as well as for symptoms and impairments, most of us can learn to experience and demonstrate warmth, interest, and spontaneity by observing mentors and role models. Without an emotional, interpersonal connection that conveys respect, genuine concern, and dignity, clinical reasoning and outcomes suffer.

ENGAGING THE PATIENT AND FAMILY IN TREATMENT

The first major challenge to those carrying out illness management is *engaging the patient and his/her family or natural supporters* in treatment and rehabilitation. Stigma, denial, and fear of being hospitalized often conspire to produce abject refusal to meet with a practitioner at worst and reluctance at best. Most commonly, engagement occurs when a practitioner or treatment team is asked to see a patient who is acutely ill. The meeting may take place in an emergency room, mental health center, hospital inpatient unit, private office, or community residential facility. Engagement may require outreach to the reluctant patient in his/her home or at a neutral locale that doesn't carry the stigma of a mental health agency.

"All stops must be pulled" at this phase to find some way to attract the patient into the treatment and rehabilitation process. If practitioners keep in mind that "the patient is always doing the best he/she can given the past and present circumstances," creative ways can be developed for a successful engagement. The most important point of departure is to help the patient see that the primary focus is on his/her personal goals and desires. The patient's personal goals for a better life should steer the conversation, not the symptoms or problems that may have led to the contact. Then, the practitioner can point out how treatment can be a means for the patient to get the necessary assistance to start moving in the direction of his/her goals. This mode of bringing a patient into treatment is called *motivational interviewing*. One can view engagement of a patient and family as a perpetual process, since the quality and success of the initial meeting start a therapeutic relationship that needs to be constantly fed, nurtured, and renewed.

CLINICAL EXAMPLE

Sarah, a 19-year-old student who had to drop out of college as the onset of schizophrenia intruded on her cognitive and social abilities, refused her family's entreaties to visit a psychiatrist or mental health center. Her parents understood that she was suffering from a mental disorder but could not persuade her to accept treatment. She was afraid that if she went to a hospital, clinic, or private office to meet a psychiatrist or other mental health practitioner, she would be railroaded into a locked unit.

She did agree to a home visit from a psychiatrist. They met together with her parents in the patio overlooking the backyard. When the psychiatrist asked Sarah, "How would you like your life to be different from the way it is right now?" she replied, "I'd like to get back to school and see my friends again." The doctor explained that these were worthwhile goals, endorsed by him and her parents.

Then he prompted her parents to say to Sarah, "We are unhappy with the way things are now, just as you are. In fact, we're scared and depressed because we don't know how to help you get back on track with school and your friends. It would be a tremendous relief for us if you agreed to meet with the doctor again, either here or in his office." Sarah agreed to one additional home visit. That session also focused on her personal goals and went into some of the ways that she was feeling stymied from reaching them. After the second session, without any mention of a psychiatric disorder or treatment, Sarah willingly met with the doctor on a weekly basis in his office to continue their conversations about the steps she could take toward her own goals.

Note that the doctor did not suggest that Sarah's parents highlight Sarah's problems, symptoms, and need for treatment. Instead, he taught them how to express their *worries, anxieties, and sadness about the family situation* and to ask Sarah to help them to feel better. This means of motivating Sarah worked because it allowed her to save face by not having to acknowledge that she was mentally ill. Since she loved her parents, it was relatively simple for her to ease her parents' unhappiness.

SUSTAINING A THERAPEUTIC ALLIANCE

A seamless transition from engagement to the development of a therapeutic alliance will facilitate the patient's progression through illness management toward recovery. Even if practitioners are well trained in delivering evidence-based services, they will encounter difficulties in sustaining their patients' attendance and adherence to treatment unless they succeed in establishing positive and trusting relationships. If the therapeutic relationship is not formed—even in a primordial fashion—at the start of treatment, why should the patient and family return? What would motivate them to follow the psychiatrist's prescription and adhere to medications over the long haul?

Conveying positive, yet realistic expectations for improvement in symptoms, helping the patient achieve his/her personal goals, and recovery are important steps for all members of the treatment team—if they are consistent as a result of team coordination. Establishing positive expectancies for the patient and family includes presenting a rationale for the effectiveness of treatment. Because many patients and families will enter a treatment episode with negative and unhappy experiences with previous treatment, it may be necessary to point out how the current treatment will differ from those of the past. This can be done in a credible fashion only if the patient and family are queried about their past experiences.

Naming a problem can be the first step to gaining control over it. Thus, one of the functions of a credible treatment rationale is to reassure patients and their families that their problems or disorders are understandable and can be effectively treated. Connected to the setting of realistically favorable expectations should be a clear description of how control or removal of symptoms with medications can clear patients' passage to achieving what they want from life—their personally relevant goals. When a positive treatment rationale is successfully communicated, by means of an interactive style, patients will experience a boost in morale, a sense of gaining control over symptoms that were mystifying and frightening, and hope for recovery.

> When patients accept a treatment rationale and hold positive expectations for the treatment, favorable treatment outcomes ensue.

Even if the patient and family members are eager to gain relief from dysphoric symptoms and to achieve a better level of functioning, the primary reinforcer for motivating continuation of treatment is the feelings of confidence, trust, respect, and comfort with the clinician. Research on treatment of outpatients with chronic schizophrenia shows that the therapeutic alliance is most consistently related to medication adherence and favorable long-term outcomes. Some of the ways you as a practitioner can build and strengthen the therapeutic alliance are described here.

- Empathically explore your patient's view of his/her situation, current life, and personal goals for the near and long-term future.
- Gain a sense of the problems or obstacles that your patients identify as interfering with their current life and with getting a better life.
- Greet your patients with a friendly smile and warm, positive regard. When entering a group, rehabilitation activity, or one-on-one interaction, unambiguously, spontaneously, and genuinely express verbal and nonverbal desire and pleasure in being with the patients. One of the best ways to counter negative symptoms is through the contagiousness of your enthusiasm, spontaneity, and expressiveness with patients.
- Rather than ask, "How are you feeling today," or "How are you today," or "Have you had any problems recently?" emphasize the positive in a greeting something like, "What have you done for yourself recently?" or "How have you been good to yourself in the last week?"
- Identify the specific obstacles to the patient's attending sessions, appointments, or programs, then assist the patient to overcome or compensate for those obstacles. Accessibility is only a buzzword unless

practitioners assume that patients will have trouble getting to the places and persons where services are offered. Some obstacles that can be remedied include transportation, child care, working hours, social anxiety and depression, medication costs, and fees.

- If your patient is having a problem meeting the requirements and expectations of the treatment, service, or program, temporarily lower your expectations until the patient has had some success and feels more comfortable in the rehab setting. When the treatment, service, and programs are tailored to each patient's needs and abilities, rather than vice versa, success will breed more success. Lowering treatment expectations can be done by:

  » Reducing the frequency of attendance or amount of time that the individual is expected to attend the program.
  » Reducing the number of planned and scheduled activities that the patient is expected to attend.
  » Allowing the patient to exit the program activities for breaks that offer opportunities for privacy, moving around, smoking, and relaxing.
  » Encouraging the patient to just watch and observe the program activities rather than actively participate. Learning of skills occurs through the process of social learning or imitative learning even when the patient is passively observing.

- Have fun with the patient and make participation in the treatment or program associated with pleasure. This can be done by changing the seriousness of the treatment scene to humor, as when a group session is begun with each person and staff member taking turns on a weekly basis in telling a joke. If that is too great a burden for some patients, they can be provided with a list of jokes that they can practice before telling in front of the other group members. Warm-up exercises, such as a simple dance, contest, or exercise, can be used to elicit humor and laughter. Practitioners can and should "go out on the town" with their patients, perhaps in rotation one at a time. This is a time for unwinding and shedding the professional–patient roles at coffee shops and fast-food restaurants, in the park, or on city streets during walks. Offering refreshments to patients during breaks in program activities also can evoke relaxation that, in turn, is experienced as a reinforcer for future attendance.

- Integrate planned and scheduled relaxation into the treatment session, program activity, or schedule of services to help patients buffer the aversive experiences that inevitably crop up in treatment and rehabilitation. Some aversive experiences are social or performance anxiety, failure to meet one's goals, having to discuss crises and problems, negative self-evaluation, and embarrassing moments.

- Demonstrate your awareness, interest, and consideration for patients' special events. Remembrances can be focused on birthdays, anniversaries of involvement in the program, and "graduation" from the program into a more independent round of life. Patients can be asked about their growing up years—where, what, and how they experienced them—and invited to bring in photos that enable them to talk about past experiences, places visited, friends, and family.

- Communicate your desire to learn as much about the patient as possible by making home visits, inviting family members or friends to sessions where they can interact with practitioners and observe their loved one actively participate and receive positive reinforcement for his/her efforts, and arranging treatment sessions in the patient's home or neighborhood. This is especially valued by patients, as it indicates that the therapist is willing to make a special, extra effort to learn more about them.

- Create and convey a policy that any patient at any time for any reason can take a break from a treatment session, whether for the bathroom or for escape from a stressful environment.

- Offer specific assistance to patients in areas of perceived needs. For example, help your patients obtain entitlements for which they are eligible from the federal, state, and local governments; find better housing; or bring about improved family relations.

Accentuate the positive and give abundant praise contingent on progress, no matter how small the steps may be. Coming to work, you should function *as though* you were wearing binoculars (to see the tiny and almost imperceptible signs of progress being made by patients) and a hearing aid (to amplify comments made by patients as they describe their progress toward their personal goals). The task for professionals is to "Catch a person doing or saying something normal, good, appropriate, or helpful to self or others . . . and tell the person how it made you feel." When you use this practical, powerful, and portable intervention, be genuine and spontaneous in communicating praise in a positive, warm tone of voice with eye contact and *praising the person's specific behavior, not the person in general* (Liberman et al. 1980, p. 113).

AVOIDING PITFALLS IN THE ENGAGEMENT EFFORT

The challenges to developing a treatment alliance are multiplied when a patient is acutely and floridly psychotic, highly anxious, depressed, ambivalent, or negative about accepting professional help. The clinician's ability to engage a patient in treatment is taxed even more when working in a busy mental health setting where time is limited by the crunch of large numbers of patients. If anticipated, the following pitfalls may be avoided.

Ignoring Where the Patient Is At

When facing an uncooperative, anxious, angry, or negativistic patient, it is not a good idea to start the conversation by asking, "How might I help you," or "What brings you to the clinic today?" Ignore the patient's thoughts, inclinations, and feelings and you jeopardize the success of the engagement process. Instead, read the patient's facial expression and tone of voice; if the patient appears angry, you might try, "If you tell me what happened to make you upset, maybe I can help you fix the situation."

Not Reading From the Same Page

Patients and clinicians may have very different agendas when meeting for the first time. Practitioners are "ready to go" with diagnostic and other evaluations that lead to treatment as efficiently as possible. Their expectations are for the patient and family to cooperate with questions and comply with professional instructions and prescriptions. On the other hand, patients are often in denial of their mental illness and want to "flee into health" and forget that their problems ever existed. They are reluctant to even consider medication, are already feeling stigmatized by virtue of visiting a psychiatrist, mental health professional, or psychiatric facility, and want to leave as soon as possible. How can these differences be resolved?

One way is for the practitioner to ally himself/herself with the patient and decompress any escalation of their divergent views of the situation. The clinician might say, "I know this is unpleasant for you and that you would prefer to be someplace else. But let me find out how you would like things to go better in your life. What would you like to be able to do 1, 3, or 6 months from now if there were no barriers in your way?" By asking questions that elicit the patient's personally relevant goals, the practitioner can then restructure the patient's attitudes by framing the evaluation and treatment in terms that hold value for the patient. This approach also shifts the focus of the meeting from adversaries to collaborators with the same mission.

Ouch! That Hurt

Patients who are in denial of their illness, have been forced by family members to seek treatment, or oppose setting goals of treatment may lash out and insult the practitioner or otherwise demean the whole process. When a clinician has had a full day of challenging patients, it is understandable that derogatory comments will have an adverse impact. But it is essential for practitioners to realize that those comments are coming from a frightened, fearful, depressed, and cognitively impaired individual. Feeling exposed, vulnerable, and powerless, the patient may try to cope by using intimidation instead of negotiation. Don't take epithets personally, and don't lose your cool. Because the patient is always right, it is up to the practitioner to identify the patient's concerns and sources of disenchantment. By exploring this with the patient while communicating with transparent candor and nondefensiveness, the clinician can often locate the source of the problem and then, remaining loyal to the therapeutic alliance, collaborate with the patient in a problem-solving process.

▶ Managing the Phases of a Mental Disorder From Relapse to Recovery

Most serious mental disorders have phases through which patients pass. Phases proceed from prodromal or early-warning signs of the onset of the disorder or relapse of the patient to the acute phase when symptoms are at their peak. Stabilizing and stable phases are next and, if all goes well, are followed by symptomatic and functional recovery. Throughout all phases, a collaborative relationship between the patient and those responsible for treatment is marked by mutual respect, shared decision-making regarding treatment, and optimal adherence to medication regimens. A simplified, graphic depiction of these phases is shown in Figure 3.1. The process of moving from one phase to another is dynamic and often unpredictable, with frequent recycling or stalling in one or another phase. Individuals will remain in each phase for different periods of time, some requiring lengthy moratoriums to consolidate their progress before moving on to the next phase, and others proceeding more rapidly through each stage. As a patient moves from the acutely ill phase to the phase of recovery, symptoms

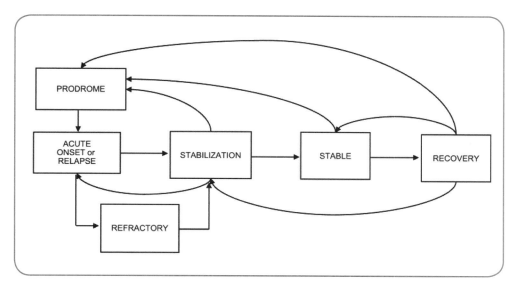

FIGURE 3.1 Phases of mental illnesses: cycling processes of improvement and relapse.

abate and psychosocial functioning improves, although functioning almost always lags behind the improvement of symptoms. The rapidity with which a patient proceeds through the various phases varies greatly, depending upon such factors as biological vulnerability, premorbid social competence, presence of stressors, family support, comorbidity with other diseases, and availability and effectiveness of treatment.

Illness management encompasses early identification of prodromes, stabilization of symptoms, and establishment of self-control of disturbing behavior often seen in the acute phase. When patients are immersed in the acute or stabilizing phases of their illness, their cognitive capacities and resilience are limited and their sensitivity to social stimulation and stressors is inordinately high. During these phases, it is important to structure, limit, and carefully titrate the amount, intensity, type, and complexity of the milieu and psychosocial interventions so as to reduce the chances of exacerbation. The psychiatrist and other members of the treatment team should take responsibility for ensuring the patient's adherence to medication, while providing education, social support, behavioral tailoring, and skills training to improve reliability in use of medication. When ushered into the stable phase, patients are able to benefit from more intensive and evidence-based rehabilitation. These modalities are personalized for improved social and vocational functioning. The task for the practitioner is to individualize the type and amount of biobehavioral treatment to fit each patient's tolerance and responsiveness. When illness management is optimal, patients will move more quickly from the acute and stabilization phases of their illness

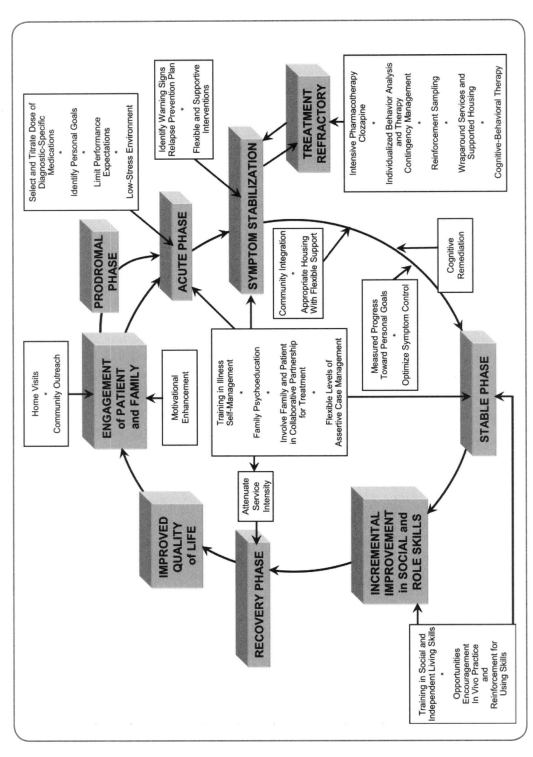

FIGURE 3.2 Phase-linked treatment of schizophrenia and related disorders.

toward stability and recovery. All of these treatments, starting in the acute phase of illness, should be developed and customized with the maximal possible collaboration with the patient. Even when the patient is in a state of acute agitation, it is possible to offer a choice in gaining self-control; for example, spending quiet time in his/her room, taking appropriate medication, taking a short walk with a staff member, or having a calming chat with his/her psychiatrist or member of the treatment team.

Even the very best, evidence-based practices should not be provided prematurely or inappropriately to patients who may not be able to participate or benefit from them. For example, supported employment would backfire as an intervention if it were offered to a patient in the acute or even stabilization phase of his/her disorder. It could very well overstimulate the recovering person and trigger an exacerbation of symptoms and demoralization because of the stress of failure to get and hold a job. On the other hand, enrolling a patient who has been stable for more than a year in a treatment program that offers only recreational activities would undermine that patient's motivation and readiness for moving forward toward the recovery phase. Some of the choices for evidence-based interventions, keyed to the phase of illness for a patient with a schizophrenia disorder, are shown in the flow chart in Figure 3.2. We describe phase-linked treatment in the following sections of this chapter, always aware of the importance of individualizing and adapting services while actively inviting the patient's collaboration in setting goals.

ACUTE PHASE: CONTROLLING FLORID SYMPTOMS

During the acute phase, when symptoms are at their peak, the highest priority is to control and stabilize the symptoms and their associated behavioral abnormalities. This is true for major depression and severe anxiety disorders as well as for bipolar and schizophrenia spectrum disorders. There are three major aims, each with recommended interventions for practitioners of psychiatric rehabilitation.

- *Identify psychotic, manic, or depressive symptoms as soon as possible after they emerge, and provide treatment as early as possible.* Accessibility to services can be achieved by providing your patients, family members, and other caregivers with emergency cards containing phone numbers to reach you, other members of your treatment team, on-call professionals, a mobile emergency team, or psychiatric consultation at an emergency room.

- *Foster symptom control by providing optimal pharmacological treatment of symptoms and signs of the disorder, reducing social and environmental overstimulation, as well as buffering ambient stressors that may be operating in the home, at work, or in other situations.* In addition, staff should offer a low-key treatment environment with planned, scheduled, and predictable activities. Whether treatment is being provided in a hospital inpatient unit, a crisis home, or a partial hospital, the patient should be clearly informed of the staff person who is on duty and designated to be available to answer questions, comfort, offer medication, or engage in problem solving. Because of impaired attention, learning, and memory during the acute phase, it is desirable to post the names of the responsible staff members assigned to each patient on a bulletin or marker board.

CLINICAL EXAMPLE

After Rosie had been hospitalized for 5 days, her symptoms were no longer intrusive, and she was taking her medication voluntarily and was looking after her personal hygiene and appearance. During two sessions of participating in a group, the *Community Re-entry Module,* she learned how to select a semi-independent apartment, and practiced, and then made, phone calls to the mental health center where she planned to receive her continuing care. She spoke with the psychiatrist who was assigned to her outpatient treatment and made an appointment. When the hospital social worker approached her for discharge planning, Rosie thanked her but said she didn't need her assistance as her plans were already settled.

- *With the patient and family, set realistic goals that are consonant with discharge readiness, the patient's current and future level of functioning, and culture.* Give feedback to the patient and family regarding progress being made toward discharge criteria. Enable the patient to maintain dignity and personal identity with attention to privacy, personal possessions, clothing, and visitors. Staff should focus on and reinforce positive, adaptive behavior of the patient, not just on symptomatic, annoying, and acting-out behavior.

Duration and complexity of verbal instructions, as well as expectations for performance, should be consistent with the patient's symptoms and cognitive capacity. As soon as practicable, the patient and family should be involved in a discussion of the criteria that will be used to determine discharge readiness. Criteria usually include control of symptoms and agitation, subsidence of aggressive behavior or suicidality, having adequate sleep, resumption of activities of daily living, and development of and participation in an aftercare program that includes a confirmed appointment with a psychiatrist and an appropriately supervised residence. With skills training technology, using video-assisted principles of learning to overcome cognitive deficits, patients can now take responsibility for managing their own aftercare.

Medication treatment of the acute and subsequent phases of severe mental illness has grown more complicated in the past decade because of the advent of new pharmacological agents. For the most part, these new antidepressant, antimanic, and antipsychotic drugs confer little or no therapeutic advantage over the earlier generation of medications, have different but not necessarily more benign side-effect profiles, and are much more expensive. There are considerable individual differences among patients in response to particular medications that frequently determine long-term adherence and protection from relapse.

When patients report that they find their prescribed medication unpleasant and dysphoric, psychiatrists should take such subjective judgments seriously, as even early adverse effects can lead to discontinuation with attendant loss of the medication's prophylactic benefits (Miyamoto et al. 2003). Considerable education of patients, families, and nursing staff is desirable so they anticipate uncomfortable side effects preceding the drug's therapeutic effects. Unless psychiatrists translate what they know about the "benefit-risk" relationships inherent in pharmacotherapy by employing visual aids and precision teaching, patients will often cease taking their medications, thereby inviting relapse and rehospitalization.

Staff responsible for planning and implementing psychosocial services must communicate and collaborate with psychiatrists and nurses whose primary role is symptom and behavioral control. Reciprocity in the provision of information on patients' progress and status can improve treatment coordination; for example, over- or undermedicated patients may function poorly in psychosocial activities. When observations are shared on a daily basis, clinicians' decision making is better informed.

Practice guidelines and algorithms for selecting evidence-based pharmacological and psychosocial treatment for the acute and subsequent phases of each disorder have been developed by the American Psychiatric Association and other organizations. Because studies have shown considerable disparities between recommended guidelines and actual practice, policies, procedures, and quality improvement standards should be implemented in hospitals and mental health centers that are consistent with best practices.

Patient and Family Education for Illness Management

Even in the acute stage of illness, patients need and can absorb some basic information about their illness and the medication being prescribed to control its symptoms. Since many patients, especially during their first episode, will be reluctant to take medication, it is important to emphasize to them that medication is the means to helping them to get back their lives, not an end in itself. Involving families in educational sessions at the time of relapses and hospitalization of their mentally ill relatives engages them at a time when their level of distress and motivation for learning coping skills are high.

Flexibility, patience, and repetition are the keys to educating acutely ill patients. The clinician must make adjustments in training illness self-management in accord with the intrusive symptoms, cognitive deficits, behavioral instability, and cultural background of the patient. To compensate for the cognitive and symptomatic impairments of acutely ill patients, educational efforts need to be simple, offered in brief segments, and repeated as often as it takes to ascertain that learning has occurred. How this is accomplished for a distractible patient with a thought disorder is shown in the example to the right.

It is always a good idea to ask patients to repeat back important points in the educational curriculum before concluding that the information has been assimilated. The admonition to keep in mind is, "Do whatever you can to facilitate patients' cognitive mastery of information about their illness and treatment." Even small increases in their grasp of knowledge are significant because they come at a time when the patients are feeling out of control.

Patients and family members will want to know how long an acute phase will last; this is an important matter to address in educational and counseling sessions. The duration of the acute phase, with its high level of symptom intensity, varies from disorder to disorder and from patient to patient. The reactivity of the patient's illness to treatment is determined by the patient's initial, subjective response to medication, the quality of the biobehavioral therapies and multidisciplinary team, the collaboration between patient and staff, and the "chemistry" of the interactions among attributes of the patient, family, staff, treatments, and environment.

An important step in the long-term management of a patient with a serious mental disorder is to involve the patient and family in a collaborative relationship. The family and patient become members of the treatment team and are encouraged to participate fully in treatment planning and evaluation. There can be little expected from treatment without relationships with patients and their families that are infused with mutual respect, confidence,

CLINICAL EXAMPLE

TRAINER: Tim, what are the two, overall types of benefits of antipsychotic medications?

TIM: What did you say?

TRAINER: Look at me, Tim. Good. I'll come closer so you can hear me while you are looking at me. Tim, tell me one of the two overall benefits of antipsychotic medication.

TIM: Antipsychotic meds help you think more clearly.

TRAINER: That's right, Tim. Great! You got one very important benefit of antipsychotic meds. When a medication reduces problems and symptoms or helps you to think and function better, we call those benefits THERAPEUTIC benefits. When a medication helps to PREVENT a return of symptoms or problems, we call that type of benefit a PROPHYLACTIC benefit. So, Tim, look at me and tell me, What is one of the overall types of benefits of antipsychotic meds?

TIM: You mean, therapeutic benefits like thinking more clearly?

TRAINER: Right on! You got it, Tim. Therapeutic benefits are one kind of benefit that you get from antipsychotic meds. For example, didn't you tell me that since you began your meds, you no longer hear voices?

TIM: Yeah, they got softer and disappeared. I'm glad because they said bad things to me.

TRAINER: Well, voices that you hear are a good example of psychotic symptoms that are removed by the therapeutic effects of medication. Once more, what are examples of the therapeutic benefits of antipsychotic drugs?

TIM: When your voices go away and when you can think more clearly.

TRAINER: Terrific! Those are two examples of the therapeutic benefits of antipsychotics. What's an example of a preventive or prophylactic benefit?

TIM: I don't know.

TRAINER: Look at me and listen closely because I'm going to ask you to repeat after me. Prophylactic benefits come when symptoms don't come back. The medication has preventive or prophylactic benefits when a person who takes the medication every day does not suffer a relapse. So, Tim, give me an example of a prophylactic or preventive benefit of antipsychotic drugs.

TIM: You mean preventing relapses?

TRAINER: Absolutely!! Prophylactic benefits prevent bad things from coming back—like relapses, voices, or trouble thinking. Now, what are the two kinds of overall benefits you get from these drugs?

TIM: Therapeutic and prophylactic.

TRAINER: You got it, Tim. Let's repeat it again.

nesty, and shared information. The psychoeducational process will also be ...ched to the phase of the patient's disorder, so in the acute phase it focuses ... the nature of serious mental disorders as stress-related, biological diseases. The clinician points out how protective factors can buffer the noxious effects of environmental stress impinging on the vulnerability of the brain.

Families are reassured to know that treatment of the acute, florid symptoms with medication and a low-stress, supportive hospital environment is the first step in reversing the pathological process and starting their relative on the path toward recovery. The purpose, services, and likely duration of hospitalization are described, and family members are given an opportunity to ventilate their worries, fears, and questions. It is often advisable to begin the education of family members separately from the education of the patient, since the latter may be too floridly psychotic to absorb information at a pace and level of abstraction that is possible for family members. In addition, an acutely psychotic person may evince behaviors that would be intrusive, distracting, and disturbing to relatives who are convened to learn about serious psychiatric disorders. There are always exceptions to this characterization, since many patients in the acute phase of illness retain good attention, memory, learning ability, and self-control. If patients cannot join the family psychoeducation, they should be involved as soon as their clinical condition permits. The educational process should be pitched to patients' cognitive and learning capacities. Specific illness management programs have been designed for this purpose: a tool kit sponsored by the Substance Abuse and Mental Health Services Administration (2004), the Medication Management, Symptom Management, Substance Abuse Management, and Community Re-entry Modules.

Patients with severe mental disorders will need assistance in becoming active partners in the treatment endeavor. Family members, personal support specialists (i.e., case managers), or other therapists can serve a key role by coaching the patient to bring useful information into his/her sessions with a psychiatrist for medication evaluation and management. Patients also need to be given coaching to ask important questions of their psychiatrists so

> Adherence to treatment is not enough. Recovery requires an informed patient who shares in decisions about treatment.

> "Shared decision-making is an ethical imperative for all patients, not a privilege for those with milder mental disorders, and is a fundamental tenet of person-centered, recovery-oriented, evidence-based medicine. People with psychiatric disabilities want some level of involvement in treatment decisions. When we move beyond medical paternalism and the related notions of compliance and coercion, innovative strategies to collaboratively engage even the most challenging patients in shared decision making often emerge."
>
> DEEGAN AND DRAKE (2006)

they can become informed consumers of medication. Face-to-face coaching with written lists of information and questions that the patient can bring to his/her doctor's appointment can overcome the nervousness, inarticulateness, and cognitive problems like forgetting that plague patients as they interact with a psychiatrist during a brief medication management session. Especially when given on the day of the appointment, coaching can be hugely effective in promoting better communication between the patient and doctor, equipping the doctor with information needed to make enlightened decisions about medication and producing greater satisfaction with treatment by the patient. Since many patients will not have access to coaches, the psychiatrist should always take on that role as his/her responsibility in fostering a collaborative relationship with shared decision making.

EXAMPLE

Some topics that are the focus for coaching and carried as a "crib sheet" by the patient into the doctor's appointment are:

- Tell the doctor how you feel about your current medication and how it's affecting your everyday life—be sure to write down the names of each of your medications and their dose.
- Describe any side effects or symptoms that may be side effects—ask the doctor to repeat the kinds of side effects that are associated with the medication being used.
- Ask the doctor, again if necessary, how the medication will be helpful to you—how you can expect to feel as a result of the medication's benefits, and how long it will take for the medication to start working.
- Tell the doctor if you're thinking of stopping the medication, and ask about the downsides to that decision.
- Ask the doctor what you should do if you forget to take a dose of medication.
- Ask the doctor how long you will need to take the medication.
- Find out how you can cooperate with the doctor to get the best effects and fewest side effects from the medication.
- If the medication doesn't appear to be working, ask the doctor when it would be time to try another medication.

The practitioner should obtain truly informed consent for treatment, which should include asking the patient to repeat back, in his/her own words, the nature of the treatment and its intended benefits and risks. It should be emphasized to the patient how important it is for all those on us/her treatment and family support "team" to be able to keep one another apprised of progress, problems, and opportunities. When natural supporters and professionals can share information, there will be more chances for treatment to accelerate progress; thus, it is in the patient's best interest to give consent to share information about progress in treatment to all those participating on the treatment team, including designated family members, with the proviso that the patient can request that any particular information be held confidential. Family education, support, and therapy should continue indefinitely. The practitioner's door should always be open to the family, with the welcome mat out. The family has a great deal more information relevant to treatment planning than does the practitioner, who may see the patient for only relatively brief sessions. Research has shown that the best "dose" of education and skills training for the family is to have weekly sessions for 3 months, biweekly sessions for 6 months, and monthly sessions thereafter for at least 2 years.

CLINICAL EXAMPLE

Jack's parents were elderly and infirm. They were also afraid of him, since he had attacked them both at a holiday celebration 3 years before. They had had absolutely no contact for 3 years. Jack had almost continuous persecutory and catastrophic hallucinations and delusions that seriously disabled him. A new psychiatrist used serial ratings on the Brief Psychiatric Rating Scale to monitor the effects of several different drugs and identified one that reduced the severity of his psychosis. A team led by the psychiatrist offered cognitive-behavioral therapy, motivational enhancement with a home-based token economy, and weekly recreational and social outings accompanied by a personal support specialist.

Jack began to make progress toward his personal goals: to reconcile with his parents, regain his interest in art history, and become more independent of his caregiver. Jack expressed sustained interest in communicating with his parents, regret about the aggressive episode, and a genuine concern about their health and well-being.

Jack's doctor met with his parents and discovered that they also wished to renew their contacts with their son; however, they were fearful of a repeat onslaught. With everyone's agreement, a plan was hatched for Jack to phone them once a week for not more than 5 minutes. Using social skills training techniques, they all learned how to structure their conversations at a mundane level, giving and asking for information related solely to their respective, current activities. Further sessions teaching communication skills were held with the parents as their exchanges with Jack gradually grew to include meetings for lunch, picnics, and birthdays. A year later, they had developed a closer and more satisfying relationship than at any time in the previous 20 years.

STABILIZATION PHASE: CONTINUING SYMPTOM IMPROVEMENT AND COMMUNITY REINTEGRATION

The functions and responsibilities of the clinician during the stabilization phase are to 1) ensure continuation of treatment, 2) educate the patient and family about the importance of giving information to the clinician on symptoms and side effects, 3) facilitate optimal pharmacotherapy, and 4) help effect a *gradual* return to psychosocial functioning. Bringing these aims to fruition requires the clinician to:

- Arrange for continuity of care from the acute phase.
- Monitor symptoms for adjusting pharmacotherapy to advance remission or stability of symptoms.
- Teach patient and family members to manage medication properly and track warning signs of relapse.
- Assist family members to continue their education about mental disorders by becoming active members of advocacy and peer support organizations such as the National Alliance on Mental Illness (NAMI), NARSAD (National Alliance for Research on Schizophrenia and Depression), and the Depression and Bipolar Support Alliance.
- Encourage family members to become active participants in their sick relative's outpatient treatment and expand the scope of psychoeducation and behavioral family management—the patient should attend these sessions as stabilization permits.
- Collaborate with patient and family in developing specific procedures for adherence to medication, avoiding notions of compliance and coercion.
- Promote the patient's adaptation to community life through supportive contacts with a personal support specialist (i.e., case manager) or assertive community treatment team. The contacts should be flexible and focused on helping the patient to learn independent living skills and use them in his/her everyday life.
- Engage natural supporters in the community to "run interference" for patients as they implement their skills in everyday life. Community

adaptation requires practice, opportunities, encouragement, and reinforcement for using skills.

Teaching Adherence to Medications

Even with persons who have medical but no mental disorders, adherence to medication regimens is notoriously poor. There are many explanations for unreliable and irregular use of medications. These include factors related to the:

- Medications themselves, such as side effects, complexities of the prescription schedule and multiple medications, and the need for sustained, long-term use.
- Patients and their characteristics, such as ignorance about their illness and the purpose of the medication, fatalism or antimedication values, and unrealistic expectations.
- Family, such as viewing medications as habit-forming and harmful.
- Doctor–patient relationship, such as inadequate education of the patient and family regarding medications and their role in the treatment of the patient's disorder.
- Treatment delivery system, such as long waits to see a doctor for medication reviews, an uncomfortably brief time with the doctor, unfriendly clinic receptionists, and uncomfortable and crowded waiting rooms.

The severely mentally ill have additional barriers to adherence, such as symptoms and cognitive impairments that interfere with memory, daily routines, apathy, and suspiciousness. The psychiatrist and other members of the treatment team are the final common denominator for helping patients to overcome the barriers to reliable medication use. When practitioners take responsibility for using the various approaches that facilitate adherence, patients will use their medication more dependably. As blaming the patient for noncompliance becomes less acceptable in the current, recovery-oriented era of treatment, psychiatrists and other clinicians will learn to become more adept at engineering medication adherence.

While the increased use of psychoeducation for patients and relatives has resulted in reliable increases in participants' knowledge about mental illness and medications, there is scant evidence that such broad-based programs have measurable effects on actual use of medication. Of course, learning about one's illness and the treatments available for it is valuable in its own right; how else will patients and their families become informed participants in a collaborative approach to treatment? There are techniques of illness management that have succeeded in improving reliable self-administration of prescribed medications, as outlined in the examples below (Mueser et al. 2002).

To compensate for the cognitive deficits, negative symptoms, and sedative side effects that interfere with remembering to follow prescribed use of medication, many techniques have been useful. These include telephone calls, beepers, and compartmentalized boxes for scheduling medication use; enlisting the assistance of family members in prompting medication use; overlearning of medication use through social skills training; home visits to attach posters, calendars, and other reminders at visible locations; and periodic monitoring of plasma levels of medication, with positive feedback to the patient for having therapeutic concentrations.

EXAMPLES

Brief descriptions are given for the following interventions that are effective in promoting adherence to the use of psychotropic medications by persons with disabling mental disorders.

- *Simplifying the medication regimen.* Using once-daily scheduling for administration.
- *Behavioral tailoring.* Placing the medication in a visible place consistent with the patient's daily routine.
- *Motivational interviewing.* Ensuring that the patient understands how the regular use of medication can facilitate achieving personal goals.
- *Training in medication self-management.* Teaching patients benefits, side effects, self-administration, and negotiation skills in collaborating with psychiatrists.
- *Assertive community treatment.* Outreach by clinicians to bring medication to the patient and supervise its proper use.
- *Behavioral family therapy.* Educating patients and their relatives in disease management plus training in communication and problem-solving skills.
- *Interpersonal therapy.* Learning how to cope with stress derived from loss of relationships, disputes, grief, transitions in life, and deficits in social skills.
- *Cognitive-behavioral therapy.* Teaching patients to challenge and reality-test dysfunctional ideas, assumptions, and perceptions about medication.

Optimizing Pharmacotherapy Through Symptom Monitoring

Prospects for recovery from a mood or schizophrenia spectrum disorder are markedly enhanced by achieving remission or optimal stabilization of symptoms. Remission or symptom stabilization is more readily achieved if the prescribing psychiatrist reliably measures and monitors patients' symptoms and side effects. When sensitive, quantitative ratings are available to the prescribing psychiatrist, decisions regarding medication type and dose can be made in a judicious manner.

The *severity* and *stability* of symptoms rated serially and objectively can help the psychiatrist and the rest of the treatment team determine when a patient may be ready for a change in medication, goals, rehabilitation regimen, psychosocial structure, support, and supervision. For example, when patients with moderately high levels of psychopathology are being rehabilitated, their skills training sessions should be shorter and have less complexity, greater structure, shorter-term goals, and more repetition. Ratings of symptoms can be made at intervals consistent with the patient's clinical stability, but are rarely needed more often than biweekly. Customarily, the ratings are made monthly or whenever the patient has a periodic visit to the psychiatrist.

Using Rating Scales to Monitor Symptoms

There are many standardized, sensitive, reliable, and user-friendly scales that can be used to inform psychiatrists about the progress of their patients. These include the UCLA expanded Brief Psychiatric Rating Scale (BPRS), Positive and Negative Syndrome Scale (PANSS), Clinical Global Impression Scale, Beck Depression Inventory (BDI), Hamilton Rating Scale for Depression, Yale-Brown Obsessive Compulsive Scale, and the Young Mania Rating Scale (see Wetzler 1989 for descriptions and references for all these measures). Because most patients have only a few target symptoms that exacerbate during periods of relapse, the clinician can economically rate only those items on a scale that are relevant to each particular patient. A *target symptom scale* is convenient to use, as any relevant, idiosyncratic symptom can be rated on a 12-point scale of severity from 0 ("not present") to 3 ("a little") to 6 ("somewhat") to 9 ("very much") to 12 ("couldn't be worse").

BRIEF PSYCHIATRIC RATING SCALE

The UCLA expanded Brief Psychiatric Rating Scale has 24 items, including positive and negative psychotic symptoms and suicidality, that are relevant to individuals with schizophrenia, bipolar disorder, and mood disorders. It also covers prodromal symptoms that have been found to arise before a full-blown relapse: anxiety, depression, distractibility, emotional withdrawal, tension, restlessness, bodily and health concerns, and suspiciousness. Therefore, the BPRS is an appropriate and flexible instrument to use for gaining information to improve decisions regarding the prescription of medications and rehabilitation modalities as well as for early identification and intervention to stave off impending relapse. Stressful life events, problems in relationships, the accumulation of daily hassles, or changes in adherence to medication may lead to warning signs of relapse that may impede a patient's progress in rehabilitation toward recovery.

Each of the 24 items is scaled from "not present" to "very mild," "mild," "moderate," "moderately severe," "severe," and "extremely severe," with each scale level anchored by operationalized, specific criteria of severity and frequency of the symptom. The manual also provides an interview guide with queries that are designed to successfully elicit responses from patients, even those who tend to deny symptoms.

CLINICAL EXAMPLE

Bill was a 38-year-old patient with long-standing schizophrenia who, after many years of struggling with relapses and rehospitalizations, finally gained a nearly complete remission of his persecutory and referential delusions and hallucinations. His good outcome was a result of developing a collaborative relationship with a psychiatrist who used the BPRS to select and titrate the dose of a second-generation antipsychotic drug. After participating for 2 months in a supported employment program, Bill got a job as a barista in a coffee shop.

One month after starting this job, Bill had a scheduled appointment with his psychiatrist. In response to the psychiatrist asking how he was doing, Bill replied that he enjoyed his job and his new identity as a worker. If his psychiatrist had asked only open-ended questions about his mental state, Bill would have left her office with a renewal of his prescription. When the psychiatrist proceeded to ask questions from the BPRS, she elicited Bill's report that he had been hearing two voices talking about him in a negative way once a day or so for the past 2 weeks. These voices were not occurring frequently enough to interfere with his work. He noticed that some of his customers were staring at him when he was making their cappuccinos. Several times in the past week, he thought that his coworkers

BPRS

Psychotic Index

	Date:	12/6	12/8	12/12	12/17	1/5	1/26	—	4/4	4/11	4/18	4/25	5/2	5/9	5/16	6/6	6/21	7/15
Unusual Thought Content	7																	
	6																	
	5																	
	4																	
	3																	
	2																	
	1																	
Hallucinations	7																	
	6																	
	5																	
	4																	
	3																	
	2																	
	1																	
Conceptual Disorganization N/A	7																	
	6																	
	5																	
	4																	
	3																	
	2																	
	1																	
Suspiciousness	7																	
	6																	
	5																	
	4																	
	3																	
	2																	
	1																	
Grandiosity N/A	7																	
	6																	
	5																	
	4																	
	3																	
	2																	
	1																	
Other Symptoms Anxiety	7																	
	6																	
	5																	
	4																	
	3																	
	2																	
	1																	
Psychotic Index	34																	
	32																	
	30																	
	28																	
	26																	
	24																	
	22																	
	20																	
	18																	
	16																	
	14																	
	12																	
	10																	
	8																	
	6																	
Drug & Dose Risperidone		6mg	6	6	6	4	4		6	6	6	4	4	4	4	4	4	4

FIGURE 3.3 Monitoring symptoms of Bill, a 38-year-old patient with long-standing schizophrenia, using the Brief Psychiatric Rating Scale.

were making critical comments about his productivity. He wasn't sure that these events were actually happening, but he ruminated about them. These thoughts frequently made him nervous, and he was worried about losing his self-confidence and his job.

As shown in Figure 3.3, Bill's hallucinations, anxiety, ideas of reference, and feelings of persecution registered "moderate" to "moderately severe" on the BPRS. Bill revealed that he had recently moved to a new residence to live closer to his job and was feeling tense because residents in his new board-and-care home weren't friendly. These major life events were undoubtedly fueling his prodromal symptoms. Bill's psychiatrist increased his dose of medication modestly and contacted Bill's personal support specialist, expressing concern about the stress that Bill was experiencing. The two of them came up with a plan to encourage Bill's job coach to meet more often with Bill and to deliver positive reinforcement for his job skills. In addition, the personal support specialist met with the manager of Bill's board-and-care home and arranged for a new roommate for Bill, a man who was more talkative and congenial than the other residents. Three weeks later, Bill's symptoms returned to their previous subclinical level and his medication was tapered back to its original dose. By carefully monitoring Bill's symptoms and modulating the sources of stress, the treatment team was able to avert a relapse and enable Bill to sustain his vocational momentum.

Establishing Provisions for Continuing Treatment and Rehabilitation

One of the most important objectives of the stabilization phase is ensuring successful continuity of care. Given the long-term and recurrent nature of serious mental disorders, continuity of services from the acute to the stabilization phases is essential. Unfortunately, coordinated care is more the exception than the rule. Unless there is a seamless transition from the hospital to community-based treatment, patients will not continue their therapeutic trajectory toward recovery.

The majority of patients do not follow through with community care, with as many as 70% failing to make even their first postdischarge appointment. Much of this tragic loss of continuity of care stems from the challenges faced by mental health authorities in bringing coherence to a patchwork system of service providers. The clinical personnel responsible for acute care versus follow-through services are almost always in different locations, under the aegis of different agencies and funding mechanisms, subject to

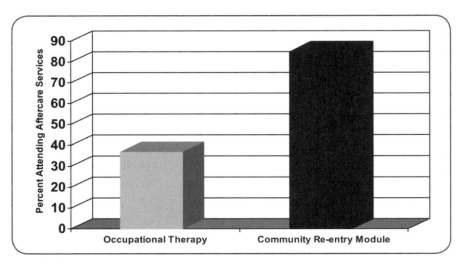

FIGURE 3.4 Fostering of continuity of care with the Community Re-entry Module. Compared with customary discharge planning, patients randomly assigned to an educational module to learn skills relevant to developing their continuing care made contact with their aftercare mental health program more than twice as often.

At one county-run hospital, inpatients were randomly assigned to eight 45-minute sessions of the module or to the same amount of time in occupational therapy using the medium of expressive arts. Sessions were held twice-daily, since the average length of stay was under 6 days. Both groups received the same assistance from discharge planners. As shown in Figure 3.4, patients who participated in the module learned almost 50% more about community reintegration and were more than twice as likely to connect with aftercare outpatient services than were their counterparts.

divergent administrative policies and procedures, and hopelessly overwhelmed with enormous caseloads and staff turnover. If patients could be escorted to the facility where they were intended to receive continuing care and introduced to the responsible staff members, the rates of continuous care would be high. Although assertive community treatment teams are successful in bridging the various phases of illness and recovery, they are operating effectively at relatively few places in the United States.

This situation places the responsibility for integrating care on the patients themselves. Patients can be taught to actively seek and obtain their own follow-up services if the curriculum and training methods take into account their learning disabilities. The *Community Re-entry Module* was designed to equip patients with the ability to make the leap from inpatient or day treatment to outpatient continuing care.

The American Association of Community Psychiatrists has developed best practices for managing transitions between levels of care. The basic assumption is that mental health teams and individual clinicians are responsible for maintaining continuity of care for persons with serious and persistent mental illness whose treatment must be sustained indefinitely. The guidelines, listed in Table 3.2, include recommendations that the use of the terms *discharge* and *aftercare* be discontinued in favor of the terms *transition* and *continuing care.*

STABLE PHASE: BUILDING SKILLS AND SOCIAL SUPPORTS WHILE MAINTAINING SYMPTOM CONTROL

The goals of the stable phase are to proceed in earnest with psychosocial rehabilitation while continuing to monitor symptoms of the disorder so that risk of relapse is minimized. When patients' symptoms have been stable for 3 months or longer, they are able to tolerate and learn from psychosocial services of greater complexity, intensity, and comprehensiveness. The stable

Controlled studies in three countries have documented the effectiveness of the Community Re-entry Module in strengthening continuity of care, improving social functioning, and increasing tenure in the community without relapse (Anzai et al. 2002; Kopelowicz et al. 1998; Xiang et al. 2006).

● EXAMPLE OF BEST PRACTICE

The *Community Re-entry Module* teaches the knowledge and skills that are needed by patients to make contact with a community-based provider of mental health services. The curriculum consists of 16 sessions, 8 of which are particularly germane for developing and implementing an aftercare plan. The learning objectives for these sessions are:

- Understanding symptoms of disabling mental disorders, such as schizophrenia, bipolar disorder, and depression—How can treatment help me control my symptoms and prevent relapse so I can live successfully in the community?
- Determining one's readiness for discharge—What improvements in symptoms and functioning are consistent with more independent functioning?
- Planning to live in the community—Where will I live? How will I get funds to support myself? Where can I receive continuing psychiatric services?
- Connecting with the community—Where and when can I meet a person who can help me to arrange my continuing care needs in a community mental health program?
- Coping with stress in the community—What coping skills can I use to manage stress and avoid relapse?
- Planning a daily schedule—How and where can I find activities that will prevent boredom, loneliness, and depression?
- Making and keeping appointments—What communication skills and resources will I need to make my own appointments for mental health, social, and recreational services?

● TABLE 3.2

Guidelines for ensuring successful transitions of patients from one level of care to another

- Transition planning should begin at the time of admission to any level of care and should be part of the treatment plan.
- Treatment plans and progress notes should demonstrate attention to issues that are likely to be encountered during transitions to new treatment settings or clinicians.
- Transition plans should be individualized and comprehensively cover all needs for service into the future, including medication services, case management, rehabilitation, housing, financial supports, and family involvement.
- Coordination and collaboration among practitioners at different agencies and levels of care should be the hallmark of communication regarding the patient. Coordination should ensure consistency in pharmacological and psychosocial treatment in support of the patient's personally relevant goals.
- Patients should not be expected to be responsible for managing complex and multifaceted aspects of their continuing care—especially during acute and stabilizing phases of their illness.
- Continuity of treatment plans, changes in clinical response to treatment, and repeated assessments should be transmitted across levels of care and from one practitioner to another.
- Transition planners should recognize the phase of illness or recovery of the patient for whom services are being developed. Treatment plans should be compatible with the phase of the patient's disorder.
- Involvement of the patient in treatment planning, choice of treatment alternatives, and decisions about transitions to other levels of care should be maximized.
- Families and other natural supporters in the community should be involved in treatment planning, the array of services, and decisions about transitions.
- Maintenance of well-being and prevention of relapse should be given prime consideration in development of treatment and transition plans. Relapse prevention plans should identify early warning signs of relapse and their "triggers" that should be transmitted across levels of care.
- Cultural sensitivity should be inherent in treatment and transition planning.
- Transition plans should be designed to include the resources that are available to the patient for continuing care and arrangements made for ensuring use of resources.
- Elements of the services system should develop clear protocols that delineate responsibility for each provision and service that is required during the transition period. The contacts that the patient must make in actualizing the transition should be written and provided to the patient in a way that ensures comprehension, transportation, child care, and other possible barriers to continuity of care.

Source. American Association of Community Psychiatrists, as published in Sowers WE, Rohland B: "American Association of Community Psychiatrists' Principles for Managing Transitions in Behavioral Health Services." *Psychiatric Services* 55:1271–1275, 2004. Used with permission.

phase is when vocational rehabilitation can be introduced and patients can be encouraged to make their own choices regarding college education, independent living, expanding friendships, dating and intimacy, initiative, and self-responsibility. However, the treatment team should be watchful and attuned to stable patients, as they may continue to be sensitive to stress, change, and challenging situations. Therefore, a major responsibility for the clinician and treatment team is to share observance with the patient and family for warning signs of relapse. When warning signs occur, temporary increases or modification of the medication regimen and/or removal or mitigation of ambient stressors are usually sufficient to keep the patient on the pathway to recovery.

Flexible levels of personal support services and frequency of visits to the psychiatrist, ranging from weekly to monthly or even longer intervals, can ensure that the patient is maintaining or improving his/her level of functioning and quality of life. Rehabilitation practitioners give positive reinforcement to their patients as the latter encounter and effectively cope with major life events, cumulative daily hassles, and any adverse effects of treatment. Family psychoeducation in this phase can shift from discussions about the course of illness and its treatments to the teaching of communication, problem-solving, and stress management skills.

This phase of services for the family is termed *behavioral family management,* reflecting its focus on management of illness through strengthening the interpersonal behavior and relationships within the family. As families gain these higher-level skills, they are able to lend support to the patient's progress toward independent functioning. The emotional and financial burden on the family lightens, freeing relatives of the mentally ill person to invest in their own goals, marriage, other members of the family, careers, recreational and social activities, and vacations.

Despite the ability to set more ambitious and demanding goals during the stable phase of illness, patients must continue to hew to the axiom that going slower is going faster. The pace toward recovery is not a race. Consolidation of one's progress before moving on to new goals must be uppermost in the minds of practitioners as well as patients and relatives as they continue to collaborate in traversing the road toward recovery. Recovery is just over the next mountain, but, as Goethe remarked, "mountains cannot be surmounted except by winding paths."

The evidence-based, rehabilitation services that satisfy the functions and goals of the stable and recovery phases of illness are described in Chapters 5 ("Social Skills Training"), 6 ("Involving Families in Treatment and Rehabilitation"), 7 ("Vocational Rehabilitation"), and 8 ("Vehicles for Delivering Rehabilitation Services").

CLINICAL EXAMPLE

"When I had my first and second breakdowns, I tried to hurry and catch up on the time I had lost when I was sick. But I learned that recovery is not a race with the clock. Getting well takes time, patience, and more than a few ups and downs. I have found the hard way that making recovery a race only puts more pressure on everyone. For me, increased pressure leads to relapse. Believe me, a person needs time to let the smoke clear and get a perspective on what is happening with him and in the world around him. With time, things will come around, even though the illness is overpowering to everyone concerned. If you go up a flight of stairs, usually you go up one step at a time. When dealing with mental illnesses, one step at a time will get you to the top without wearing you out."

Dylan Abraham, consumer member of a mental health team

RECOVERY PHASE: ACHIEVING AND MAINTAINING PERSONAL GOALS AND A NORMAL LIFESTYLE

As new treatment and rehabilitation services are developed and empirically validated, more and more patients with serious mental disorders are able to enjoy lives that can be considered within the normal range. Of course, this depends upon services that are *comprehensive, continuous, coordinated, collaborative, consumer-oriented, consistent with the phase of the disorder, competency-based with evidence-based techniques, connected with the patient's skills and deficits, compassionate,* and *cooperative.* While treatment and rehabilitation programs of excellence that meet these criteria are still sadly limited in availability, we can expect wider accessibility to such programs with the persistent advocacy of stakeholder organizations, consumers, and family members, together with the increasing acceptance by mental health professionals of recovery as a legitimate goal for clinical intervention.

The services that are keyed to the recovery phase must be highly individualized to meet the long-term goals of patients whose symptoms are in abeyance and psychosocial functioning enables them to work, study, actively socialize, and enjoy recreational activities and family ties—all within normative venues and relationships. The case example below highlights one patient's experience of recovery and the continuing services she sought to maintain herself in a state of wellness.

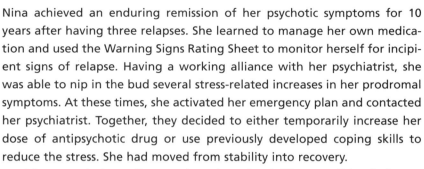

CLINICAL EXAMPLE

Nina achieved an enduring remission of her psychotic symptoms for 10 years after having three relapses. She learned to manage her own medication and used the Warning Signs Rating Sheet to monitor herself for incipient signs of relapse. Having a working alliance with her psychiatrist, she was able to nip in the bud several stress-related increases in her prodromal symptoms. At these times, she activated her emergency plan and contacted her psychiatrist. Together, they decided to either temporarily increase her dose of antipsychotic drug or use previously developed coping skills to reduce the stress. She had moved from stability into recovery.

After completing college and nursing school, Nina was living independently, working full-time as a school nurse, and participating in environmental organizations. Her hobbies were bird-watching and hiking. At this point, her goal was to develop friendships and date, but she had always been shy and unassertive. After 8 months of weekly social skills training, she had acquired friendship and dating skills that she practiced on hikes sponsored by the Sierra Club. After a year of dating, she met a man with whom she had much in common. Ultimately, they decided to live together, and some years later, they married. Her wedding celebrated her marriage and her recovery.

TREATMENT-REFRACTORY ILLNESS

While psychotropic drugs and psychosocial treatments for major mental disorders have been scientifically documented as effective, there are still many mentally ill individuals for whom even competently delivered, evidence-based treatments are relatively ineffective. Estimates of patients with treatment-refractory illness have ranged from 15% to 25% of persons with schizophrenia, mood disorders, and anxiety disorders, depending upon the criteria used to define *refractory*. Suboptimal treatment outcomes lead to persisting symptoms, disability, restrictions on one's opportunities to participate in community life, and a dismal quality of life.

We must guard against using misguided language that stereotypes and stigmatizes persons who do not respond to customary treatment. Labeling suboptimally responsive patients as "treatment resistant" is pejorative and suggests that they would respond if they only wanted to. Terms such as *treatment resistant* can restrict our therapeutic creativity and interfere with our ability to provide novel, effective treatments. "The customer is always right" means that it is our responsibility as researchers, clinicians, and administrators to respond to the challenges posed by treatment refractoriness. We must dedicate ourselves to finding, adapting, combining, or creating treatments that will be more effective for these individuals.

Just as for other medical problems that seem unresponsive to standard care, specialized and unique services are available for those patients whose illness is refractory to customary treatments. Clozapine has been used for this purpose for over 17 years in the United States. There are many notable examples of individuals who were lost in their psychoses but then recovered after receiving clozapine. But it is a rare patient who recovers with clozapine alone. Patients cannot *learn how to live* a normal life solely with medication.

Clozapine can evaporate some or all of a patient's positive psychotic symptoms. This sets the stage for psychosocial treatments to teach the person how to use a computer, develop friends, get and hold a job, and learn to play games. One large randomized controlled trial of patients with treatment-refractory schizophrenia compared clozapine with haloperidol with or without concurrent psychosocial treatment and activities. Results indicated that there was a reciprocity between clozapine and the psychosocial activities. Clozapine facilitated participation in psychosocial treatment and enhanced participation led to improved quality of life.

Behavioral therapies also can make a dent in the disabilities experienced by persons with refractory schizophrenia. Unfortunately, behavioral techniques are not widely available and are effective only in the hands of well-trained and experienced specialists. Behavioral strategies for managing refractory illnesses include:

- *Cognitive-behavioral therapy* for attenuating delusions and hallucinations.
- *Token economy* and other contingent reinforcement programs for increasing adaptive behavior.
- Individualized *behavior therapy* combined with *social skills training* for strengthening personal effectiveness.
- *Planned and scheduled positive activities* that have the effect of displacing persistent, psychotic symptoms.
- *Behavioral and environmental prostheses, such as those in cognitive adaptive therapy,* that enable the individual to *compensate* or sidestep persisting symptoms and cognitive impairments.

These techniques are described more fully in Chapter 9 ("Special Services for Special People") of this book.

▶ From Compliance to Collaboration for Adherence to Treatment

The terms *treatment compliance* and *noncompliance* misdirect the responsibility for proper use of pharmacological and psychosocial treatments to patients. The terms imply that if patients really wanted the treatment, they would take it. This view of treatment perpetuates the misconceptions that adhering to treatment derives primarily from the patient's motivation or resistance. The term compliance stems from the paternalistic mind-set that the clinician is the altruistic expert with the right prescription for treatment. If the prescription isn't followed, the fault lies with the patient who refuses to follow the prescription.

But the truth lies somewhere else. Rather than the patient being viewed as a passive receptacle for treatment, it is the practitioner's responsibility to mobilize the patient as a cooperating partner in treatment. In this collaborative approach, the practitioner and patient share the responsibility for proper participation in treatment. To have success in achieving collaborative relationships in treatment, it is necessary for the clinician to understand and respect the reasons why patients don't take medication or don't elect to join psychosocial treatment programs. From the very start, patients' participation in treatment is always in balance between factors that favor or nullify it. Roadblocks to collaboration may originate in the treatment techniques used, the patient's perceptions and cognitive capacities, the patient's family or other caregivers, the relationship between the patient and clinician, and the treatment delivery system. As shown in Figure 3.5, all of these factors carry weight in determining whether the patient accepts or rejects treatment. In the example above, one all too commonly overlooked problem illustrates the failure in the patient–doctor relationship.

Low literacy is rife in our society, but doctors, associated mental health professionals, and health educators often write information for patients—including prescription labels—that are much above the eighth-grade level or too high for many adults to understand. Most doctors are not adept at detecting reading problems or knowing what to do when such individuals are identified. We need to give more time for office visits and more support from nurse educators and reading specialists. Our patients need a simpler, "one-stop shopping" approach to their health care, such as clinics or mental health centers that offer accessible and low-cost lab tests that will enable psychiatrists to have the basic information they need to provide effective treatment.

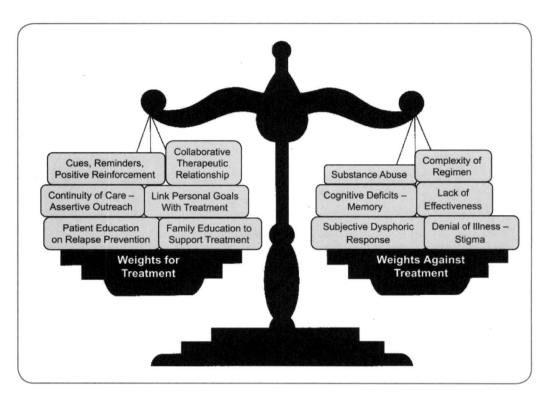

FIGURE 3.5 Balancing of factors that determine adherence to treatment.

CLINICAL EXAMPLE

Joseph, a pleasant and cooperative 57-year-old with a 30-year history of manic depression, suffered multiple relapses and rehospitalizations. When Joseph was hospitalized, his lithium serum levels were brought into the therapeutic range by titration of his daily dose of lithium, and his symptoms rapidly improved. When transitioned to community care, he quickly destabilized despite his psychiatrist's best efforts at prescribing lithium and other drugs. One problem stood out; Joseph never got his lithium laboratory tests done. It was not for lack of effort from his psychiatrist, who gave Joseph bus routes and maps and wrote down directions to the lab as well as reminding him by phone when his laboratory appointment was scheduled. Some might blame Joseph for being "noncompliant," but the real reason he never got the lithium levels done was something else, something he will never admit: he can't read.

MOTIVATIONAL ENHANCEMENT TO GAIN AND MAINTAIN PATIENTS' PARTICIPATION IN TREATMENT

After patients and families are successfully engaged in treatment, as described earlier in this chapter, most patients will accept and participate in treatment. Being flexible is as important at this stage of illness management as it is throughout; aim for the smallest amount of participation that a reluctant patient is willing to try. For patients who stall after initial engagement, the practitioner can use techniques of motivational enhancement. Insight into one's illness is not necessary for persuasion to motivate a patient to accept treatment. Here are examples of motivational enhancement that have been effective in gaining patients' cooperation in treatment.

- Find out what is nearest and dearest to the patient's immediate and longer-term desires and then engage the patient in a dialogue that conveys how treatment can facilitate the attainment of those desires. *"I know how much you want to get back to college and that you think you can do it all by yourself, but what if we meet a few times to do some planning on what steps you can take to move in that direction?"*

- Give patients a choice in selecting among alternative treatments, any and all of which would be effective. Offering choices to patients for their treatment is consistent with the findings of surveys that patients with schizophrenia express stronger desires to participate in decision making regarding their treatment than primary care patients without mental illness. *"There are several ways to start feeling better; antidepressant medication is just one of them. We can discuss other treatments like cognitive-behavioral therapy, interpersonal therapy, acceptance therapy, and behavioral activation. I want you to share with me the decisions about your treatment."*

- Gain a consensus and a united front among those whom the patient trusts and join them in presenting the treatment as important to the entire cohort. *"Your parents and brothers, grandparents, and best friend all agree that taking medication, at least for now, is very important to them. We all want you to give it a chance."*

- Especially when the stigma of a mental illness is weighing against the decision to accept treatment, use a different term to describe the person's problems. *"You're not schizophrenic or psychotic. It's like you say, you have trouble concentrating, reading, keeping a job, and socializing. It's like a learning disability."*

- Or change the conceptualization of what the therapeutic experience will be like. *"You've told me how and why you can't come to a mental health center, but the activities here are educational, not therapy. In fact, you'll be taking classes and learning how to be more personally effective in reaching the goals you have for improving your life. This is really like a school, and you'll be learning ways to get ahead in your life."*

- Put your patients in charge of the treatment experience, empowering them to start or stop when they wish. *"I want you to be the person in charge of the medication. You can take it for 2 weeks and decide for yourself whether it has been helpful in improving your concentration and allowing you to feel more comfortable around your family and friends. I'll just be your consultant, answering any questions that you have about side effects or any problems that you may experience."*

- Connect patients and their family members with peer-directed educational and motivational programs, such as those sponsored by NAMI, such as *Peer-to-Peer, Family to-Family,* and *In Our Own Voice,"* which are offered by many local affiliates of NAMI.

- Join with the patient's view of the noxiousness of the treatment and use analogies to other treatments that are unpleasant but important for having a better life. *"I certainly agree that taking medications and coming to a clinic are annoying, time-consuming, and unpleasant, but just think about when you had to start wearing glasses, get the injections of antibiotics, and wear a cast when you broke your leg. None of those treatments were pleasant, but they did help you get what you needed— better vision, rid of your infection, and back on your feet again. All of us would prefer not to take treatment, but sometimes it can do a lot more good than bother."*

- Find sources of motivation in the person's everyday life and, with the family's help, use its incentive value to reinforce accepting treatment. *"Your parents have told me that they are worried about your using the family car until you can become calm, relaxed, and not irritable. I think the medication will help with those things so you can drive again."*

PSYCHOSOCIAL TREATMENT ROLE INDUCTION

For psychosocial treatments that seem foreign, strange, and anxiety-provoking because of social or performance demands, patients can acquire more accepting attitudes, reassurance, reality-testing, and greater comfort through in vivo exposure to the treatment. Inviting a patient to sit in on a skills training or cognitive-behavioral therapy group or attend orientation sessions for supported employment or supported living programs often results in a change in the patient's weighing the pros and cons of participation.

It's important to keep the performance expectations very low; thus, for new patients entering a social skills training group, simply observing the group process for the first few sessions is followed by asking them to give positive feedback for the role plays of more veteran patients. Performance expectations increase incrementally with genuine and spontaneous positive feedback made for each of the steps taken by the patient toward full participation.

- Consider employing peers who have benefited from treatment as role models for the reluctant patient. *"Would you be willing to meet with a young woman who has been through the same type of experiences that have interfered with your life? I'll have her come to our next appointment and introduce you, and you both could go out for coffee instead of having the session."*

- Engage the patient in a role reversal during behavioral rehearsal of a physician attempting to persuade a reluctant patient to accept treatment. The patient takes the role of a doctor attempting to persuade a reluctant patient to accept treatment. The doctor takes the role of the reluctant patient. By playing the role of the doctor giving a rationale for the benefits of accepting medication or other treatments, cognitive dissonance is created and attitude change often ensues.

- Involve families in motivating patients' acceptance and participation in treatment. This can be done by teaching family members to make a "positive request." A positive request refocuses the family's communication on how the patient can help them with their problems rather than putting the spotlight on the patient's problems, which are often denied or stigmatized. *"As your parents, we are very worried about the tension in the family. We are having daily headaches and stress and often lose sleep. You can help us feel better if you come with us to see Dr. Brown. We really need help, and you can help us work out our problems together."*

- Maintain adherence to treatment by developing and sustaining a collaborative partnership in treatment decisions with the patient. *"You know, we have to work on solving the problems you're describing with your treatment. You will make the final decisions, and I can only consult with you while you are trying out one or two alternative medications and rehabilitation options. You'll be in charge as the captain—I'll be your navigator and technical adviser."*

Once you and your patient have developed a positive, therapeutic relationship, the collaborative alliance is the most important means of encouraging adherence to treatment. As shown in the example below, the practitioner predicts that discontinuing treatment will be a natural reaction at some point, thereby detoxifying anticipated displeasure or criticism from the practitioner when these times arise. Often, predicting that problems will occur has a paradoxical effect.

EXAMPLE

"As you go along in your treatment, there will be times when you will get tired of taking the medication and attending the social skills group. You'll want to stop, and I can understand that. It's really important that you to tell me how you feel about your treatment and let me know that you want to stop before you do so. I believe that you should only continue with your treatment for as long as you feel it's beneficial. So, when you feel like stopping, let's talk about it and maybe we can figure out what went wrong."

Given the impairments that accompany severe mental disorders, *flexible levels of intervention* have a key role in maintaining adherence to treatment. In using this basic principle of rehabilitation, counterbalance the patient's cognitive, symptomatic, and emotional deficits by reducing the complexity and simplifying the organization of the treatment environment.

- Medication adherence can be improved by simplifying the medication regimen (e.g., having fewer medications and having the patient take all meds at one time each day) or by engaging family members to assist the patient's participation in treatment.
- Starting with simpler regimens and increasing their complexity in gradual increments can maintain better levels of adherence, especially if the clinician and family give positive reinforcement for successful adherence. Eliciting the patient's participation in simplifying excessively complex treatment gives the patient greater identification with and "ownership" of the use of the treatment.
- Adherence to treatment and appointments can be improved by using adaptive techniques in the patient's home environment, such as cues, posters, telephone reminders, daily calendars, medication dispensers with alarm clocks, beepers, and cell phones. Having medication placed in locations where it is seen automatically each day can help to

compensate for memory deficits. Medications should not be hidden from sight behind the doors or drawers of cabinets.

- Shifting to higher levels of community-based intervention such as assertive community treatment or other modes of intensive case management will often aid adherence to all forms of treatment.

- Involving peer supporters, self-help programs, and natural support persons such as friends, storekeepers, and operators and staff of group homes offers opportunities, encouragement, and reinforcement for the patient to participate in treatment and complete community assignments.

DEALING WITH SIDE EFFECTS OF TREATMENT

Most psychiatrists and allied mental health professionals are sensitive to the noxious side effects of medications and how these can weigh against adherence. But even those who are vigilant about identifying side effects may miss those that are subjective and not visible. Akathisia is one of the most troubling side effects of antipsychotic drugs—even of the atypical medications. Unless practitioners periodically inquire with "side-effect checks," it may be too late to deal with troublesome side effects once the patient has fled from treatment. Sexual side effects are another reason for discontinuing antipsychotic and antidepressant drugs; unfortunately, few psychiatrists regularly inquire about the sex life of their patients.

Side effects are associated with dropouts from psychosocial as well as medication treatment. Periodic debriefing sessions for patients participating in psychosocial programs can be very helpful for catching negative feelings and attitudes toward the psychosocial program. If patients are bummed out by failing to achieve their personal goals in social skills training, they may quit before discussing this openly in the group. It's understandable for patients to become demoralized during a lengthy job-seeking process or, after securing employment, to have problems on the job. They may not voice their feelings to their employment specialist, psychiatrist, or case manager; in fact, side effects from problems experienced in supported employment may explain much of the less-than-desired job tenure found in this form of vocational rehabilitation. Regardless of whether the treatment is pharmacological or psychosocial, a proactive approach is required for identifying side effects and collaborating with patients to overcome or cope with them. Holding periodic individual sessions with patients to elicit dissatisfactions, much as professors hold office hours for students in their lecture classes, gives opportunities for such dissatisfactions to be aired.

CLINICAL EXAMPLE

Alan did very well in his supported employment program and had a good relationship with his employment specialist and psychiatrist. He had worked for 6 months as a ticket taker at a movie theater when the manager of the theater asked him to become assistant manager. This position required a considerable increase in responsibilities and performance expectations. Alan was proud of his success on the job and did not want to disappoint his manager, psychiatrist, or employment specialist. He kept the offer of a promotion to himself but was increasingly distressed with anxiety, insomnia, and depression, which were warning signs of psychotic relapse. Alan was prepared to quit his job to avoid his quandary. Because his employment specialist routinely debriefed her clients about their experiences, symptoms, and job satisfaction, she caught wind of his worrisome symptoms. She and Alan worked out a compromise with his boss that added some new responsibilities with a salary increase but did not require Alan to get in over his head. Together with a temporary increase in his antipsychotic medication, Alan's symptoms resolved with no absenteeism from his job.

▶ Teaching Illness Self-Management

By learning illness self-management skills, patients are empowered to feel more in control of their symptoms, instead of being controlled by them. While simple interventions such as behavioral tailoring may improve compliance with medication, the patient is still placed in a passive position and may not continue with the plan once the overseer departs. Better compliance doesn't purvey empowerment or a better-informed consumer of medication and other treatments. Teaching patients the knowledge and skills of illness management offers a broader foundation for coping with their illnesses over a lifetime.

Three categories of skills contribute to patients' progress through the phases of their disorder to achieve stability and recovery:

1. Achieving informed and reliable use of medication and psychosocial treatments
2. Developing and implementing a relapse prevention plan in response to emergence of prodromal symptoms
3. Avoiding relapses of a mental disorder and substance use disorder among individuals with dual diagnoses

Acquiring the knowledge, mastery, and use of skills to control one's illness is not limited to adherence to medication. Some programs have been developed to improve adherence to medication, but they are delimited in their scope and primarily serve as mediators of the paternalistic, doctor–patient relationship.

Teaching skills for illness self-management goes beyond discussion with one's psychiatrist and educational programs, because such programs, while effective in conveying knowledge, have not demonstrated carryover into the acquisition of skills that can be used in patients' everyday lives. The aims of teaching these skills include 1) transferring what professionals know about managing psychiatric disorders and their treatment to the patient and family for their autonomous use; 2) switching from hierarchical doctor–patient roles to educational, student–teacher roles; and 3) improving the collaborative relationship between patient and practitioner by empowering patients to control and direct their own treatment.

The Medication and Symptom Management Modules are highly structured and thoroughly specified curricula that teach individuals the skills needed for illness self-management (Liberman and Wallace 2006). Each module is divided into *skill areas* that focus on the requisite skills that patients need to learn. The modules can be used with groups, individuals, and families and are designed with video-assisted training manuals for practitioners and workbooks for patients. Each skill area contains specified educational objectives that are achieved through *learning activities* that compensate for the cognitive deficits and symptoms that might interfere with patients' acquisition of skills. Because the session-by-session lesson plans are user-friendly, the curricula can be taught with accuracy by practitioners and nonprofessionals with diverse educational backgrounds and practical experience. When the training manuals have been used, the skills have been taught effectively by recovered consumers as well as family members who have a bent for teaching.

EARLY IDENTIFICATION OF PRODROMAL SYMPTOMS AND PREVENTION OF RELAPSE

Progress has been made in averting the full-blown relapse of major mental disorders because of the growing awareness of the role of *prodromal* symptoms of major mental disorders. Prodromal symptoms are those that occur just prior to the onset or relapse of a mental illness. For example, it's common for individuals to experience an increase in anxiety and insomnia just prior to the onset or development of a major depression. Before the relapse of florid psychotic symptoms in persons with schizophrenia, individuals

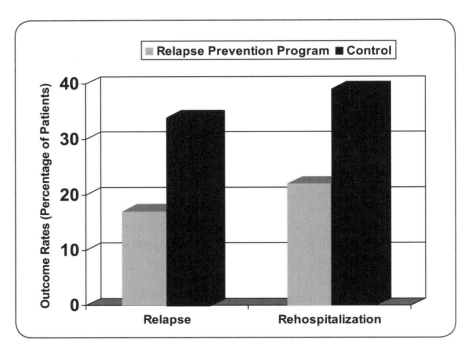

FIGURE 3.6 Effectiveness of teaching relapse prevention skills to patients and families. Effectiveness of teaching relapse prevention skills to patients and families was revealed in significantly fewer rehospitalizations among patients with schizophrenia than among patients offered customary care.

customarily show prodromal signs and symptoms: irritability, social withdrawal, less interest in activities, worrying, preoccupation with religion, and difficulty concentrating and completing tasks.

A strategy using prodromal symptoms has been shown to be effective in reducing the frequency of *relapses* of major mental disorders. This *secondary prevention* strategy teaches patients, their families, and other caregivers to identify the warning signs of relapse and create a *relapse prevention plan.* As can be seen in Figure 3.6, relapse rates are reduced substantially when patients and family members are schooled in recognizing warning signs of a relapse and urged to immediately make contact with a psychiatrist, mental health center, or emergency room for assistance (Herz et al. 2000).

The modules have been rigorously evaluated, and their effectiveness has qualified them as evidence-based. Even chronically ill and disabled patients and those with severe symptoms of their illness can learn the know-how and skills of the modules. When the training is done twice weekly in groups of 4 to 12, robust learning effects are found after 3 months. Learning proceeds faster when the training is done individually with a patient and with families. Training can be effectively carried out in hospitals, clinics, mental health centers, private offices, psychosocial rehabilitation programs, residential care homes, and patients' homes. Controlled studies show that the learning of skills doubles by the end of training and endures for even up to 2 years of follow-up. Failing to teach patients to become informed participants in using their antipsychotic medication has serious, adverse consequences. For example, in a multimillion dollar national study testing four different antipsychotic medications in which patients were not educated about their medications, over 60% of the 1,493 involved patients discontinued their assigned drug treatment—an atrociously high rate that could have been avoided if the project psychiatrists had offered their patients psychoeducation on benefits, coping with side effects, and negotiating with prescribing doctors (Lieberman et al. 2005).

MEDICATION MANAGEMENT MODULE

The five skill areas of the Medication Management Module are:

- Learning about the purposes of medications and the therapeutic and prophylactic benefits of medication.
- Knowing correct self-administration and evaluation of medication.
- Identifying side effects of medication.
- Negotiating medication issues with health care providers.
- Understanding the benefits of long-acting, injectable antipsychotic medications.

The structure of this module is presented diagrammatically in Figure 3.7, including the specific verbal and nonverbal skills that are the educational objectives for one of the skill areas. The module aims to promote adherence but addresses much more than that. Using techniques akin to Socratic questioning and cognitive therapy, patients learn to value their medications while anticipating the realistic problems that occur when taking medications.

Education and skills training should also include a focus on stigma, cultural attitudes toward treatments, financial problems in purchasing medications, concerns about addiction, reluctance to use medications "for the rest of my life," and frustrations in discussing their medications in the limited time they have with their psychiatrists. The role of knowledge and attitudes toward medication has been shown to be significantly associated with adherence to medication, insight, and positive relationships with psychiatrists. This module is most effectively taught by psychiatrists, as they have the greatest credibility with their patients. The learning activities of the

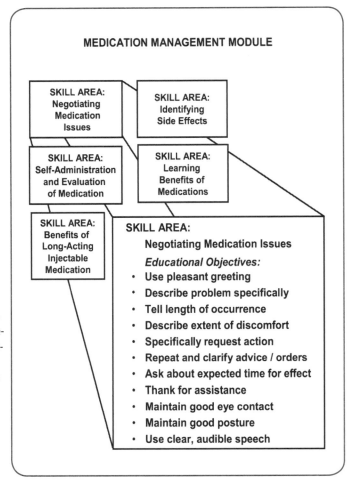

FIGURE 3.7
Structure of the skill areas in the Medication Management Module includes specific behaviors that define the educational objectives for the training process. Educational objectives of one of the five skill areas, "Negotiating Medication Issues," are shown in the foreground.

module amplify the strength of the therapeutic relationship and the quality of the psychiatrist's communication. Nurses and other mental health professionals are also effective teachers of the skills in the module.

A problem-solving approach is taken in the training to prepare patients for the unpredictable exigencies they will encounter as informed and reliable users of medication. For example, in the skill area on side effects, a problem is posed that involves a patient who is prescribed medication three times a day. Shortly after taking his midday dose, he feels drowsy, and this interferes with his alertness in a vocational rehabilitation program. His supervisor notices his drowsiness and says, "If you're not alert, we won't be able to keep you on the job." The patients participating in the module then go through a problem-solving process that prompts them to consider each of a sequence of possible solutions and determine each option's feasibility, advantages and disadvantages, and prospects for solving the problem.

The module uses a Socratic or cognitive therapy approach to encourage patients to learn through their own reasoning about the importance of adherence. To instill collaboration with their prescribing physician for an informed grasp of the effects and side effects of their medication, patients are taught to use a *Self-Assessment Rating Sheet* (see Figure 3.8) and to bring the completed sheet to each appointment with their psychiatrist. The module's impact is not limited to the patients, since the role-plays and homework assignments teach patients to discuss medication issues with their psychiatrists and family members.

Relapse Prevention

Several features of prodromal signs and symptoms make a relapse prevention plan feasible:

- People who have had several relapses of schizophrenia, bipolar disorder, depression, or other recurrent mental disorders can reliably describe the very same profile of signs and symptoms that preceded each of their acute episodes. For example, if a person with several depressive episodes had irritability and social withdrawal as early indicators of his episodes, those same two early warning signs would likely surface as prodromal symptoms of subsequent relapses.

- Prodromal signs and symptoms are best discovered by combining the subjective experiences of the patient with observations of close friends and relatives. Thus, the individual with the mental disorder is more likely to be sensitive to private events such as unwanted thoughts, insomnia, and anxiety, while observers might more rapidly detect changes in behavior such as hostility, ritualistic behavior, or talking about unfounded fears.

- It is possible to identify prodromal signs and symptoms days to weeks before they lead to a full-blown relapse, thereby permitting time for the implementation of an emergency or relapse prevention plan.

- Not all symptoms are actually prodromal to an episode of psychosis as are those listed in Table 3.3; rather, some represent "false alarms." However, from the point of view of preventing relapses, it's better "to mistake a stick for a snake than a snake for a stick" or "to be safe than sorry."

- Preventive action to head off a relapse when symptoms appear prodromal may comprise temporarily increasing medication, providing social support, assisting the person to cope with stressors that may be triggering the symptoms, or recommending to the patient that he/she

Self-Assessment Rating Sheet

Your Name: _____   Physician's Name: _____

Name of Medications: _____   Address/Phone: _____

Month/Year: _____

Instructions: Use daily; check each item that applies to you. List any side effects you experience and check them daily if applicable.

Day of the Month		1	2	3	4	5	6	7	8	9	10	11	12	13	14	15
Took Meds	Yes															
	No															
Slept Well	Yes															
	No															
Appetite Good	Yes															
	No															
Concentration	Yes															
	No															
Feel Alert	Yes															
	No															
Feel Tired	Yes															
	No															
Feel Restless/Uneasy	Yes															
	No															
Feel Irritable/Grouchy	Yes															
	No															
Side Effects	Yes															
	No															
	Yes															
	No															

FIGURE 3.8 Self-Assessment Rating Sheet from the Medication Management Module.

withdraw from the source of stress until the warning signs dissipate. Some common prodromal signs are listed in Table 3.3.

SYMPTOM MANAGEMENT MODULE

The Symptom Management Module has two skill areas that engage patient, family, and treatment team in a collaborative and cooperative enterprise, leading to the development and implementation of an emergency plan to head off relapses at the "prodromal pass." In the first skill area, the clinician, patient, and family or other caregivers who are familiar with the patient meet together to watch a video that features a young man who goes through the steps of identifying warning signs of relapse. After joint consensus nails down two to four warning signs that have reliably preceded each of the patient's prior episodes of illness, the collaborators work together to give specific anchor points to the severity of each warning sign: mild, moderate, and severe. Then, the patient and family are taught how to monitor up to four of the identified warning signs on a daily basis by using a chart. Each warning sign is rated nil, mild, moderate, or severe. When one or more of the warning signs go up two scale levels or more and remain elevated for more than 1–2 days, the patient and family are urged to call their responsible clinicians for emergency assistance.

● **TABLE 3.3**

Commonly noted prodromal warning signs of relapse

- I don't have much interest in doing things that were enjoyable.
- I have trouble thinking and concentrating.
- Religion has become so meaningful for me that I can't think of anything else.
- I have trouble sleeping.
- I'm busier than usual with a lot of plans for new projects.
- I have been feeling drained of energy.
- I'm having trouble getting things done at work (or school).
- I feel tense, nervous, and worried all the time.
- I'm not getting along with my family or friends and don't want to be around people.
- I sometimes think that maybe people are looking at me and talking about me.
- I feel angry about little things.

In the second skill area, the patient and family learn to distinguish warning signs—which flare up only prior to illness episodes—from persisting symptoms and the normal ups and downs in mood and behavior of everyday life. The patient is reassured that he/she does not have to make those distinctions; rather, after the patient and family make contact with a mental health professional, the decision can be made about the nature of the upsurge in symptoms. Finally, an emergency plan is worked out that has five steps to take when the Warning Signs

CLINICAL EXAMPLE

The Warning Signs Rating Sheet and emergency plan are shown in Figures 3.9 and 3.10, completed by a young man who had recovered from schizophrenia. He was working full-time after completing the Plan for Achieving Self-Support, a work incentive program of the Social Security Administration. He was supporting himself, living independently, and managing his income and medication. He and his parents completed the Medication and Symptom Management Modules, which led directly to his monitoring his warning signs of relapse and having an emergency plan ready for use.

The Warning Signs Rating Sheet completed by this patient (Figure 3–9) shows an upsurge of warning signs after each of three stressful experiences. In the first stressful event, the patient was knocked off his bike by a car but did not sustain serious injury. The second episode occurred shortly after the patient bought a used car that was in good condition for commuting to work. This purchase used most of the funds he had saved during his Plan for Achieving Self-Support. His car was rear-ended by another car. Although the patient was not injured, he had to deal with insurance, police reports, and estimates for his car repairs. A third stress developed when the patient was stymied by the difficulties in performing a job he had obtained in a welding shop. He had taken a yearlong welding course at a local occupational center but discovered that the employers with the only available jobs expected journeyman skills, rather than offering him an opportunity as an apprentice.

The patient's medication dose was increased slightly for a few days in response to the first two stresses. This adjustment in dose brought the prodromal symptoms under control rapidly. In response to the stressful job that was beyond his level of experience, he and his psychiatrist decided it would be the better part of valor if he quit and found another job in a less stressful occupation. Together, they decided not to increase his medication dose, as he appeared much relieved that he would not have to persevere in the welding job that had proved too much for him. He obtained work as a picture framer at an art store and has maintained that job and his recovery for over 8 years.

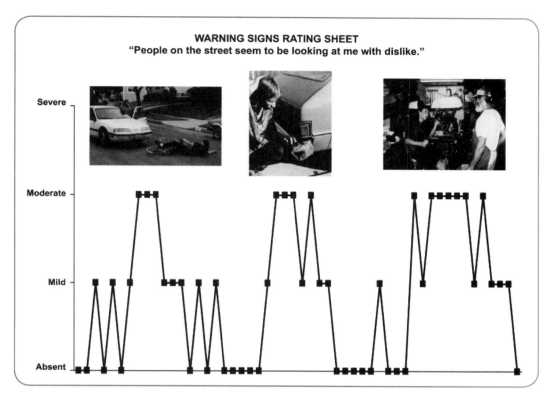

FIGURE 3.9 Warning Signs Rating Sheet for a patient whose stressful life events triggered prodromal symptoms of relapse. The young man had recovered from schizophrenia and was working full-time after completing the Plan for Achieving Self-Support, a work incentive program of the Social Security Administration. He was supporting himself, living independently, and managing his income and medication. See example on page 140 for case description.

Rating Sheet indicates that it is time for seeking help (Figure 3.10):

1. Review the Warning Signs Rating Sheet with a close family member or support person who can help decide whether the changes noted are sufficient to make contact with a professional.
2. Contact one's therapist, clinical case manager, treatment team, or psychiatrist and describe the symptoms that have increased on the sheet.
3. Decide with professional consultation whether a trip to see the psychiatrist is called for.
4. If yes, proceed to the clinic, hospital, mental health center, or doctor's office and request an evaluation and possible intervention.
5. If the warning signs flare at night or on a weekend, go to an emergency room that has a psychiatrist on call.

Name: __Joe D.__   Clinician: __Danica Brown__

Emergency Plan

Session 15: Developing an Emergency Plan

Step 1: Review Warning Signs Rating Sheet with support persons to determine whether a health care provider should be notified.

Names of Support Persons	Telephone Numbers
Mother	310-794-1060
Roommate	cell: 818-254-1771

———————— If support persons are not available, go to **Step 2.** ————————

Step 2: Contact a health care provider to determine whether the doctor should be notified.

Names of Health Care Providers	Telephone Numbers
Danica Brown MSW	323-769-1555
Tim Kuehnel PhD	323-769-2419

———————— If health care providers are not available, go to **Step 3.** ————————

Step 3: Contact doctor to determine whether a clinic visit is necessary.

Names of Doctors	Telephone Numbers
Dr. Robert Liberman	323-769-4286
Dr. Alex Kopelowicz	818-832-2405

———————— If doctors are not available, go to **Step 4.** ————————

Step 4: Go directly to clinic and ask to see a doctor or someone who can do an immediate evaluation.

Names of Clinics	Telephone Numbers
Hollywood Mental Health Center	323-769-2400
Westside Mental Health Center	310-245-3566

———————— If clinic is closed, go to **Step 5.** ————————

Step 5: Go directly to a hospital emergency room and ask to see a doctor who is familiar with psychiatric symptoms.

Names of Hospital Emergency Rooms	Telephone Numbers
UCLA	310-206-1455
County Emergency Team - 24hr	323-856-7000

Personal Warning Signs:

Feeling uncomfortable in public. Worried that people are thinking bad things about me.   Trouble sleeping...

Current Prescriptions:

Medication	Dose	Frequency
Perphenazine	4mg	daily

Doctor's Name: __Robert Liberman MD__   Phone: __323-769-4286__

Doctor's Signature: __Robert Liberman MD__   Date: __6/10/06__

FIGURE 3.10 Emergency plan for relapse prevention that is activated when warning signs reach a moderate or severe level for 2–3 consecutive days.

● EXAMPLE OF BEST PRACTICE

Stable outpatients with schizophrenia were randomly assigned to supportive group therapy or participation in the Medication and Symptom Management Modules. Patients in both psychosocial treatment conditions received low doses of fluphenazine decanoate and either placebo or oral fluphenazine as temporary adjuncts during periods when warning signs became evident (Eckman et al. 1992; Marder et al. 1996). Figure 3.11 reveals the expected, substantial differences in the levels of skills acquired by the patients in the modules versus those in supportive group therapy. The skills remained durable even after 1 year following the end of training. In addition, patients in the skills training condition experienced significantly greater improvement in their social adjustment in the community. In terms of relapses, skills training plus placebo provided as much protection against exacerbations as did time-limited, adjunctive oral antipsychotic medication plus supportive therapy.

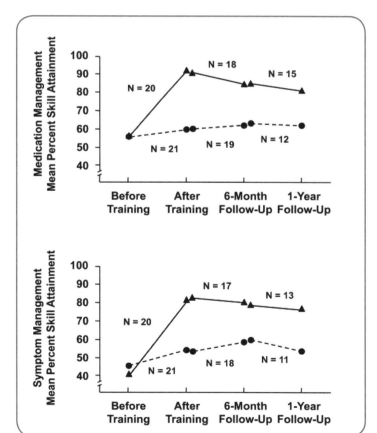

FIGURE 3.11

Effectiveness of Medication and Symptom Management Modules on acquisition of illness management skills in patients with schizophrenia. The effectiveness of these modules was found immediately after training, with durability of the skills demonstrated for 1 year.

The emergency plan is finalized when the patient shows his/her Warning Signs Rating Sheet to the various mental health providers who are listed on the emergency plan and obtains their assent to be listed along with their phone numbers.

▶ Management of Co-occurring Medical Illness

Illness management is for all diseases afflicting the severely mentally ill, not just their psychiatric disorders. Upward of 60% of the severely mentally ill have co-occurring medical diseases, including cardiovascular disease, respiratory diseases, musculoskeletal disease, HIV/AIDS and other sexually transmitted diseases, hepatitis, dental diseases, diabetes, and diseases of the gastrointestinal and renal systems. The mortality rate among persons with severe mental disorders is approximately twice that of the general population, and their life expectancy is 10 years less. Lifestyle problems such as crowded living conditions, poor diet, sedentary routines, poor dental hygiene, lack of exercise, obesity, and high rates of smoking, drug, and alcohol abuse contribute to this disproportionately elevated comorbidity. Unfortunately, mental health clinicians often fail to recognize these complications, and this lack of recognition in turn generates greater levels of disability among the mentally ill.

What, then, can be done to improve the diagnosis and management of the medical illnesses of our psychiatric patients? Psychiatrists and other mental health practitioners can ensure that their patients have a physical examination and appropriate laboratory tests at least once a year. When a co-occurring medical disorder is diagnosed, the patient's responsible psychiatrist should maintain liaison with the treating primary care physician. Plans for managing the medical disorders of the mentally ill should include the actions listed in Table 3.4 to improve continuity, adherence, and response to treatment.

The very same motivational and educational interventions used to manage psychiatric disorders can be fruitfully applied with patients with medical comorbidities. Promising results for the diagnosis and treatment of comorbid psychiatric and medical disorders are now within grasp. Integrating psychiatric professionals and expertise with primary care teams—as described in Chapter 8—provides reciprocal benefits for the professionals and cumulative benefits for the patients. "One-stop shopping" for medical and psychiatric services not only leads to better diagnosis and treatment of comorbidities but also offers a less stigmatizing and more accessible setting for patients to receive services.

● TABLE 3.4

Management of co-occurring medical disorders in the mentally ill

- Education of the patient regarding the type, severity, consequences, and acute and maintenance treatment of the disorder
  » The psychiatrist or allied mental health professional is more likely to have time and success in communicating this information to the patient than the primary care physician or nurse.
- Motivational interviewing of the patient to promote attendance at appointments for physical exams and lab tests
- Referrals to primary care and specialist physicians made in writing regarding the particular medical concerns about and information on the patient's psychiatric disorder and medications
- Arrangements for ensuring that the person gets to medical appointments, with escorts, taxis, phone and note reminders, and other assistance from family members, friends, or case managers
- Collegial phone conferences with the primary care physician about diagnosis and requisite medical treatments so that communication and education with the patient can be effectively carried out by the responsible psychiatrist and other members of the patient's treatment team

Because of the serious problems of weight gain, diabetes, and lipodystrophies with many of the commonly used atypical antipsychotics, expert consensus recommends that laboratory tests be done every 3–6 months. By weighing our patients at each visit and charting those weights, we both monitor problems produced by obesity and create motivation to adopt more nutritious eating habits and exercise. When patients are shown a graph of their weekly or monthly weights, the graphs and our verbal encouragement and praise provide positive reinforcement for their making healthy changes in selecting, preparing, and eating food and in building exercise into their everyday lives. Weight control cannot be achieved in a time-limited wellness program. It must be built into the longitudinal doctor–patient relationship through frequent monitoring of the patient's weight, individualized approaches to eating and exercise habits, and contingent social reinforcement for adherence to the weight management regimen.

Wellness centers are now being established by community mental health agencies. A major role for these centers is to engage seriously mentally ill patients in education and activities that are aimed at healthier lifestyles. Groups for discussion of the adverse or positive consequences from diet, nutrition, exercise, weight, alcohol and drug abuse, and smoking are unlikely to produce behavioral changes. Talking about wellness, health, and sickness has minimal impact on persons without mental disorders, so the prospects of talk being converted into action are slim indeed for the severely mentally ill. Action-oriented, behavioral therapies are more effective for modifying lifestyle habits.

The fields of behavioral medicine and health psychology, utilizing principles of learning theory, have a much better track record in achieving healthier outcomes in persons with problems such as obesity, diabetes, hypertension, and smoking. Many of the advances in behavioral medicine can be implemented in wellness centers located in mental health centers. For example, training in relaxation and meditation has documented efficacy for stress disorders and hypertension. Goals of more realistic weight stabilization within 5%–15% of a person's current weight can be achieved by behavioral techniques such as eating smaller portions, leaving food on the plate, putting utensils down between bites, not washing food down with beverages, monitoring caloric intake with food diaries, and using opaque instead of transparent containers for storing food in the refrigerator. Also effective are group walks that are scheduled during meetings of the wellness center, with homework assignments to find "buddies" for daily walks from among the participants in the center.

Smoking cessation programs, adapted for the level of awareness, comprehension, and capabilities of persons with mental disabilities, have been shown to be helpful, including those sponsored by the American Lung Association. Very few heavy smokers among schizophrenia patients are able to become abstinent, but many are able to reduce their amount of smoking. Just as with graphic reinforcement for weight, the patient and clinician must work out some way for frequent feedback on cigarettes smoked each day. Positive reinforcement for cutting back on cigarettes can be mobilized with "community reinforcers" such as tickets to movie theaters, coupons for free dinners or lunches at local restaurants, and gift certificates for coffee shops and stores. Reinforcement for abstinence from smoking must be a long-term effort just as in weight loss.

Because patients with schizophrenia and related disorders are at high risk for contracting sexually transmitted diseases, they have a critical need for education and skills training for safe sex. The *Friendship and Intimacy Module* (Liberman and Wallace 2006) was specially designed for this population as a video-assisted educational program. This module, using the same techniques as those in the Medication and Symptom Management Modules

(Liberman and Wallace 2006), compensates for the cognitive deficits of the severely mentally ill through procedural memory and learning.

▶ Summary

Most serious mental disorders persist throughout a lifetime, with continuous vulnerability, episodic relapses, or varying levels of symptom disability. Learning how to control these disorders is of overriding importance if recovery is to be a reality and not just a dream. Managing one's illness is not simple and straightforward. It cannot be accomplished by the patient alone, nor by clinicians and the multidisciplinary team, nor by families and other natural caregivers, nor by evidence-based treatments. Only a collective of all of these people and treatments can confer the protection from relapse and disability that makes recovery possible. Illness management is by definition a collaborative enterprise that stands or falls with the competence of practitioners in developing and maintaining cohesive working relationships.

Translating professional knowledge, expertise, and experience to the comprehension and abilities of patients and family members is a critical step in illness management. Patients and their families are empowered by practitioners and mental health teams that successfully engage and maintain their consumers as partners in treatment and rehabilitation. If patients are to successfully travel down the road to recovery, they will require knowledge, skills, training, and support to pass through the gates that mark the acute, stabilizing, stable, and recovery phases of mental disorders.

Surviving the passage to recovery is graphically represented in Figure 3.12; the involvement of patients in collaborative and informed relationships encourages patients to:

- Adhere to their medication and psychosocial treatment programs.
- Engage in shared decision-making about treatments.
- Remember their enduring vulnerability to stress.
- Use skills to manage stress.
- Build protection against stress and vulnerability by

  » Acquiring community, family, and professional supports.
  » Actively participating in evidence-based treatments.

What can't be cured must be endured. By learning how to manage their illnesses themselves, with collaboration, support, and training from professionals, patients can acquire the endurance to overcome their disability and achieve their goals for a better life.

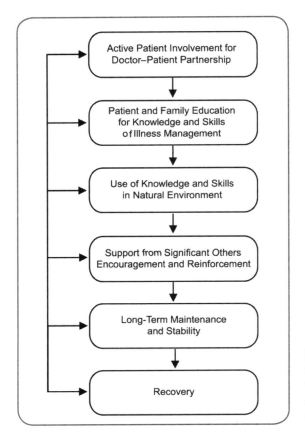

FIGURE 3.12
Outline of procedure for obtaining skills of illness management.

▶ Key Points

- In collaborating for the long and arduous march to recovery, patients and their professional practitioners must first learn how to effectively manage a disabling mental or developmental disorder. Gaining control over the symptoms and cognitive disturbances of a mental or developmental disorder is a prelude to provision of services that bolster a person's social skills and orchestrate needed supports and resources for independent living.

- Illness management comprises
  » Controlling symptoms.
  » Preventing relapses.
  » Overcoming demoralization, passivity, and stigma.
  » Acquiring skills for self-management of one's illness.

» Becoming an active participant in developing and pursuing personally relevant goals.

» Gaining realistic optimism and hope for recovering a valued daily life in the community.

- Successful engagement of the patient and family in treatment starts the process of illness management and is followed by their active collaboration with practitioners to bring the acute phase of the disorder under control. It is essential for practitioners to become competent in establishing and maintaining a partnership with patients and their caregivers in setting goals, selecting interventions, and evaluating progress. Collaboration, not compliance, is the key to illness management.

- Collaboration and adherence to treatment are in the service of successful illness management and they emerge from:

» Using motivational enhancement to connect illness management with each patient's personal goals and to engender hope and empowerment for the patient.

» Providing psychoeducation and personal rapport for induction of a therapeutic alliance.

» Teaching patients and their caregivers to understand the value of medication and psychosocial services as a means to reach patients' personally relevant goals.

» Teaching patients and their caregivers how to deal with side effects of medication and become assertive and reliable consumers of medication.

» Developing a relapse prevention plan, focusing on agreed-upon recognition of early warning signs of relapse, and establishing an emergency system to obtain intervention before a full-blown relapse.

- Illness management requires individualized assessment that identifies the stage of a person's illness and then links type and intensity of treatment to the needs of the patient as he/she moves through the stages of disorder: acute relapsing, stabilization, stable, recovery, and refractory.

- Effective management of serious psychiatric illness requires not compliance but an active and shared decision-making process that includes both the technical expertise of the psychiatrist and the personal experience of the patient.

- Agreement on the value of any treatment—pharmacological or psychosocial—for its capacity to bring stability and self-control of a serious mental disorder emerges from joint consideration of its advantages, disadvantages, acceptability, and feasibility. Patients and family members must be educated and empowered to share in setting goals and making decisions regarding treatments.

- Patients, family members, and mental health professionals are partners in embarking on treatment and rehabilitation in the context of recovering a life with meaning, purpose, and personal satisfaction after contending with the symptomatic and cognitive impairments that characterize severe mental disorders.

▸ Selected Readings

Amador X, Johanson A: I Am Not Sick: I Don't Need Help. New York, Vida Press, 2000

American Psychiatric Association: Practice guideline for the treatment of patients with schizophrenia, 2nd edition, in Practice Guidelines for the Treatment of Psychiatric Disorders: Compendium 2006. Arlington, VA, American Psychiatric Association, 2006, pp 565–746

Azrin NH, Teichner G: Evaluation of an instructional program for improving medication compliance for chronically mentally ill outpatients. Behav Res Ther 36:849–861, 1998

Corrigan PW, Liberman RP, Engel J: From noncompliance to adherence in psychiatric treatment: strategies that facilitate collaboration between practitioner and patient. Hosp Community Psychiatry 41:1203–1211, 1990

Deegan PE, Drake RE: Shared decision making and medication management in the recovery process. Psychiatr Serv 57:1636–1639, 2006

Gingerich S, Mueser KT: Illness management and recovery, in Evidence-Based Mental Health Practice: A Textbook. Edited by Drake RE, Merrens MR, Lynde DW. New York, WW Norton, 2005, pp 395–424

Harding CM: An examination of the complexities in the measurement of recovery in severe psychiatric disorders, in Schizophrenia: Exploring the Spectrum of Psychosis. Edited by Ancill RJ, Holliday S, Higenbottom J. New York, Wiley, 1994, pp 153–170

Herz MI, Marder SR: Schizophrenia: Comprehensive Treatment and Management. Baltimore, MD, Lippincott Williams & Wilkins, 2002

Herz MI, Lamberti JS, Mintz J, et al: A program for relapse prevention in schizophrenia: a controlled study. Arch Gen Psychiatry 57:277–283, 2000

Hogarty GE: Personal Therapy: A Guide to the Individual Treatment of Schizophrenia and Related Disorders. New York, Guilford, 2002

Kemp R, Hayward P, Applewhaite G, et al: Compliance therapy in psychotic patients. BMJ 312:345–349, 1996

Kopelowicz A, Liberman RP: Integrating treatment with rehabilitation for persons with major mental disorders. Psychiatr Serv 54:1491–1498, 2003

Koran LM, Sox HC, Marton KI, et al: Medical evaluation of psychiatric patients. ArchGen Psychiatry 46:733–740, 1989

Lukoff D, Ventura J, Nuechterlein K, et al: Integrating symptom assessment into psychiatric rehabilitation, in Handbook of Psychiatric Rehabilitation. Edited by Liberman RP. Boston, MA, Allyn & Bacon, 1992, pp 56–77

Mellman TA, Miller AL, Weissman EM, et al: Evidence-based pharmacologic treatment for people with severe mental illness: a focus on guidelines and algorithms. Psychiatr Serv 52:619–625, 2001

Psychiatric Rehabilitation Consultants: Community Re-entry Module, Medication Management Module, and Symptom Management Module, 2006. Available from Psychiatric Rehabilitation Consultants, PO Box 2867, Camarillo, CA 93011–2867 or www.psychrehab.com.

Rosenheck R, Tekell J, Peters J, et al: Does participation in psychosocial treatment augment the benefit of clozapine. Arch Gen Psychiatry 55:618–625, 1998

Strauss JS, Hafez H, Lieberman P, et al: The course of psychiatric disorder, III: longitudinal principles. Am J Psychiatry 142:289–296, 1985

Substance Abuse and Mental Health Services Administration (SAMHSA) program materials on illness management can be found at: http://www.mentalhealth.samhsa.gov/cmhs/communitysupport/toolkits/about.asp.

Wellness Recovery and Action Plan (WRAP) program materials available at: www.mentalhealthrecovery.com.

▶ References

Anzai N, Yoneda S, Kumagai N, et al: Training persons with schizophrenia in illness management : a randomized, controlled trial in Japan. Psychiatr Serv 53:545–546, 2002

Eckman TA, Wirshing WC, Marder SR, et al: Technique for training schizophrenic patients in illness self-management. Am J Psychiatry 149:1549–1555, 1992

Halpern J: From Detached Concern to Empathy: Humanizing Medical Practice. New York, Oxford University Press, 2001, p 25

Kopelowicz A, Wallace CJ, Zarate R: Teaching psychiatric inpatients to re-enter the community: a brief method of improving continuity of care. Psychiatr Serv 49:1313–1316, 1998

Liberman RP, Wallace CJ: Modules for Training Social and Independent Living Skills, 2006. Available from Psychiatric Rehabilitation Consultants, PO Box 2867, Camarillo, CA 93011–2867 or www.psychrehab.com.

Liberman RP, Wheeler EG, de Visser LAJM, et al: Handbook of Marital Therapy: A Positive Approach to Helping Troubled Relationships. New York, Plenum, 1980

Lieberman JA, Stroup FS, McEvoy JP, et al: Effectiveness of antipsychotic drugs in patients with chronic schizophrenia. N Engl J Med 353:1209–1223, 2005

Marder SR, Wirshing WC, Mintz J, et al: Two-year outcome of social skills training and group psychotherapy for outpatients with schizophrenia. Am J Psychiatry 153:1585–1592, 1996

Miyamoto S, Stroup TS, Duncan GE, et al: Acute pharmacological treatment for schizophrenia, in Schizophrenia. Edited by Hirsch SR, Weinberger D. London, Blackwell Publishing, 2003, pp 442–473

Mueser KT, Corrigan P, Hilton D, et al: Illness management and recovery: a review of the research. Psychiatr Serv 53:1272–1284, 2002

Substance Abuse and Mental Health Services Administration, Center for Mental Health Services: Evidence-Based Practices: Shaping Mental Health Services Toward Recovery. Toolkit for Illness Management and Recovery. Washington, DC, Department of Health and Human Services, 2004. Available at: http://mentalhealth.samhsa.gov/cmhs/communitysupport/toolkits/illness/. Accessed September 10, 2007.

Wetzler S (ed): Measuring Mental Illness: Psychometric Assessment for Clinicians. Washington, DC, American Psychiatric Press, 1989

Xiang Y, Weng Y, Li W, et al: Training patients with schizophrenia with the Community Re-entry Module: a controlled study. Soc Psychiatry Psychiatr Epidemiol 41:464–469, 2006

CHAPTER **4**

Functional Assessment

4

Functional Assessment

If you don't know where you're going, you may never get there.

ASSESSMENT OF how mentally disabled people *function* in their current living environments begins a collaborative process that leads to the formulation of personal goals and a rehabilitation plan. Each individual's personal goals for social, vocational, educational, family, spiritual, and residential roles are the point of departure for psychiatric rehabilitation. But to achieve desired social roles, individuals must have the requisite skills and community supports to progress from where they are to where they want to be. Comparing the person's current strengths and limitations with the abilities and resources needed for desired role functioning is the major task of functional assessment. Together with the psychiatric diagnosis and symptom assessment, functional assessment provides the wherewithal for developing a rehabilitation plan. In short, functional and symptom assessment enable practitioners and patients to develop a road map for recovery, while rehabilitation empowers patients to follow that map to a full life with quality and dignity.

> "A physician is obliged to consider more than a diseased organ, more even than the whole man. He must view the man in his world."
>
> HARVEY CUSHING
> (1869–1939)

Identifying individuals' abilities and deficits allows practitioners to determine the psychosocial services that are needed to perform everyday activities in pursuit of their personal goals while meeting community norms and expectations. Thus, functional assessment is a prelude to rehabilitative services for building skills, supports, and resources for successful living in the community. In Chapter 3 ("Illness Management"), the importance of assessment, management, and control of symptoms was highlighted for developing rehabilitation plans. In this chapter, we focus on patients' past and present performance of social roles in the environments where they live. Only with both types of evaluation can a comprehensive rehabilitation

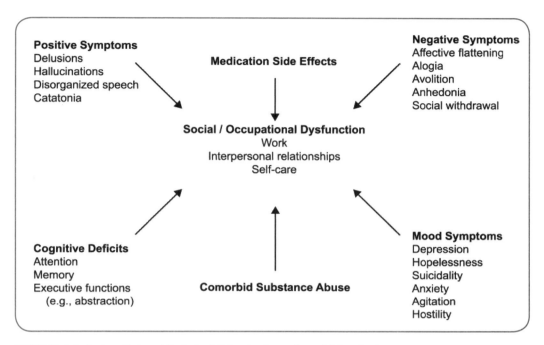

FIGURE 4.1 Factors that contribute to deficiencies in psychosocial functioning.

plan be formulated. Illness management involves educating and empowering patients and families to actively participate in removing the roadblocks to recovery posed by symptoms of mental illness. Functional assessment pinpoints the types of social skills training, family supports, vocational rehabilitation, and community supports needed by patients to travel down the road to recovery.

Figure 4.1 presents an overview of the symptoms and cognitive impairments that contribute to poor psychosocial functioning. Other barriers to functioning include poor premorbid adjustment, inadequate services for skills training and support services, inadequate community resources, complexity of the social roles available in society, and lack of family support. Psychosocial functioning is the starting point for functional assessment and rehabilitation planning, since all mentally disabled individuals are more or less subject to the factors that contribute to their disability. The purpose of functional assessment is to identify each person's 1) goals, skills, supports, and resources; 2) deficiencies in psychosocial functioning that interfere with the individual's desired roles and goals; and 3) services available for psychiatric treatment and rehabilitation that might compensate for the identified deficiencies.

Functional assessment is a planned, organized, and individualized process starting with empathic and consumer-oriented interviewing to identify patients' aspirations for improving their lives. When successful, this process creates a starting point for planning rehabilitation that pinpoints each person's unique wishes for an identity anchored in family, friends, work, education, residence, and spiritual fulfillment. The wishes and hopes of individual patients for a better future are translated into specific and realistic goals by functional assessment through the use of 1) semistructured interviews with the patient; 2) communication with family and other informants who know the patient; 3) past school, vocational, psychological, and medical records; 4) clinical and naturalistic observation; and 5) neurocognitive tests. For planning treatment and rehabilitation, functional assessment is the process of collecting, integrating, and interpreting information related to patients' past and present psychosocial adaptation. If not done in an individualized manner, functional assessment and rehabilitation become mechanical, standardized, and irrelevant. When conducted in a systematic and comprehensive manner, functional assessment can provide a road map to eventual recovery.

▶ Framework for Functional Assessment

Functional assessment is carried out to plan rehabilitative interventions by identifying the individual's:

- *Personal goals* that are relevant to the individual's social, occupational, educational, family, recreational, and independent living *roles* to which the individual aspires.
- *Psychiatric, cognitive,* and *motivational impairments* that may impede acquisition or use of skills and competencies, thereby blocking progress toward desired goals and roles.
- *Skills, competencies, values,* and *motivation* needed by the individual to fulfill the desired roles.
- *Deficits in social and instrumental behavior* as well as any *deviant or dangerous behaviors or habits* that would be considered intolerable by the community for normal social life.
- Professional and naturally available *resources for providing supports* and *teaching skills* that can be harnessed for the use of the patient in reaching his/her personal goals and desired social roles.

Resources include family assistance; financial capacities and disability benefits; professional services such as supported education, employment, and housing; and the full panoply of treatment programs that can facilitate the patient's reaching his/her goals. For any given set of personal goals, the individual's skills, strengths, interests, and resources need to balance the environmental demands and role complexities that are inherent in the person's desired roles.

PERSONAL GOALS AND ROLES

The process of functional assessment begins with the identification of goals that are congruent with the patient's desired life roles. This first step of role definition serves to guide future assessment and interventions. It provides the patient with a road map that makes clear the connections between his/her personal goals and rehabilitation interventions. Without this map, there is a risk that patients will not see the benefits of addressing their deficits of skills and needs for family, social, and professional supports in the community. Thus, right from the start of functional assessment, the patient is infused with motivation to participate in rehabilitation. Personally relevant goals fuel motivation to pursue rehabilitation.

CLINICAL EXAMPLE

John, a 26-year-old single man with a disabling form of bipolar disorder, insisted that his goal was to return to the Ivy League college from which he had dropped out at the start of his illness. After a third hospitalization for manic episodes, he agreed to take his mood stabilizer drug but refused rehabilitation, saying, "I don't need rehab, I just need to get back to college." Rather than refer him to some rehabilitation program, an occupational therapist met with him for a functional assessment. She agreed that his goal to return to college was admirable and offered to assist him. Having gotten his attention, she invited him to specify some intermediate goals that would be necessary for gaining the experience and confidence to return to college and to persuade the college that he was indeed prepared to rematriculate. Among the goals he identified was taking a course at a local community college. When he encountered problems concentrating, completing homework, and attending all of the class sessions, he agreed to work on study skills and note taking with a personal support specialist, who helped him establish incentives to improve his concentration and attention. The methods used to enhance John's ability to sustain his attention on making eye contact with the teacher, note taking, homework, and studying for tests included:

- Giving positive feedback to John for increasing periods of concentration.
- Demonstrating for John how to use outlining for taking notes in class.

- Supervising and giving positive feedback to John for retyping lecture notes using word processing after each class.
- Teaching John to highlight salient information from the text and then use word processing to outline the highlighted information.
- Encouraging John to study in the mornings, when he was most alert.

As his residual mood symptoms stabilized and his neurocognitive impairments improved, John was referred to a supported education program at the local community college. Given the supports of tutoring for a course that did not burden his cognitive functioning—as well as positive reinforcement from his family and personal support specialist for incremental progress in the course—John successfully passed the course, thereby taking one step toward his personal goal of completing college.

Roles define one's place among peers, family, community, and society. They determine the attitudes, expectancies, tasks, rewards, and self-esteem that give structure and meaning to daily life. We see ourselves in relation to others in terms of the roles we occupy in the spheres of work, school, family, friends, and residence. It is often necessary to invest considerable time and effort in helping mentally ill individuals to articulate realistic and feasible roles and interim goals to be attained en route to their desired long-term roles. The desired attributes for effective goal setting are listed in Table 4.1.

There is much to be learned by mental health professionals in eliciting and listening to the personally meaningful goals of patients. Asking open-ended questions such as "What goals do you have for the future?" will not yield many personal goals, in contrast with more specific probes by the clinician for the various areas of life functioning that are common to all: work, education, family life, friendships and dating, recreation and leisure activities, physical health, and spiritual involvement. For example, in one study of the concordance between goals selected by patients and services offered to them, the primary areas of overlap were on symptom relief and reduction of aggressive, self-destructive, and other inappropriate behaviors in the community that often result in hospitalization. However, patients identified a much broader array of goals that carried value for them: achieving better physical health, improving financial situation, attending school or obtaining employment, improving interpersonal relationships, attaining spiritual or religious goals, improving living conditions, and gaining more autonomy in money management (Lecomte et al. 2005). Rehabilitation specialists should systematically assess patients' goals in accord with their subjective views and by using structured interviews that do not presume that the clinicians' values are the same as those of their patients.

● **TABLE 4.1**

Guidelines for helping patients set attainable goals

- Make your goals functional to help you with your everyday life; link them to your longer-term, desired roles that will motivate you to make efforts to reach them.
- Write down your goals, as this makes them real, allows you to show them to others, and adds commitment.
- Make your goals specific and measurable so you will know when you have achieved them.
- Visualize your goals in terms of how you would feel when you reach them, as this adds motivation.
- Make your goals achievable—break down longer-term, more challenging goals into small steps.
- Give yourself realistic deadlines to achieve your goals; set short-term goals that can be attained within a week and that occur often.
- Anticipate obstacles that you will encounter as you attempt to achieve your goals and engage others in problem solving to remove those obstacles or choose new goals.
- Periodically review your goals to make sure they are still relevant and to determine how well you are progressing toward attaining them.

COGNITIVE IMPAIRMENTS THAT INTERFERE WITH PSYCHOSOCIAL FUNCTIONING

Research has accumulated that has documented the importance of cognition in the learning, performance, and retention of psychosocial skills. The cognitive capacities that are dysfunctional in serious mental disorders, reflecting basic neurophysiological abnormalities in the brain, include sustained attention, concentration, information processing, verbal and nonverbal learning and memory, working memory, perception of emotion and meaning, visuospatial skills, social judgment, insight, goal-oriented planning, initiative, and problem solving.

Evaluation of cognitive abilities as part of a functional assessment leads to recommendations regarding the types of work, schooling, and social relationships with which a mentally ill individual would likely have success or difficulty. For example, research has documented that severely mentally ill persons who have significant deficits in working memory as well as psychotic symptoms require the coaching, encouragement, job development, and frequent contacts of an employment specialist. With this assistance they are much more likely to succeed in supported employment. On the other hand, patients with the same diagnosis but with fewer symptoms and better working memory tend to succeed at independent employment without the help of an employment specialist (McGurk and Mueser 2003). As with all facets of rehabilitation, the byword is "play to your strengths." As you will read in Chapter 10 ("New Developments for Rehabilitation and Recovery"), new techniques are being devised to "train the brain" to help patients to overcome their cognitive deficits.

CLINICAL EXAMPLE

Melvin had made a reasonable recovery from schizophrenia. He was able to control occasional "voices" and beliefs that TV personalities were talking directly to him. He had worked throughout his adult life and was particularly gifted in repairing and servicing cars. He gave up a job in a tire store to take a better-paying position driving long-distance rigs. On the long hauls, he enjoyed the solitude and the scenery; however, because of short-term memory and visuospatial deficits, he would often get lost after he made a delivery and not be able to find his way back to the highway. After discussing the problem with his father and psychiatrist, he decided to apply for a truck driver's job with a local, standard route that he could remember through repetition. He was employed by a food distributor and had no problems delivering the products to the stores on his well-defined route. Seven years later, he has had several promotions but continues to make his local deliveries along with work assignments in the company warehouse.

Cognitive deficits should not consign individuals with severe psychiatric disorders to lifelong disability. For example, certain jobs can be selected for side-stepping a person's cognitive deficits: a person with autism or Down's syndrome with limited verbal learning and memory can perform repetitive psychomotor tasks such as bagging groceries or washing dishes extremely well. Jobs that offer the accommodations of quiet and subdued office or factory environments can support the employment of persons with schizophrenia for whom social overstimulation would burden their cognitive capacities.

Overcoming Motivational Deficits

Amotivation or volitional dysfunctions—also referred to as *negative symptoms*—are particular types of cognitive deficits that reduce the physical activity level, desire to participate in events, interest in socializing, and curiosity for new experiences of individuals with schizophrenia, depression, and bipolar disorder. If potential correctives to this problem are not identified, the rehabilitation plan will falter no matter how carefully it is crafted. Most practitioners fall back on empathic encouragement, exhortation, and suggestions to remedy lack of motivation, usually with limited response.

As described in Chapter 2 ("Principles and Practice of Psychiatric Rehabilitation"), reinforcement theory is a powerful means of influencing behavior. *Reinforcers* are consequences of behavior that increase the probability that the desired behavior will increase in frequency or strength in the future. For the mentally disabled, it is very important to have reinforcers that can strengthen attendance and participation in rehabilitation services, abstinence from illicit substances, socialization, exercise, and completion of goal-oriented assignments. Therefore, it is important to include a *reinforcer survey* as part of the functional assessment. The most generalized reinforcer is the attention, interest, concern, warmth, praise, compliments, and positive feedback given to a patient *contingent* on some appropriate and adaptive behavior. These forms of interpersonal responsiveness are called *social reinforcement.* Social reinforcement is portable, free, and usable anywhere and anytime and has the additional virtue of strengthening the therapeutic relationship.

Individuals are motivated by interactions with other people, places, things, and activities. In persons who have negative symptoms, it is useful to know what reinforcers were effective prior to the person's mental illness, because when these reinforcers are offered as part of the rehabilitation plan, they often regain their motivating quality. The *Psychiatric Reinforcement Survey* identifies motivating experiences in five categories, as shown in Table 4.2 (Lecomte et al. 2000).

Reinforcers can be used in the rehabilitation plan two ways: 1) as incentives to reward adaptive behavior that is instrumental to progress toward personal goals and desired roles, and 2) for strengthening the incentive value of people, places, things, activities, and consumables by exposing the patient to them. This latter purpose, called *reinforcer sampling,* is exemplified by "Try it, you'll like it." Many things that have no initial motivational value for us can acquire it through sampling—for example, test drives in cars, trying on clothes in a store, tasting food samples in a market, and going out on a blind date.

> ● **TABLE 4.2**
>
> **The Psychiatric Reinforcement Survey**
>
> ●
>
> | People | Who are preferred as friends, relatives, and acquaintances and with whom you spend much time or would like to spend more time |
> |---|---|
> | Places | Where you spend a lot of your time, where you would like to spend more time, and where you prefer to visit when you have time and a choice (shopping, movies, museums, recreational locations, church, homes of friends and relatives) |
> | Things | That you prefer to use, would like to have, or spend time with (computers, TV, CD player, hobbies) |
> | Activities | That are enjoyed, preferred, and engaged in regularly or that you would like to do more often (walking, bicycling, driving a car, dancing, reading, talking on the phone, playing sports, taking naps) |
> | Consumables | That you enjoy eating or drinking, prefer to eat or drink when given a choice, or would like to eat or drink more (steak, French fries, fish, omelets, milkshakes, ice cream, candy, lobster, champagne, beer, soda) |
>
> *Source.* Lecomte et al. 2000.

SKILLS AND COMPETENCIES AS BUILDING BLOCKS FOR ATTAINING GOALS

The next phase of functional assessment is an analysis of abilities, coping skills, and personal competencies that individuals already have demonstrated and those still needed to successfully enact their chosen social roles. Clinicians, in league with their patients, take an inventory of each person's social and independent living skills in the areas of life that are relevant to reaching his/her desired goals and roles. These include personal hygiene, appearance and clothing, care of personal possessions, transportation, money management, purchasing and preparing food, maintaining one's living space, recreational activities, consumerism abilities, friends and family, job seeking and employability, learning and studying, health maintenance, management of one's mental illness, and dealing with social agencies.

Just as specification is essential for setting rehabilitation goals, describing a person's skills or behavioral deficits in operational and measurable terms is necessary in functional assessment. Unless skills are delineated clearly, it is difficult to design a rehabilitation plan with skills-based educational objectives that are specific enough to be taught and evaluated. In conducting the functional assessment, the practitioner determines which skills are currently being used, given the expectations and requirements of the social environment in which the patient lives. For instance, patients living at home may not be expected to wash and dry their clothes or prepare their meals. Patients living in residential treatment facilities may not have opportunities to manage their own medications. Practitioners should also be sensitive to cultural differences regarding normative expectations for behavioral functioning in the home and community. For example, among Asian Americans, work is valued very highly even for their mentally ill family member. A strong predilection for work would point the clinician in the direction of those social and instrumental skills relevant to work environments, community resources available for job finding, and an emphasis on work when crafting the rehabilitation plan.

The *Independent Living Skills Survey,* pictorially presented in Figure 4.2, covers the full range of personal skills and abilities and is ideal for functional assessment (Wallace et al. 2000). Practitioners who use this tool as part of the functional assessment can determine which skills are currently being used, have been used in the past, and may be needed in the future when the patient is functioning at a higher level in a new social role. If skills that are required for functioning at a higher level are deficient, they are readily apparent and can be integrated into a skills training program as part of the rehabilitation plan. The questions in this survey are phrased in such a way to elicit "yes" or "no" answers that demarcate reliably the specific skills that are being used, not the skills that the individual might hypothetically be capable of deploying. Examples of information regarding deficits of skills that may be useful for planning rehabilitation are "attended a self-help or community group once or more in the past month," "carried wallet with identification and money daily," and "bathed or showered at least twice a week."

DEVIANT BEHAVIORS INCOMPATIBLE WITH COMMUNITY FUNCTIONING

A functional assessment also identifies disturbing behaviors that are not tolerated by family members and the community at large. Of great importance for a behavioral or functional analysis of the objectionable conduct, its antecedents and consequences must be identified. A behavioral analysis proceeds by obtaining answers to questions such as:

- What is the sequence of events that precede and follow the problem behavior?

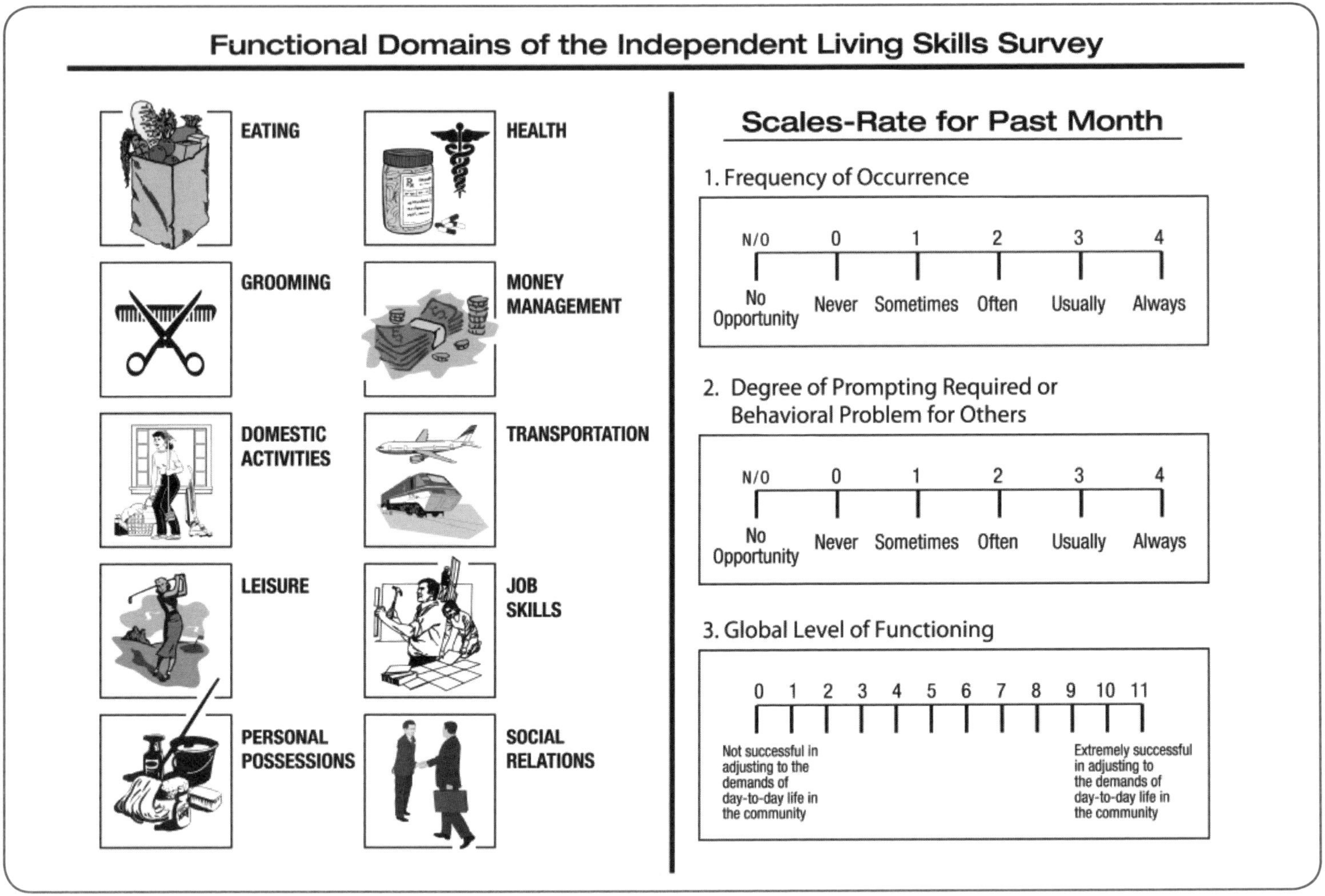

FIGURE 4.2 Pictorial display of areas of functioning measured by the Independent Living Skills Survey. Ratings are made for each of the specific behaviorally defined items within each of the 10 domains on the basis of the degree of independence (vs. supervision needed) exercised by the patient. Ratings are also made for the degree to which deficits from each item cause problems for the patient and/or family and caregivers.

- Are there events that often trigger the deviant behavior or start an escalating cycle that leads to the outburst?
- What do people do immediately after the provocative or abnormal behavior occurs?
- Does the individual draw attention, concern, discussion and remonstrances, emotional reactions, or punishment after the problem behavior occurs?

Examples of intolerable behaviors that often lead to hospitalization or referral to other types of locked facilities include aggressiveness in certain situations with certain people, incontinence, insufferably poor personal hygiene, inappropriate sexual behavior, and polydipsia. Often these behaviors reflect a lack of learning opportunities in the person's natural, everyday

CLINICAL EXAMPLE

Jerry caused quite a stir at his board-and-care home because he would engage in public masturbation. This behavior was unfortunately maintained by the staff of the home who would shout and bring others to the scene of the impropriety. A consulting psychologist set up a behavioral program that 1) encouraged Jerry to masturbate privately behind closed doors in his room or bathroom and 2) provided points exchangeable for special treats and privileges for every day that there was no inappropriate sexual behavior. Within 2 weeks, Jerry learned to enjoy sexual stimulation behind closed doors, thereby preventing a regrettable hospitalization.

living environments, combined with emotional responses by caregivers that inadvertently reinforce the very behavior that is objectionable.

Aggression is commonly directed at family members, often in response to a family member criticizing, making demands, or nagging the individual to complete tasks that are beyond the individual's capacity. Alternatively, vituperative communications often erupt into destructive or aggressive behavior when the patient is frustrated in obtaining some need, privilege, or desire. When family members and the patient have opportunities to learn communication skills—such as those described in Chapter 6 ("Involving Families in Treatment and Rehabilitation")—aggressive episodes can be avoided. For example, compliance with a request often occurs in the absence of aggression when a family member makes a "positive request" (e.g., "I'm so busy now and my back is hurting. It would be a big help to me if you could take out the trash") instead of a demand (e.g., "You don't have anything to do now, so I want you to take out the trash"). Further examples of dealing with disturbing behaviors will be given in Chapter 9 ("Special Services for Special People") in the section on effective management of patients with treatment-refractory illness.

SOCIAL SUPPORTS AND COMMUNITY RESOURCES

At this point, the process of functional assessment has elicited the patient's desired roles and the personally relevant goals that give impetus to reaching the roles. The practitioner has identified the cognitive and motivational deficits that may interfere with the patient attaining his/her goals. Social and independent living skills that are either already part of the patient's behavioral repertoire or in need of training have been inventoried. The next task for functional assessment is to ascertain the supports and resources available to the individual that can be mobilized to assist the patient in reaching his/her goals. Social supports and community resources are extremely important because they can compensate for deficits in cognitive, motivational, and social skills by providing patients with the wherewithal to achieve their goals. While "independent living with the least amount of professional supervision necessary" is an ideological goal for rehabilitation, no one can function effectively in a community without making use of resources that enable us to survive and enjoy a good quality of life. Thus, it is axiomatic that the availability of a broad spectrum of community resources makes optimal levels of functioning possible.

Patients with severe mental disorders need a judicious combination of skills training and supports to make headway with their goals. When functional assessment is done competently, it is possible to recruit a minimum effective number of resources that need to be added to efforts at skills training so the patient can see positive movement toward his/her goals. Table 4.3 lists the types of social supports and community resources that are more or less available in many communities. Informed selection of the supports and resources for the patient's individualized rehabilitation plan depends upon the person's unmet needs for attaining goals and moving forward toward recovery.

The single most important source of emotional, social, and financial support for the patient is the family. Practitioners, mental health agencies, and community programs come and go, but the family remains as the single continuous thread in the patient's life. Families that are educated about mental illness and how to cope with it are a vital resource for reinforcing the patient's progress for reaching personal goals and eventually recovery. Therefore, the functional assessment and rehabilitation plan must include services that meet the needs of the family: information and training for coping with the

● TABLE 4.3

Social supports and community resources available for rehabilitation planning

Vocational services	Adult education	Colleges with disabled student services offices
Residential care homes	Crisis services and homes	Supported and subsidized housing
Psychosocial clubhouses	Psychiatric inpatient services	Day treatment and partial hospital programs
Peer support and self-help	Peer-run businesses and services	Affiliates of NAMI, DBSA with support groups
Protection and advocacy	Police and court diversion	Psychiatric services in jails
Homeless outreach	Integrated dual-diagnosis services	Assertive community treatment teams
Wraparound services	Integrated service programs	YMCA/YWCA with discounts for disabled persons
Child care	Parent training	Recreation and parks districts
Family psychoeducation	Social clubs and computer dating	12-step abstinence support programs
Social Security office	Bus discount passes for disabled persons	Veterans benefits and mental health services

Note. DBSA = Depression and Bipolar Support Alliance; NAMI = National Alliance on Mental Illness.

ill family member's behavior; knowledge about medications and relapse prevention; access and referral to the full range of services from crisis intervention to case management, psychiatrists, and vocational rehabilitation; and involvement in treatment planning and ongoing reevaluations.

▌ Development of the Rehabilitation Plan

Because of the many facets of functional assessment and the complementary information from psychiatric and symptom-based assessment, it is customary for the rehabilitation plan to be developed by a multidisciplinary treatment team. The participation of the patient and family in the planning process and their endorsement of the plan are essential, as these things give them "ownership," empowerment, and hope and set the stage for their continued involvement as active members of the treatment team. The rehabilitation plan results from the integration, organization, and interpretation of the information collected during the functional assessment. Each rehabilitation plan should be individualized and personalized by attending to the specific strengths, deficits, symptom profile, phase of illness, and social and community resources that are relevant to the patient's needs. Table 4.4 provides an outline for the construction of a rehabilitation plan for a patient whose desired role is to move into his/her own apartment and live independently.

Unless the relevant elements of psychosocial functioning and their influences are assessed and incorporated into the rehabilitation plan, provision of services is relegated to trial-and-error guesswork. To the extent that functional assessment leads to informed and judicious goal setting and treatment planning, the individual can get and stay on the road to recovery.

MONITORING PROGRESS TOWARD GOALS

Once the rehabilitation plan has been activated, periodic monitoring is essential if deliberate and consistent progress is to be made toward the patient's personal goals and desired roles. Monitoring requires a continual focus on the patient's personal goals and the interventions and services that are being used to promote progress toward those goals. Monitoring progress is done jointly with the patient and, when possible, with the family. Multiple contributions to the monitoring process permit different views of progress to be included with greater informational validity. Even more importantly, a collaboration in reviewing progress provides a wonderful opportunity for the practitioner to offer abundant positive feedback to the patient for attaining goals and actively participating in planned interventions and services. This use of positive reinforcement, contingent upon constructive effort and problem solving, maintains a steady march toward personal goals.

The writing of narrative progress notes does not lend itself to good-quality monitoring of progress in rehabilitation. Inadvertently, practitioners enter information related to current problems and concerns without noting the positive progress that is occurring and how the various problems may need to be resolved to reestablish progress. Having overprinted forms for entering progress can facilitate goal-oriented monitoring. These forms can be quite simple and straightforward, with spaces for entering and indicating

● TABLE 4.4

Organization of the rehabilitation plan

What are the long-term goals and social roles that have been identified?

Independent living in own apartment.

Is this goal congruent with the patient's phase of illness, psychiatric symptoms, and cognitive and motivational capacities?

Patient is stable and has few, nonintrusive symptoms and has normal cognitive functions except for questionable social judgment and problem-solving skills. Motivation for the long-term goal is very high. He will meet with his psychologist weekly to learn social problem-solving skills, and psychologist and occupational therapist will communicate with each other and with his parents.

What are the skills and supports that the patient will need to live independently and to succeed?

Patient is currently able to maintain his living space, care for his clothing and personal possessions, and use public transport. He has obtained a subsidized apartment that he can afford, but he will need to learn money management and to shop and prepare meals, and to reassure his parents by calling them at least once per week.

How will the patient learn these needed skills?

Occupational therapist will make home visits to teach shopping, cooking, and cleaning-up skills and to check on his use of medication to ensure that he is taking it reliably. She will serve as his representative payee until he demonstrates ability to manage his funds. At each visit, she will prompt him to call his parents and will do modeling and role-playing to teach him telephone etiquette.

How will the patient get his medication and psychiatric needs met?

He will continue to meet with his psychiatrist at the local mental health center with whom he has a good relationship. He will use a medication dispenser to facilitate regular use of his medication.

Does the patient know anyone in the neighborhood where he will be living? If he desires friends, can he establish interpersonal contact?

Patient has friends across town and can use public transport to meet them. He does not have good social skills and would like to get training in conversation and friendship skills at the local mental health center. He is willing to join a peer-support self-help club to structure his week and enable him to participate in social and recreational activities and meet prospective friends.

(continued)

TABLE 4.4 (*cont'd.*)

What services will be needed and desired for improving the patient's relationship with his family?

Parents and older brother want to assist patient in apartment living but are worried about his ability to function on his own. Patient's personal support specialist will conduct biweekly behavioral family management sessions at the apartment. Family agreed to attend Family-to-Family seminar sponsored by local National Alliance on Mental Illness organization.

Does the patient want access to vocational services?

Not until after he is well established in his apartment. He has agreed to assist his parents with chores at their home once a week.

Who will coordinate his rehabilitation plan?

His personal support specialist from the mental health center will maintain contact weekly with patient, family, occupational therapist, psychiatrist, and psychologist. Home visits for special services or crisis intervention can be provided, and a mobile team is available after hours and on weekends. The personal support specialist will review progress and problems weekly with the multidisciplinary team.

successful completion of the patient's short- and long-term goals, participation in treatment sessions, and use of community supports. The progress note should also include a timeline for attainment of each goal and indicate the person responsible for the monitoring of the progress of the patient.

Assessment and treatment reciprocate in a continuing fashion over time. Functional assessment is not a lockstep procedure, nor is it implemented in a sequentially linear fashion. Rather, assessment of assets and deficits, selection of goals, and goal attainment are overlapping and require recurrent administration during the course of treatment and rehabilitation. While clinical decision making is informed by assessment of the individual and environment, interventions proceed and are revised by regularly scheduled reassessments.

If a goal has been attained, the clinician and patient together can decide whether enough progress has been made to place a "hold" on further goal setting while the patient consolidates his/her progress, or whether new goals can be identified for moving forward. If progress toward a goal is stymied, then consideration can be given to the completeness of the initial assessment, appropriateness of the goal, or the relevance and efficacy of treatment. Goals are sometimes chosen by overeager patients, by those whose desires for change outran their personal abilities, or by patients whose wish fulfill-ment was not tempered by realistic optimism. Perhaps the goals were set too high, beyond the limitations of the patient's functional state or treatment resources available. Of necessity, functional assessment is dynamic and open-ended, with reevaluation performed as indicated by the monitoring of progress toward short- and long-term goals.

How will a disabled person and those who are in family and profes-sional support roles have any confidence that the services being provided are actually bringing about improvements relevant to recovery? Feed-back of clear and credible information on progress is the most powerful form of positive reinforcement and motivation for the treatment team—including the patient and family—to push on and on toward recovery. It is the information provided from continuing functional assessment that fertilizes patients' self-esteem, self-efficacy, empowerment, hope, and per-sistence in overcoming adversities and setbacks. Conducting treatment and rehabilitation without regularly obtaining and sharing systematic informa-tion on a person's progress toward improved psychosocial functioning is tantamount to clipping the wings of the collaborative effort to reach per-sonal goals and a better quality of life.

Functional assessment is not limited to the initial evaluation of a patient; rather, it is a recurring process that gives patients opportunities to revise their personal goals, choose different rehabilitative services, and gain empowerment and decision-making skills. Because the road to recovery is marked by detours, obstacles, potholes, and breakdowns, functional assess-ment should be repeatedly administered to identify the patient's current status for *flexibly* modifying goals and rehabilitation services. Assessment and treatment are inextricably linked in clinical decision making; interven-tion proceeds most effectively when it is redirected by periodic infusions of assessment information. Clinicians often meet with failure in their thera-peutic efforts with patients because a lack of assessment information makes it difficult to create new treatment plans to take the place of those that fail.

▶ Client's Assessment of Strengths, Interests, and Goals (CASIG)

Assessment is properly performed as a means of treatment planning. Func-tional assessment that is not merged with goal setting and decisions regard-ing treatment is like a sailboat without sails. CASIG (Client's Assessment of Strengths, Interests, and Goals) is a multidimensional assessment tool that helps practitioners plan, document, and evaluate psychiatric rehabilitation

(Wallace et al. 2001). The acronym uses the terms "strengths, interests, and goals," which reflect the empowerment of the patient in identifying treatment goals, priorities, and service needs. The functional assessment and plan for services solicit the active participation of the patient, family, and clinician that confers greater validity on the direction of the resulting rehabilitation. As shown in Figure 4.3, CASIG assesses performance in 10 areas of functional living skills, 11 areas of subjective quality of life, key symptoms, medication side effects, adherence to medication, satisfaction with mental health professionals, and acting-out behaviors that are unacceptable for community tenure.

Until the development of CASIG, there were no instruments with documented psychometric properties that seamlessly integrated assessment with planning, monitoring, and evaluating treatment and rehabilitation for individual patients. Most attempts at measuring psychosocial functioning have been limited to ratings of overall dimensions of patients' community living. Rather than being put in the service of individualized assessment for treatment planning, extant scales are used to summarize average changes in groups of patients from one point in time to another in research and program evaluation. Administration and scoring of assessment tools are typically insulated from the program's practicing clinicians by having the work done by specialized staff responsible for research, quality assurance, or program evaluation. The results are primarily of interest to program managers to justify the value of the program and to defend budgets; results are aggregated across large cohorts of patients and are too general to pinpoint the specific services that need to be included in an individualized treatment plan.

CASIG permits functional assessment to become utilitarian for clinicians and their patients. With CASIG, information on the changing functional capacities of patients is embedded in the routine clinical procedures for planning and evaluating services for each patient. Although CASIG is primarily an instrument for developing individualized rehabilitation plans, the information obtained with CASIG also can be aggregated across all the individuals in a program for purposes of quality improvement and program evaluation. Aggregated data for a mental health unit, program, or facility are sufficiently descriptive to inform program managers of the distribution of needs, personal goals, level of functioning, and effectiveness of treatment as identified by patients and staff. Such information can be helpful in modifying and prioritizing services to better respond to patients' needs. Obtaining program evaluation data would require little additional cost, since individual patients would have been assessed during their participation in routine clinical services. The dual use of CASIG for assessment of individual patients and for program evaluation is shown in Figure 4.4.

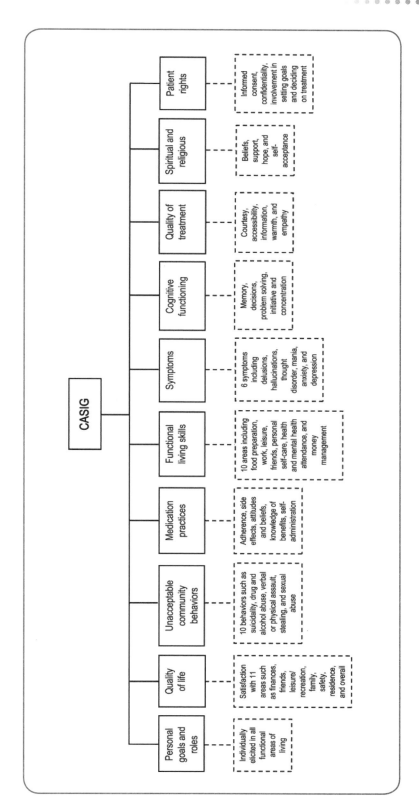

FIGURE 4.3 Areas of personal functioning assessed by CASIG (Client's Assessment of Strengths, Interests, and Goals).

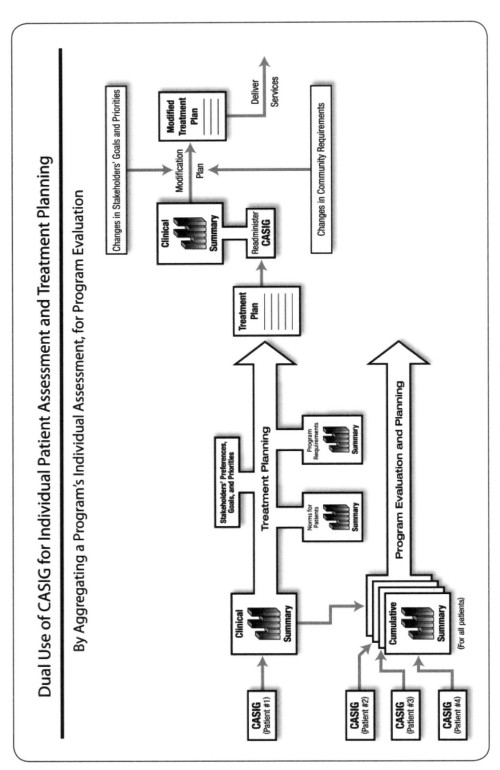

FIGURE 4.4 Dual use of CASIG for individual patient assessment and program evaluation.

In summary, CASIG is a patient-driven and user-friendly assessment tool for clinicians to use in their everyday work as they connect patients' needs with treatment and rehabilitation plans. CASIG can be administered repeatedly at clinically meaningful intervals to inform the clinician in making decisions for updating the rehabilitation plan. It has been used in hospital and community-based programs with diverse staffing patterns, clinical populations, and resources. When used in a system of care, CASIG can bridge the many facilities in which patients are served.

BASIC PLAN FOR CASIG

Designed for functional assessment of persons with mental disabilities, CASIG is a method for gathering information that enables clinicians to:

- Collaborate with patients in selecting areas for rehabilitation and personal goals that are realistic, relevant, and meaningful to the patient and significant others.
- Use functional assessment to identify deficits, strengths, interests, and resources for attainable goal setting.
- Enhance the motivation of patients to participate in treatment planning by highlighting the gap between current and desired functioning and quality of life.
- Construct a treatment and rehabilitation plan based on available mental health services, skills training, and social and community supports that can be mobilized to bridge the gap between current and desired functioning.
- Establish a baseline of functioning for making judgments about progress.
- Monitor progress toward recovery and provide informational feedback on progress that reinforces continuing efforts of patients to participate in treatment.
- Foster a continuing relationship between patient and practitioner based on periodic use of CASIG to review and revise the treatment plan based on the patient's progress.
- Evaluate treatment outcomes for both individual patients and entire programs.

ORGANIZATION OF CASIG: AREAS OF ASSESSMENT

CASIG is a 60-minute structured interview that is so well specified that it can be administered by recovered patients as well as all levels of paraprofessional and professional staff. It surveys individuals' desired improvements in social functioning, personal factors, and community supports that will result in greater satisfaction with their quality of life. Family members, various clinicians working with the patient, or other informants who are familiar with the patient can provide additional and confirmatory information to add to that obtained from the patient. An alternative version of CASIG is available for clinical staff and family members to use for providing relevant information to supplement that given by patients who are cognitively impaired, unreliable in their responses, or otherwise unable to participate fully in an interview.

Treatment planning with CASIG begins by involving patients in identifying their personal goals and desired psychosocial roles, as shown in Figure 4.5. The types of goals and roles that are the key points of departure for treatment planning with CASIG were drawn from needs assessments obtained through numerous surveys of patients with mental disabilities. The individual's goals are elicited by open-ended questions for improvements in daily functioning, housing and residence, social and family relationships, financial resources, vocational activities, religious and spiritual activities, and physical and mental health. Mental health goals that are elicited include attitudes toward medication, psychiatrist, and other mental health service providers. The initial question asks about the individual's expectations and wishes for improvements in the next year; for example, "Would you like to improve your ability to work in the coming year?" If the patient answers in the affirmative, follow-up questions elicit the patient's positive assets, expe-

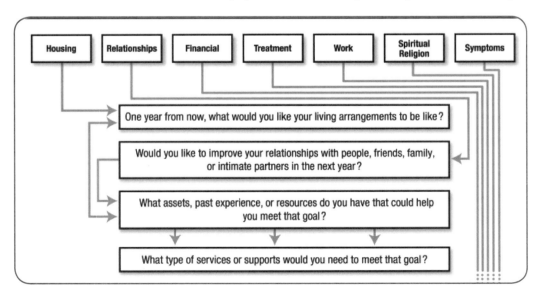

FIGURE 4.5 Use of CASIG to identify patients' personal goals.

riences, and resources that can be used to make the desired changes, and the services and supports that would be needed to meet that goal.

Once the patient expresses a desire for change in an area of community functioning, follow-up questions obtain very specific information about the patient's current functioning and status, since these are the positive roots from which a treatment program can grow and take shape. Questions to further nail down the ways that the goal might be reached are asked and collaboratively discussed regarding the amount and type of treatment that might be needed to achieve the goal—for example, skills training, family assistance, supportive services, community resources, and medication adjustments.

Questions that tap the patient's current level of functioning are very specific, answered in a yes/no format to simplify the administration and increase the reliability of the assessment. Exemplifying the structure of each question in Figure 4.6 are six items from money management, one of the functional living skills that is elicited and rated by CASIG.

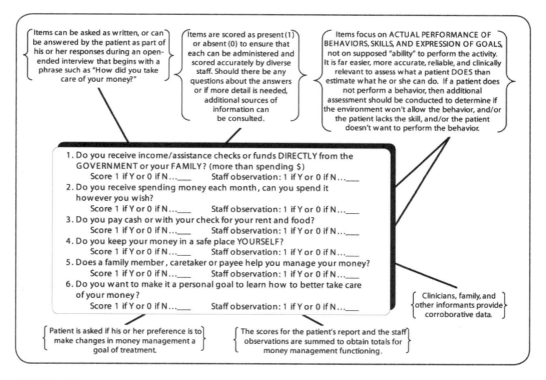

FIGURE 4.6 Structure of questions from the CASIG interview to elicit patients' skills. The questions from the CASIG interview are exemplified by a sample of questions used to assess money management skills. Questions are well structured to more easily elicit reliable responses from the patient. Questions can be answered during an interview with the patient, by having the patient respond by using CASIG as a questionnaire, or by means of a computerized interview. Responses to questions should be confirmed by obtaining all sources of relevant information from past and current treating clinicians, family members, and other caregivers.

The specific and direct nature of CASIG enables clinicians to determine, for each patient, the presence of a goal, problem, strength, desire for change, or community resource; in addition, for every question, the respondents are encouraged to give more details, qualifications, comments, or observations. Thus, a combination of open-ended and yes/no questions elicits information to clarify areas of interest and concern. Collaboration between patient and clinician is built into the CASIG interview by questions that explore the patient's goals and the skills and supportive resources needed to achieve them. Summarizing the results of the initial assessment empowers patient and clinician to identify the gaps between the individual's current and desired functioning. Services are selected to close the gaps, and continued measurement gives feedback on the efficacy of the services.

Given the answers to the questions embedded in CASIG, a service plan is constructed on the basis of four "rules" or criteria:

1. If a change in the patient's personal functioning, medication practices, cognition, symptoms, or behavior is required for improved adaptation to the community, life, health, safety, or quality of life, then provide services.
2. If the patient doesn't have the skills to function as needed to reach his/her goal, then offer skills training or supportive services that can compensate for lack of skills.
3. If the environment doesn't permit, encourage, or reinforce the skills, then modify the environment through such means as assertive community training, family psychoeducation, or consultation to appropriate agencies.
4. If the patient wants to use or learn the skills to function better in the community, then offer training or opportunities and encouragement to use the skills.

The process by which the rules are utilized for setting goals that lead into a treatment plan is illustrated in Figure 4.7.

Because CASIG is designed to provide information on patients' progress, it can be readministered at appropriate intervals to monitor positive or negative changes that inform the process by which the clinician and patient consider modifications in services or goals. If desired changes are occurring, the treatment plan may remain in place. If improvement is not moving at a realistically expected rate, if the patient's goals change, or if the supports and resources in the patient's environment shift, the plan can be modified. Additional information will need to be obtained from the knowledge base or awareness of the clinician or mental health team of resources, stigma, and constraints in the community, family, peers, and

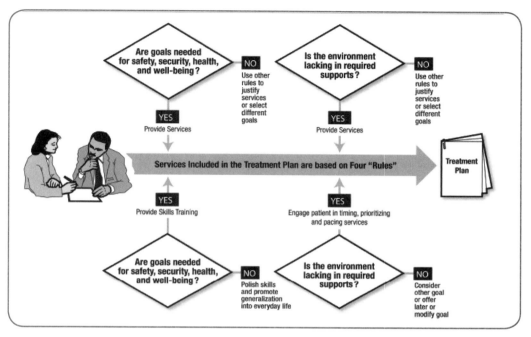

FIGURE 4.7 Rules for setting goals that lead to the rehabilitation plan.

residence to answer the question "Why is the service plan not effective?" Modification or addition of new services, motivational enhancement, involvement of family, or mobilization of other community agencies may be necessary for the service plan to enjoy greater success.

When CASIG is readministered to patients who are already known through a previous assessment and clinical experience, the interview is streamlined in focus and duration. The way repeated administrations of CASIG are used to inform decision making for changes in treatment plans is shown in Figure 4.4. The comparisons of the repeated CASIGs reveal the changes that have been accomplished and those that are yet to be achieved. For example, after 3 months of treatment a patient may have demonstrated progress in the areas of friendship and use of leisure time but little or no progress in two other personal goals—namely, housing and finances. His/her quality of life may have improved moderately over the 3-month period. Cumulatively over months and years, these summaries can guide the clinician or mental health team in maintaining or modifying the service plan in ways to bring about greater improvement and attainment of personally relevant goals.

The case example described below illustrates how CASIG is used for functional assessment, treatment planning, and monitoring of progress over time.

CASE EXAMPLE OF CASIG

Melinda was 22 years old when she had her first psychotic break. When her episode occurred, she had to drop out of her university studies and lost the part-time job she held to defray her tuition costs. At the time of her breakdown, she was living in an apartment with a roommate and had just begun dating. Her family was close-knit and supportive but also emotionally overinvolved with her, and had been so even before her psychotic episode. Her psychotic symptoms were delusions of reference and persecution, auditory hallucinations, social and emotional withdrawal, and poverty of speech. Her psychotic symptoms were accompanied by deep depression, elicited by her tormenting hallucinations.

In response to command hallucinations that told her to kill herself to save her family and herself from horrendous tortures, she made two life-threatening suicide attempts while driving her car. After her second hospitalization she began steady improvement with clozapine. Despite the subsidence of her hallucinations and delusions, Melinda had persisting negative symptoms and was demoralized. Because of their understandable fear of another sudden psychotic break and suicide attempt, the family took turns keeping her under observation, shadowing her wherever she went. As would be expected, this surveillance elicited hostile dependence on her part. Living at home with her parents, Melinda had successfully traversed from the *acute* to the *stabilization phase* of her illness.

Setting Personal Goals and Taking Inventory of Strengths, Supports, and Resources

Melinda was next referred for psychiatric rehabilitation at a local mental health center and began the process with a CASIG interview, administered by Tracey, an occupational therapist who was also Melinda's personal support specialist, the term preferred at the mental health center instead of "case manager." Melinda's parents were invited to participate in this interview that would lead to Melinda's treatment plan.

Personal goals

Beginning the CASIG evaluation with setting personal goals, Melinda indicated that she wanted to move back into her apartment (housing goal area), which was a condo her parents owned; live independently of her parents (family relationship goal area); regain a social life with peers, including dating (relationships with peers); and return to college (education). "I have to keep well and not slip back into my psychosis with the terrible thoughts and voices that make me feel hopeless and desperate." In response to the question "Would you like to improve your health and mental health in the next year?" Melinda stated that she was determined to stick with her clozapine and avoid a relapse. She complained about having gained over 25 pounds since starting clozapine and wanted help in losing the weight (illness management goal area).

Through the CASIG interview, Melinda articulated her goals but felt confused and in the dark regarding how she could get from point A to point B. With so many goals but still burdened by apathy, she didn't know how she could even begin the process. Tracey, her personal support specialist, acknowledged her frustration but told her that completing the evaluation would give them both ideas for her treatment and rehabilitation. Melinda was told that the mental health center sponsored learning-based rehabilitation that would put her into a student's role right off: "We will work together so you can gain the skills and confidence to begin moving toward your goals. You need to know, Melinda, that we'll have to go slowly so you'll be more likely to achieve each of the steps that you take toward your long-term goals."

In the next part of the CASIG interview, Tracey asked her, "Based on your current skills and past experiences, what could help you meet these goals? Let's start with what you already have going for you in taking steps toward each of your goals, one at a time." Melinda was able to identify a number of personal attributes, social supports, skills, and positive experiences that were relevant to her goals:

- Educational accomplishments—completed 2 years of college with good grades
- Brief period of successful independent living and desire to get back her independence
- Past success and satisfaction in making and maintaining friendships, including some dating (In addition, two of her friends had kept in contact with her throughout her illness and hospitalizations and were continuing to be supportive.)
- Loving and supportive parents who owned a condo where she might eventually live on her own
- Persistence and determination to work hard on reaching her goals
- Feeling a lot better since her symptoms were mostly gone thanks to clozapine
- A good relationship with her psychiatrist at the mental health center with whom she had weekly sessions

Strengths, supports, and resources

Melinda was then asked, "OK, you've mentioned a bunch of things that you already have under your belt; now, in addition to those positive things, what type of help, services, and resources would you need to meet each of your goals? Let's start with your desire to keep well and not have a relapse." After a brief pause, Melinda replied, "I know I have to continue with my clozapine indefinitely. If I'm going to return to college, live on my own, and resume a social life, I'll need to maintain control over my illness. My psychiatrist has convinced me of that. And I'll need to have regular appointments with him for a long time to come."

Tracey asked Melinda what she would do if her symptoms came back and she once again developed thoughts of harming herself. Melinda said that she had hoped that the clozapine would continue to keep her well but that she'd be able to tell her psychiatrist if she started to slip. Tracey described the mental health center's illness management program and recommended that Melinda participate in the Medication and Symptom Management Module groups that met once a week, where she would learn effective ways to communicate with her doctor and how to develop a relapse prevention plan. Melinda agreed but then asked, "But what about my weight? I'm getting fat and can't stand the way I look. I can't even fit into my clothes anymore." Tracey told her that she could help her with that problem. "We have a wellness program here that teaches healthy nutrition and exercise. Our center also has a volunteer instructor from a local Weight Watchers club that you could join."

Moving to her goal of independent living, Tracey asked Melinda to identify the kind of assistance she'd need to get to her eventual goal of living on her own. Melinda said, "I can count on my parents to help me. They own the condo where I used to live, but now they insist that I live with them at their home. Not only that, but they take turns staying with me 24 hours a day. I feel like they're babysitting me." Melinda's parents were encouraged to consider their daughter's goals from her perspective, taking into account that the mental health center's spectrum of treatment services would be backing up Melinda as she participated in its rehabilitation program. Her parents said they agreed with the goals that Melinda identified; however, they were worried that she would be stressed by taking on too much. They also worried about her suicidality in the past and said that they felt they needed to watch her closely for the time being.

After discussing each of her goals and the services and supports she would need to attain them, Melinda, her parents, and Tracey agreed on a treatment plan that would give priority to her living arrangements. At the same time, she would learn ways to maintain her remission by self-administering her clozapine and developing a plan to quickly deal with any return of psychotic symptoms and suicidal thoughts.

Surveying Social and Independent Living Skills

The next phase of CASIG turned to the skills that Melinda had or did not have but that she needed in order for her to live independently with less supervision from her parents. With each area of functioning, Tracey asked Melinda and her parents if it was relevant for achieving her personal goals. When patients like Melinda see the connection between improving their personal skills and using those skills for more independent living, they are motivated to pursue the arduous, incremental effort required to achieve their mastery. If any of the skills can't be readily learned, supports would be sought as substitutes for achieving her goal.

Melinda, with confirmation from her parents, told Tracey that she had no serious trouble performing adequately the following skills: care of personal possessions, personal hygiene, money management, friendships and dating, and food preparation. However, she did need help in a number of skill areas, including those in which she had been capable prior to the intercession of her illness. Together, they identified the skill areas, the troubles that Melinda was having, and the services and supports that she would need.

SKILL AREA	PROBLEMS	SERVICES AND SUPPORTS
Nutrition	Obesity	Wellness program, Weight Watchers
Lesiure time	Shadowed by her parents	Participation in consumer-run activities
Education	Lacked confidence and initiative	Social skills training
Mental health	Did not have a relapse prevention plan	Symptom Management Module
Medication side effects	Was not aware of metabolic syndrome	Medication Management Module
Cognitive functions	Had deficits in concentration and memory	Remediation exercises, practice
Patient rights	Did not know about confidentiality	Discussion with quiz, booklet
Transportation	Lost her driver's license after suicide attempts	Follow Department of Motor Vehicles procedures; parents will provide transportation

In the CASIG session, Tracey explained to Melinda and her parents the HIPAA provisions on privacy and suggested, "You know, the clozapine by itself can't get all of your goals; the doctor, myself, and the other staff and programs here in the mental health center added to the medication won't be enough to help you control your illness and move on to recovery. You'll need your parents to be on our treatment team, too. They are the single, continuous thread in your life and the ones who can provide you with the most important sources of support. Therefore, I want you to give permission for the doctor and me to provide them the same progress reports that we give you, to inform them of problems that we've discussed with you, and to encourage them to work together with us for your benefit." "That's fine with me," said Melinda, "but what if something comes up that I want kept private?" Tracey responded, "You just tell me or the doctor that you don't want a particular matter shared with your parents and we'll honor that." Melinda then signed the informed consent to involve her parents as integral members of the treatment team along with Melinda.

Addressing Symptoms and Unacceptable Community Behaviors

Since Melinda's positive symptoms, depression, and suicidality were in remission, the interventions required were to maintain her clozapine, regulate its dose and maintain her adherence through periodic blood levels, and have her psychiatrist conduct a quarterly interview rating her symptoms with the Brief Psychiatric Rating Scale. She had already agreed to participate in the illness management program in which she and her psychiatrist would create a relapse prevention plan. The only behavior that might be considered incompatible with community living was her past history of suicide attempts. Presently, this was being dealt with by her remission of psychosis, by continuous monitoring by her parents, and, eventually, by her relapse prevention plan.

Formulating a Treatment and Rehabilitation Plan

The centerpiece of Melinda's treatment plan was her five personal goals. If achieved, these would enable her to meet criteria for recovery. Attaining these goals would also be consistent with her fitting into the normal roles of student, friend, family member, and citizen of her community. A central feature of her rehabilitation plan was to recognize the importance of prioritizing her focus and efforts on each of her goals, work on them in sequence of their importance, and not attempt to accomplish too much too fast. Figure 4.8 depicts how the assessment information from CASIG flows into an individual's rehabilitation plan.

Her personal support specialist had the responsibility to 1) monitor her progress toward her goals, 2) organize the skills and supports that she needed, 3) ensure that the planned treatment and rehabilitation services were implemented, and 4) conduct problem-solving as needed while maintaining frequent and good-quality communication on her progress with all service providers, Melinda, and her parents.

Skills and supports that would smooth the way to each of her goals are listed on pp. 185–186 under each goal. These are connected to the treatment and rehabilitation services that would mediate her obtaining the skills and sup-

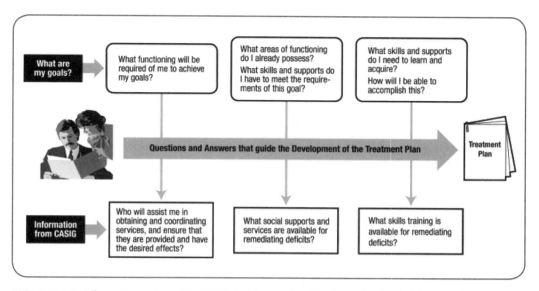

FIGURE 4.8 Information gathered by CASIG that is organized for the patient's rehabilitation plan.

ports she needed. A bulwark against relapse would be her continuing ability to actively control her enduring vulnerability to psychosis. As she made progress toward her long-term personal goals, acquiring the skills and supports contributing to her progress, she increasingly would experience empowerment, hope, and responsibility.

- Maintain her remission of psychosis and prevent a relapse.
  - » Build a collaborative and informed relationship with her psychiatrist.
  - » Learn medication and symptom self-management, with emphasis on relapse prevention and an emergency plan to activate when early signs of relapse or suicidal thoughts emerge.
- Lose weight, reach an appropriate weight, and maintain it.
  - » Learn about metabolic syndrome from psychiatrist.
  - » Develop healthy nutrition and exercise through participation in wellness center.
  - » Participate in Weight Watchers, with realization that participation will be long-term.
  - » Weigh self daily each morning and then review weights with personal support specialist.
- Achieve independent living in her own apartment.
  - » Learn communication skills for negotiating with her parents how to gradually demonstrate her ability to remain alone safely for increasing periods of time without their supervision (by attending weekly social skills training group).

» Participate in family sessions for problem solving and negotiating, gradually increasing autonomy without observation by parents (led by personal support specialist).

» Demonstrate and practice home maintenance and nutritional food preparation skills with personal support specialist during home visits and with parents.

- Reactivate her social life and leisure-time pursuits with friends and, eventually, start dating.
  » Refresh her friendship and dating skills by participating in the module for training friendship and intimacy skills.
  » Participate in a consumer-run, peer-support social club.
  » Learn how to initiate meetings and hold conversations with her current and former friends through participation in the weekly social skills training group and the Basic Conversation Skills Module.

- Return to college and complete her education.
  » Visit college with letter from psychiatrist indicating readiness to resume studies.
  » Practice communication skills for interactions at college in the social skills training group.
  » Consult with counselor at the college's disabled students office for special accommodations in test taking, studying, reports, and tutoring.

In addition, subsidiary goals that included improving Melinda's cognitive functioning and coping with her lack of a driver's license would be dealt with as conditions required. The skills and supports that she would need as she progressed in her rehabilitation plan were not static, nor were her personal goals. This made it even more vital for Tracey to conduct repeat CASIG interviews every 3–12 months, depending upon Melinda's progress, the problems encountered, and the need to change her goals. Tracey would also meet with Melinda on a weekly basis—at least initially—to review progress, engage the patient in problem solving, and run interference for her in obtaining services, supports, and community resources.

Making Progress Through Rehabilitation

Melinda's treatment was guided by the information collected through the CASIG interview. Because Melinda had just emerged from the acute and stabilization phases of a severe psychosis, it was important for Tracey to ensure that Melinda and her parents were educated about the nature of her illness and drug treatment she was receiving. In addition to the illness management that was offered at the mental health center, Tracey suggested that the parents attend the National Alliance on Mental Illness's *Family-to-Family* educational seminar on mental illness and that Melinda attend that organization's similar *Peer-to-Peer* seminar.

Tracey introduced Melinda to the nurse who led the mental health center's weekly sessions using the Medication Management Module, and Melinda agreed to join the group. During Melinda's first 3 months at the mental health center's rehabilitation program, her psychiatrist spent time during each session informing her about the scope of clozapine's side effects as well as the prophylactic benefits of its long-term use. He also spent a number of sessions describing the metabolic syndrome and why Melinda would be getting periodic blood tests for glucose, hemoglobin A1c, and lipids. Given Melinda's close relationship, frequent contacts, and shared stress with her parents, it was important for all three to obtain information from her psychiatrist. Her parents were invited to attend these sessions and they often did.

Because of the high priority that she and her parents accorded prevention of relapse, Melinda's initial treatment plan gave priority to relapse prevention. Her psychiatrist explained the value of Melinda's gaining personal control over her illness and of all three working collaboratively with him to identify the early signs of psychotic relapse and suicidality. Together, they helped one another to identify likely warning signs of relapse. For Melinda, these included insomnia, depression, preoccupation with worries about the future, and a voice calling out her name. The psychiatrist taught them how to monitor these symptoms using a Warning Signs Rating Sheet. By the end of eight sessions, Melinda and her parents had developed an emergency plan that included a list of two professional persons in addition to her psychiatrist whom they could contact if and when her warning signs kicked up.

Entering the Stable Phase of the Disorder

By the end of 3 months, Melinda had entered the stable phase of her illness. Her negative symptoms had ebbed, and she was participating more actively in her group and individual sessions. She completed homework assignments given to her for the Medication Management Module and was conscientious about daily monitoring of her warning signs of relapse. Melinda slowly acquired confidence in her ability to keep her illness under control. Melinda also noticed that as she got into the swing of regularly scheduled, structured learning activities, her concentration and memory improved. These improvements buoyed her hope and confidence in achieving her personal goals. She was now on the road to recovery. However, she had made little progress in her desire to gain greater independence.

As her level of functioning improved, Melinda became more and more frustrated with the round-the-clock observation that her parents maintained with her. They argued frequently. Melinda said that she was well enough to move back to the condo. Her parents had been so traumatized by her two serious suicide attempts that they were scared that she might relapse and commit suicide. As the family emotional temperature rose, family negotiation was recommended to thrash out this quandary. A problem-solving session with Melinda and her parents, mediated by Tracey and Melinda's psychiatrist, resulted in a compromise. Melinda initially would spend 2 hours alone in her apartment each day and would call her parents every half hour so they would be relieved of worry. Each week that she demonstrated that she could take responsibility for her own safety, the amount of time apart from her parents would be extended another 2 hours. When she was on her own for 6 hours, she would need to call them only once per hour.

As she moved further into the stable phase of her illness, it became clear that she was ready to engage in a more normal social life. Until then, she had occasional visits to her apartment by her two friends and attendance at a consumer-run self-help club. In line with recommendations from the wellness center, she began working out in a gym located in her condo complex. There, she met other residents and enjoyed exchanging small talk. She wanted to start dating but lacked the confidence and felt "rusty" after 2 years of being out of circulation. When a young man who also lived in her condo complex asked her out for dinner, she demurred but felt badly afterward.

After discussing her mixed feelings about dating with Tracey, Melinda asked, "You mentioned something about a friendship and dating program here at the mental health center. What's that?" Tracey gave her an overview of the Friendship and Intimacy Module, the skill areas of which included finding people who share the same interests and activities, making positive requests for getting together, giving compliments, maintaining a conversation using matched levels of self-disclosure, and learning how to be successful on a date. Melinda joined this skills training group and attended faithfully each week. After 1 month of training, Melinda got up the courage to contact some of her former friends and go out with them to dances and clubs. After 2 more months, she completed the training and felt ready to engage in dating. She met men through introductions by her friends, through meeting them at the gym and swimming pool at her condo complex, and by using dating services. Within a few months, she was going out on dates almost every week and enjoying leisure-time activities two or three times a week with her friends.

Reviewing Progress and Reprioritizing Goals With Repeat CASIG

A repeat CASIG interview was conducted 6 months after she began her rehabilitation. The assessment indicated that she had attended the wellness center, but not Weight Watchers, and had lost very little weight. She felt better with regular exercise but was having a hard time quelling her appetite, even though her diet was more nutritious. She and Tracey took a realistic view of the weight problem and reframed a new goal, which was to keep within 5 pounds of her current weight. A review of her progress to date revealed numerous accomplishments. She was now living on her own without any supervision from her parents; socializing actively in age-appropriate places with non–mentally ill people; using her car for transportation, having regained her driving privileges; and continuing to keep her Warning Signs Rating Sheet for her relapse prevention plan.

In reprioritizing her goals, Melinda stated that getting back to college was now her most important goal. She and Tracey developed a series of steps that were necessary for Melinda to take as she readied herself for college-level studies. These included gathering her transcripts; obtaining a letter from her psychiatrist clearing her for readiness to return to college; meeting with the admissions counselor, disabled students counselor, and registrar; and obtaining application forms. Tracey suggested that Melinda practice each of these subgoals in her weekly social skills training group and achieve them sequentially as homework assignments. Melinda agreed with Tracey that it might be wise to start with a single course before taking on a full load. She made use of the disabled students office, where she received special supportive counseling and accommodations for test taking and tutoring.

Entering the Recovery Phase

Melinda began attending college a little more than a year after discharge from the hospital. Because many of the academic credits from the courses she had previously completed were accepted by her college, she was able to graduate with a major in art after 2 years. Shortly thereafter, with supports from her mental health center team and an employment specialist, Melinda obtained and successfully maintained a part-time job teaching art in a preschool.

The weight gain associated with clozapine bothered Melinda a great deal, especially making her self-conscious with friends and dates. She made use of the assertiveness that she learned in the social skills training group to persuade her mother—who was also overweight—to attend Weight Watchers with her. She also got her father, an inveterate jogger, to take her on fast walks three times a week. She lost 25 pounds and was able to maintain her new figure with Weight Watchers' maintenance program. She considered switching to another medication but, at a conference with her parents and psychiatrist, decided to stick with clozapine given the seriousness of a possible relapse.

Her life now was full, and she felt proud of her ability to set her own goals and accomplish them. She was taking responsibility for herself, making her own choices, and in control of her illness. Her schizophrenia was no longer an obstacle to her recovery, although she realized continued vigilance was essen-ial with her medication and appointments with her psychiatrist. Over time, her sessions with her psychiatrist were faded to once every 2 weeks, once a month, and then once every 3 months. When asked to say a few words as an alumna of the rehabilitation program at one of the program's graduation ceremonies, Melinda said, "During the past 4 years I've learned that you can only climb a mountain by using a winding path. By participating as a full partner in your treatment and taking advantage of the great programs here at the mental health center, you too can recover from your mental illness."

▶ Summary

Restoration of functioning is the cornerstone of rehabilitation. In collaboration with the patient and family, the rehabilitation practitioner draws on evidence-based services to assist the patient to reach 1) the highest feasible level of functioning and participation in the community, 2) with the best quality of life, 3) in the least restrictive setting, and 4) as free of symptoms as possible. In conducting functional assessment, the practitioner gathers information that is relevant to the patient and this four-part mission of rehabilitation:

- Goals, preferences, and desires
- Skills, values, resilience, initiative, persistence, and other personal attributes
- Phase of illness, symptoms, warning signs of relapse, attitudes, adherence to medication, and medication side effects
- Relationships with family, professional and nonprofessional caregivers, and social network
- Requirements for acceptable living in a preferred residence and in the community
- Elimination of unacceptable, harmful, bizarre, or disturbing behavior
- Available resources and supports in the community

Assessment is intertwined with treatment and rehabilitation through an individualized, jointly developed plan that empowers and motivates patients to proceed on the road to recovery. Severe mental disorders are associated with lifelong vulnerability to relapse and disability; thus, assessment must be ongoing to guide goal setting and therapeutic decision making as the patient's preferences, needs, and well-being require.

GATE is an acronym that enables mental health professionals to capture the information needed for a rehabilitation plan.

- **G** is for treatment **GOALS** that are established by a collaboration between patient and practitioner. Goals are consistent with desired social and vocational aims of the individual.
- **A** is for functional **ASSESSMENT** of patients' current skills and strengths, cognitive and symptom impairments, medication attitudes and practices, available resources and supports in the environment, quality of treatment, and quality of life.
- **T** is for **TREATMENT** and rehabilitation services selected on the basis of assessment information and jointly planned by patient and practitioner to achieve short-term goals that are the stepping-stones for reaching desired long-term social and vocational goals.
- **E** is for **EVALUATION** to determine whether the chosen services are "hitting the mark," enhancing the patient's desired social and vocational roles.

Goal setting, assessment, treatment, and evaluation are continued until, through a process informed by functional assessment, the patient and practitioner agree that services have succeeded in opening the GATE for achieving optimal progress toward desired goals and roles.

LEARNING EXERCISE

In this exercise, you will write a patient's rehabilitation plan, based on a real person with whom you have worked. Your task is to identify the patient's personally relevant goals that, when attained, can cumulatively enable the person to assume desired social or vocational roles. The patient's realistic goals and the rehabilitation plan that you establish are linked to the functional assessment of the patient. Finally, you will decide on a way to measure or evaluate the progress or lack of it that is being made by your patient.

1. Specify two or three *long-term goals* that you and your patient have decided on. Long-term goals are those that will bring about desired changes in the person's roles at work and school, with family, and in recreational, residential, financial, and disability areas within 6 months to 2 years.

2. Identify several *short-term goals* that can be stepping-stones to one of the long-term goals. Short-term goals are set at 1- to 4-week intervals and should be achieved if progress is to be made in reaching personally relevant long-term goals.

3. For your functional assessment, pinpoint two or three obstacles that may stand in the way of your patient attaining his/her long-term goals. These can be in domains such as symptoms, deficits of social and independent

living skills, cognitive impairments, inadequate motivation, and lack of social, family, and community supports and resources.

4. Select a rehabilitation plan with services that can remove or attenuate obstacles such as impairments and symptoms, build skills, and mobilize professional, social, family, and community supports.

5. How will you, your patient, and the patient's family know that progress is being made? Design a means of measuring or evaluating progress that has been leveraged by the rehabilitation services you have set into motion.

▶ Key Points

- The major task of functional assessment is to identify the discrepancies between the individual's current abilities, limitations, and social supports and those needed to achieve that person's desired personal goals and role functioning.

- Functional assessment is a recurring process that provides feedback to the patient and practitioner on progress being made to achieve personally relevant goals. Ongoing assessment of the individual's strengths, limitations, family and community support, and resources informs the treatment process so that appropriate interventions can be brought into play as well as decisions regarding possible changes in goals.

- Inherent in recovery from mental disabilities are the person's social roles that define his/her place among peers, family, community, and society. These roles determine the individual's identity—attitudes, expectancies, tasks, rewards, and self-esteem—that gives structure and meaning to daily life. In measuring progress toward the goals and associated roles of the individual, functional assessment provides a barometer of treatment and rehabilitation.

- A dynamic and changing individualized rehabilitation plan requires periodic assessment of each person's strengths and limitations, motivational deficits, cognitive impairments, social supports, and community resources. Clinical justice can be given to these requirements only when a structured, user-friendly, valid, and reliable instrument is used. CASIG (Client's Assessment of Strengths, Interests and Goals) offers a means to establish, monitor, modify, and evaluate each person's unique rehabilitation plan.

❱ Selected Readings

Adams N, Grieder DM: Treatment Planning for Person-Centered Care. London, Elsevier Academic Press, 2005

Caldwell B: Assessment in psychosocial rehabilitation, in Best Practices in Psychosocial Rehabilitation. Edited by Hughes R, Weinstein D. Columbia, MD, International Association of Psychosocial Rehabilitation Services, 2000, pp 145–184

Client's Assessment of Strengths, Interests and Goals (CASIG). Available from Psychiatric Rehabilitation Consultants, PO Box 2867, Camarillo, CA 93011-2867 or www.psychrehab.com.

Cubie S, Kaplan K: A case analysis method for the model of human occupation. Am J Occup Ther 36:645–656, 1982

Ishak WW, Burt T, Sederer LI (eds): Outcome Measurement in Psychiatry. Washington, DC, American Psychiatric Publishing, 2002

Kennedy JA: Fundamentals of Psychiatric Treatment Planning, 2nd Edition. Washington, DC, American Psychiatric Publishing, 2003

Lecomte T, Wallace CJ, Perreault M, et al: Consumers' goals in psychiatric rehabilitation and their concordance with existing services. Psychiatr Serv 56:209–211, 2005

Miller WR, Rollnick S: Motivational Interviewing, 2nd Edition. New York, Guilford, 2002

Mueser KT, Tarrier N (eds): Handbook of Social Functioning in Schizophrenia. Needham Heights, MA, Allyn & Bacon, 1998

Peck DF, Shapiro CM (eds): Measuring Human Problems: A Practical Guide to the Assessment of Adult Psychological Problems. Chichester, UK, Wiley, 1990

Smith GR, Manderscheid RW, Flynn LM, et al: Principles for assessment of patient outcomes in mental health care. Psychiatr Serv 48:1033–1036, 1997

Vaccaro JV, Pitts DB, Wallace CJ: Functional assessment, in Handbook of Psychiatric Rehabilitation. Edited by Liberman RP. New York, Macmillan, 1992, pp 78–94

Wallace CJ, Liberman RP, Tauber R, et al: The Independent Living Skills Survey: a comprehensive measure of community functioning of severely and persistently mentally ill individuals. Schizophr Bull 26:631–658, 2000

Wallace CJ, Lecomte T, Wilde J, et al: CASIG: a consumer-centered assessment for planning individualized treatment and evaluating program outcomes. Schizophr Res 50:105–119, 2001

❱ References

Lecomte T, Liberman RP, Wallace CJ: Identifying and using reinforcers to enhance treatment of persons with serious mental illness. Psychiatr Serv 51:1312–1314, 2000

Lecomte T, Wallace CJ, Perreault M, et al: Consumers' goals in psychiatric rehabilitation and their concordance with existing services. Psychiatr Serv 56:209–211, 2005

McGurk S, Mueser KT: Cognitive functioning and employment in severe mental illness. J Nerv Ment Dis 191:789–798, 2003

Wallace CJ, Liberman RP, Tauber R, et al: The Independent Living Skills Survey: a comprehensive measure of community functioning of severely and persistently mentally ill individuals. Schizophr Bull 26:631–658, 2000

Wallace CJ, Lecomte T, Wilde J, et al: CASIG: a consumer-centered assessment for planning individualized treatment and evaluating program outcomes. Schizophr Res 50:105–119, 2001

Social Skills Training

5

Social Skills Training

The field of psychiatry is the study of interpersonal relations. . . . A personality can never be isolated from the complex of interpersonal relations in which the person lives and has his being.

HARRY STACK SULLIVAN CONCEPTIONS OF MODERN PSYCHIATRY *(1947)*

RECOVERY FROM a serious mental disorder is synonymous with having the ability to participate as a member of the community in meaningful and satisfying ways. "Meaningful and satisfying" must be defined by individuals according to their personal goals, needs, priorities, preferences, and interests. In addition, an individual's values, family, and cultural influences and the norms of society shape each person's sense of satisfaction with life. The principal goal of persons with mental disabilities, fostered by rehabilitation practitioners, is to function in social roles that bring quality to their lives.

Participation in society through pursuit of one's desired goals in life requires interpersonal and social skills. Our purpose in this chapter is to define social skills and describe the educational technology for training social skills. Practitioners who are competent in using social skills training are in a stronger position to promote the recovery of their patients.

"The rubber hits the road toward recovery" in social skills training when patients' interpersonal abilities result in their achieving their personal goals and favorable responses from the social environment. Empowerment is a natural outgrowth of acquiring social skills, because skilled patients gain more control over their lives, enjoy greater self-efficacy, and develop the ability "to do more for themselves" instead of depending on others "to do for them." Social skills training is an active therapy of *learning by doing,* not by talking about what to do.

▶ What Are Social Skills?

Social skills are all of the behaviors for communicating our emotions and needs to others in a manner that allows us to negotiate the pathways of

● TABLE 5.1

Broad range of important interpersonal relations that are mediated by social skills

- Ability to love and work
- Intimacy and reciprocal attachments
- Kindness, generosity, and nurturance
- Social and emotional intelligence
- Empathy and genuine concern for others
- Tolerance for others with different views, customs, and backgrounds
- Capacity for a variety of mutually fulfilling and enduring relationships
- Loyalty to family, friends, and teams at work and play
- Effectiveness in solving problems in league with others
- Concern for others
- Appropriate goals and expectations for oneself in the context of social norms

everyday life and achieve our personal goals. We are indeed "social animals," with most of our daily needs for food, shelter, work, recreation, and relationships bound up with others. A recovery-oriented approach to rehabilitation focuses us on *mental health* rather than mental illness. Definitions of mental health are embedded in a social matrix and require social skills to actualize. A quick perusal of Table 5.1 illuminates how much of adaptive functioning is mediated by our interpersonal communications and quotidian social routines. Because most personally relevant needs and goals derive from the realms of human relationships, social skills training is a direct means of enabling mentally disabled persons to bring satisfaction and quality into their lives. Skills vary according to the nature of the situation, the respective aims of each person in the situation, the appropriate social norms and expectations, and the type of relationship that exists between the individuals who are interacting.

Because our basic survival needs, as well as the even more valuable friendships and ties with family and workmates, are all rooted in the realms of human relationships, personal effectiveness with others is the prerequisite for successful living. Of course, there is no one single formula for personal effectiveness in establishing and maintaining relationships. Normality casts a wide net on acceptable social communication; for example, we often make allowances for foreign accents, stuttering, hearing impairments, sign language for the deaf, and baby talk—as long as the responder can make sense of the communication. Some countries and some individuals are more or less tolerant of variations in attempts by others to make greetings, ask questions, or make requests for their needs.

EXAMPLE

An otherwise educated and articulate American tourist attempted to get directions from a person staffing an information kiosk at the Paris East railway station to get to the Paris West station. The person at the kiosk was less than helpful, all but ignoring the request for information. The individual tried to get instructions from many others in the train terminal, including taxi drivers. No response was forthcoming. In exasperation, the American began to cry in the terminal. Quickly a francophone woman came to the rescue, using sign language and a few words of English to understand the problem and then helpfully accompanying the stranded tourist to her destination. This anecdote reveals two principles of social competence: (1) it is possible to attain one's goal with what superficially appears to be a deficit of social skills but is actually a universally understood appeal for assistance; and (2) the French woman possessed a high level of social perceptiveness, empathy, and personal humanitarianism.

Accommodations even are made by mental health professionals and family members for patients whose speech is not fully coherent; however, the rewards of a satisfying and rewarding life are more readily available to persons whose social and emotional communication are understandable, appropriate for the context and expectancies of the other, and conveyed with relevant nonverbal and paralinguistic skills.

Social skills that are effective in helping the person reach his/her needs vary according to the nature of the situation; the respective aims of each person in that situation; appropriate social norms, standards, and expectancies; and the type of relationship that exists between the individuals who are interacting. It can be readily understood, then, how important social skills training is for those individuals with mental disabilities who may lack the rudimentary capacities to express themselves effectively to others. What may be accepted by nurses and psychiatrists in a hospital setting does not gain reciprocity and responsiveness on the streets, in stores, in school, or on the job.

While many individuals with mental disorders naturally learn good or even outstanding social skills, given their favorable genetic endowment and role models in the family and among friends, the cognitive and other premorbid impairments of the vast majority of the seriously mentally ill have interfered with developing these skills. Moreover, after an illness like schizophrenia occurs, patients encounter new difficulties in social communication. The reasons derive from lengthy periods of social and emotional withdrawal from others, negative symptoms of the illness, disuse from lack of practice, and deficits in verbal learning and memory, working memory, reciprocity, social perception, and executive skills. Because of the many obstacles to the learning or relearning of social skills, such skills cannot be acquired through conventional methods of "talk therapy" such as are used in individual or group therapy. Medications, while they may reduce or even eliminate symptoms, are not able to teach social skills to those who never acquired them or whose illness has intruded upon them. For our patients with psychiatric symptoms and cognitive impairments, social skills must be learned through systematic, planned, and structured training relying on principles of human behavior.

Whether persons have natural social skills or have arduously learned them over many years, social skills training is a direct means of enabling mentally disabled persons to bring satisfaction and quality into their lives. Social skills training is also a normative experience that builds on each patient's strengths. It does not focus on symptoms or psychopathology. In addition, social skills training is used broadly in society to improve the communication ability of salespersons, company executives, diplomats, and medical students.

A variety of specific skills are involved in any successful social encounter: initiating conversations; giving and asking for opinions, assistance, and feelings; giving and asking others for information and facts in a specific situation; making and complying with requests; giving and accepting affection and compliments; and untold other interpersonal skills. What is communicated and how it is communicated will of necessity vary according to the situation, personal and social context, and cultural norms.

For example, requesting assistance from a physician for a medical problem will require different communication skills than a request to a sales clerk in a store. Expressing condolences to the widow of one's brother will differ from a condolence to a person whom one knows at work. The truly skillful individual can flexibly adapt his/her communications to the specific requirements of the situation. Because skills must be demonstrated in a wide variety of interpersonal contexts, the individual must be attuned to the social, cultural, and ethnic norms and expectations of the situation and other persons. Hence, sensitivity to social rules and expectancies is a key element in social skills training.

AFFILIATIVE AND INSTRUMENTAL ROLE SKILLS

Social skills may be divided into two dimensions of human behavior that overlap to a certain extent: affiliative skills and instrumental role skills. These two arenas of roles and relationships are pictorially represented in Figure 5.1. *Affiliative skills* are communications that enable people to develop and maintain relationships—with peers, family members, neighbors, schoolmates, and coworkers. They are the basis of friendship, affection, dating, cohabitation, marriage, and family relations. Affiliative skills are essential for gaining social supports, affection, camaraderie, membership in groups, and reciprocity in relationships. Because our personal identity is defined in large measure by our family and group membership, affiliative skills are highly relevant to recovery and a meaningful life.

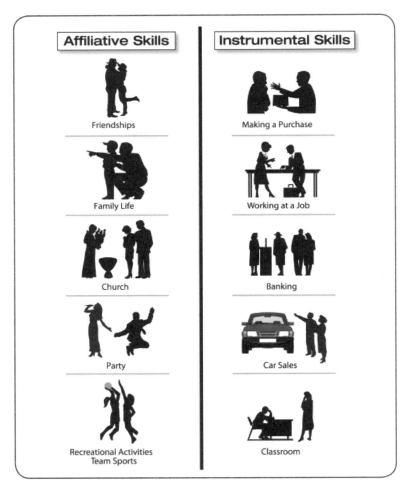

FIGURE 5.1 Two realms of social functioning: affiliative and instrumental skills.

Instrumental role skills are used for obtaining material and tangible needs of everyday life that are pegged to self-maintenance. The skills involved in using transportation, money management, obtaining a job, or securing Social Security entitlements are instrumental in obtaining income for self-support. Being able to negotiate medication issues with one's psychiatrist is instrumental to disease management and stability in one's mental illness. The ability to interact with store clerks in purchasing food and clothing, as well as in securing housing, is in the realm of instrumental role skills. There is a functional connection between affiliative and instrumental skills; if one is endowed with mutually satisfying and supportive relationships, it is possible to obtain assistance in times of need for surviving financial, employment, housing, and medical crises.

THREE-STAGE PROCESS OF SOCIAL COMMUNICATION

Social communication and social skills can be subdivided into three stages of information processing, each of which has its own specific attributes and requirements: *social perception*, or receiving information; *social problem solving and decision making*, or processing information; and *expressiveness*, or sending information. Figure 5.2 depicts the three stages of social commu-

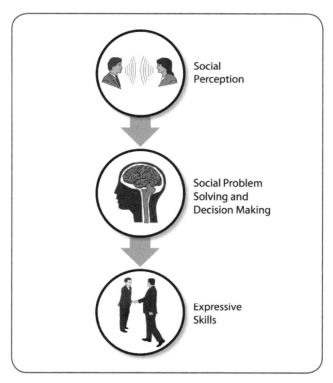

FIGURE 5.2
Three stages of social communication: social perception, social problem solving and descision making, and expressive skills.

nication. *Social perception* is the accurate recognition of what is being said by others and the social and environmental cues, norms, and expectations of the social situation. This stage also incorporates accuracy in recognizing the emotions shown by others with whom one is communicating.

Social information is often processed quickly without conscious thinking and effort, but will be a key element in teaching patients whose social perception is poor. Individuals whose illness produces distractibility and problems with focused attention will likely have difficulty interpreting the quality and meaning of others' communications. Incoming verbal, nonverbal, and contextual information must be absorbed as the "raw material" for deciding on how and what to express in a social situation. Social intelligence begins with decoding the social cues and social rules that are embedded in a situation. For persons with serious mental disorders, social perception is an important focus of training.

While it is often the case that we enter a social situation with a particular goal in mind, flexibility in goal setting is important, since our goals may change based on the information received from others in the immediate situation. Once a situation has been accurately "sized up" by good social perception, we must choose a response that is most likely to be successful in achieving our short- and long-term goals. This stage of communication is the *decision-making* or *problem-solving stage,* in which we consider a variety of alternatives for achieving our personal goal in the situation. To succeed in an interpersonal encounter, we need to decide which alternative among many would be best to use. Alternatives include what will be said, how it will be expressed, and when the timing of the response would best mesh with others' communications in the situation.

After we accurately perceive social information and decide how and what to say, the third stage of communication requires the use of effective *expressive skills.* Choosing appropriate words and putting them together into phrases and sentences gives meaning to our interactions with others. But how one talks is often as important as what one says. Choosing our words may make us more articulate, but our style of communicating engenders the critical social perceptions and judgments of others. Their evaluations and reactions to our verbal and nonverbal communications will determine our personal effectiveness. The components of effective social expression are listed in Table 5.2.

SOCIAL SKILLS VERSUS SOCIAL COMPETENCE

Social skills may be viewed as the coping process by which social competence is achieved. The skills of social perception, decision making, problem

● **TABLE 5.2**

Components of the expressive stage of social skills

Verbal	Content of speech or semantic level of communication—the alternatives selected to communicate one's needs, opinions, thoughts, desires, and emotions, as well as empathy and concern for others
Nonverbal	Facial expression, gestures (kinesics), eye contact (gaze), posture, and interpersonal distance and body language (proxemics)
Paralinguistic	Intonation, pitch, and loudness of voice; pacing of speech; latency of response; fluency; turn-taking in conversation

solving, verbal and nonverbal communication, and expression of one's feelings, attitudes, and thoughts mediate successful outcomes of social interactions. When social communication creates a favorable impression and results in achievement of one's goals, social competence can be said to occur. Social competence can be equated with a high frequency of successful social outcomes and a satisfying quality of life—in other words, personal effectiveness for successful living. Social competence is sometimes referred to as "social intelligence" or "social IQ." It is likely that genetics, as well as early life experiences, has a considerable role in determining social skills and social competence.

Because persons with serious mental disorders are commonly low on social competence, social skills training has great importance and relevance for treatment and rehabilitation. However, it should be understood, by practitioners and patients alike, that acquiring and applying high levels of social skills does not always translate into social competence. There are simply too many other factors that determine the outcome of any one social interaction beyond any one person's level of social skills. To reduce the demoralization of patients when they fail to achieve a specific homework goal set in a social skills training session is to point out that the world is unpredictable in its response to socially skillful persons. By participating in social skills training, patients will increase the probability that their social skills will have favorable consequences, generate positive reinforcement, and empower them to move farther along the road to recovery.

In summary, gaining social competence through social skills training is influenced by a host of personal, clinical, and environmental factors, as

● **TABLE 5.3**

Factors that influence the acquisition of social skills and the effectiveness of those skills in attaining personally relevant goals and social competence

PERSONAL FACTORS	ENVIRONMENTAL FACTORS	CLINICAL SERVICES
Cognitive impairments	*Stigma*	Medication
Symptoms of mental disorders	Community supports	Supported employment
Medication side effects	Family support	Supported education
Motivation to perform a role	*Social stressors*	Case management
Social role complexities	Realistic goals	Therapeutic alliance
Traits of personality disorders	*Social isolation*	Motivational enhancement
Substance abuse	*Complexity of social roles*	
Social intelligence—empathy, tact	*Demoralization*	Competent trainers
Self-reinforcement	Social reinforcement	Positive feedback

Note. Factors that impede the learning and utilization of social skills are shown in italics.

listed in Table 5.3. Actual transfer of social skills into everyday life depends upon the extent to which a person's social and community supports provide opportunities, encouragement, and reinforcement for using the skills in relevant situations. The empowerment of patients is a vital aspect of recovery, and social skills training provides the engine to drive greater efficacy in everyday life, promote success in meeting one's needs and achieving autonomy, and facilitate choice in setting and prioritizing goals.

▌ Social Skills Training

Social skills training encompasses a broad swath of psychosocial treatment methods, but all of these methods have certain features in common:

- An educational approach to strengthening skills
- Targeting of skills so that the training will be focused and its results measurable
- An initial assessment of a person's skills to ensure that only those that are deficient and desired by the individual are selected for training and to determine the specific cognitive and behavioral deficits that will be the targets for training

● TABLE 5.4

Principles of human learning and precision teaching that are translated into procedures for social skills training

- Specifying attainable goals in observable and measurable terms
- Repetition in training the skills and overlearning
- Instructions
- Social modeling
- Prompting, coaching, and fading of these interventions
- Behavioral rehearsal or role-playing
- Positive reinforcement for improvements in skills
- Schedules of reinforcement, including
  » Continuous and intermittent reinforcement
  » Differential reinforcement of appropriate social behavior
  » Differential reinforcement of any behavior other than that which is disruptive to the training situation
- Negative reinforcement
- Extinction or ignoring maladaptive behavior to reduce its frequency
- Corrective feedback, emphasizing skills that the individual can improve rather than the individual's deficiencies
- Shaping and chaining
- Problem solving as a means of removing obstacles to learning skills
- Homework assignments and other means of generalizing the skills learned in training sessions to a person's everyday life

- A focus on the *cognitive* underpinnings of interpersonal competence, including accurate social and emotional perception, awareness of social norms, flexible responsiveness in accord with situational and interpersonal requirements, and understanding the differences among passivity, assertiveness, and aggressiveness
- Use of principles of human learning (as outlined in Table 5.4)

Social skills training engenders motivation for active participation through highlighting the functional value of learning the skills in each person's life in order to teach participants how to acquire the knowledge and skills that are essential for a particular domain of life, to promote durability of the skills over time, and to foster generalization of the skills into participants' natural environments and interactions. When patients have participated in social skills training for long enough to have achieved several personal goals, they are able to function more autonomously, with less professional and family supervision. Independent living is a key criterion for recovery from serious mental disorders.

▶ Rationale for Teaching Social Skills to Mentally Disabled Persons

In our society, there are schools and educational opportunities for almost every conceivable human skill, from cooking and foreign languages to sports, dancing, and computer programming. Systematic training and apprenticeships are available for people who want to learn how to become a carpenter, a truck driver, or a dental technician. However, for mentally disabled people who lack social and emotional skills, there is a void of learning opportunities. Moreover, studies have documented that social skills deficits in schizophrenia do not change over time. There is little evidence that participating in otherwise effective treatments, such as intensive case management, psychosocial clubs, or supported employment, or living in the community for many years serves as a corrective to social skills deficits.

> "Give a man a fish, feed him for a day. Teach a man to fish, feed him for a lifetime."
>
> OLD CHINESE PROVERB

With a growing awareness of the failure of insight-oriented and other psychotherapeutic techniques to improve the psychosocial functioning of persons with schizophrenia and other mental disabilities, the author pioneered the use of behavioral learning principles to teach social skills to mentally disabled patients in 1968. At that time, the field of behavior therapy was in its infancy. Almost all of the early clinical studies focused on the use of reinforcement and other learning principles for reducing bizarre behavior and improving adaptation of chronically hospitalized patients to the requirements of wards and units in large psychiatric hospitals. With a research background in social psychology and a realization that behavioral learning principles could be used to improve social communication, the author began to apply reinforcement and other techniques to teach social skills to his patients in group and individual therapy.

The prototypes for social skills training were carried out by the author with group and individual treatment formats in large psychiatric hospitals, in community mental health centers, and at the Harvard–Massachusetts Mental Health Center. Early research studies showed how learning principles could enhance cohesion and social interaction in groups and accelerate symptom improvement (Liberman 1970, 1972). In subsequent studies and clinical elaboration, the group remained the preferred venue for training of the personal goals of each individual attending a day treatment center (Liberman et al. 1974). Within 7 years, social skills training had become an active area of treatment development and research that permeated services for numerous psychiatric disorders (Curran and Monti 1982).

Initially, social skills training was met with disdain by mainstream psychiatry. Based on the psychodynamic approaches in ascendance in the 1960s, conventional wisdom suggested that efforts to modify social behavior would be ineffective and that if behavior did change, it would lead to symptom substitution. When research demonstrated that patients with schizophrenia could learn social skills and that symptom substitution did not transpire, the proponents of traditional psychotherapy acknowledged that "social skills could be learned, but these changes were superficial and of no value to patients." Finally, when evidence was forthcoming of the rehabilitative impact of social skills training on the lives and community experiences of severely mentally ill persons, the old guard reluctantly responded with "social skills training is effective and valuable, but we've been doing that all along." That was the signal indicating that social skills training had "arrived" as an evidence-based practice.

While many psychosocial programs pronounce that social skills training is carried out as a component of the program, it is important to distinguish between informal group activities that engage patients in "socialization" and methods that deliberately and systematically use behavioral learning techniques in a structured approach to building skills. Socialization activities are valuable, of course. People meet people, find commonalities, develop relationships, make contributions to the group effort, enjoy the sense of identification with group membership, and have meaningful activities for what would otherwise be a barren existence.

Unfortunately, socialization without specific training procedures has little or no impact on acquisition and utilization of new social skills that can raise one's social functioning. Formal and focused educational techniques are required to compensate for cognitive deficits and to mobilize patients with requisite skills for community reintegration. Everyday interactions with family, neighbors, shopkeepers, friends, and non–mentally ill individuals require effective social communication that is appropriately linked to the social environment. The one rehabilitation service that can remediate the social inadequacies of patients is social skills training.

In summary, there is a difference between *doing activities with patients* and *teaching patients to do activities for themselves.* In this chapter, we shall limit our definition of social skills training to those methods that harness the specific principles of human learning to promote the acquisition, generalization, and durability of skills needed in interpersonal situations.

● **TABLE 5.5**

Rationale for social skills training, with examples of benefits accruing to patients who learn social and independent living skills

- Skills are acquired that enable patients to communicate with others—particularly patients whose process schizophrenia is of insidious onset, beginning in adolescence, and whose social skills are poorly developed and stunted.
- Regaining the social competence that was acquired prior to intercurrent episodes of severe mental disorder—such as major depressive episodes or psychotic illnesses—during and after which skills are lost, often for lengthy periods of time.
- Reestablishing relationships after long years of institutionalization in hospitals or on community backstreets, during which time one's social and emotional skills withered from disuse.
- Participating in an active and structured learning process that permits mastery and success associated with improved self-esteem, optimism, hope, and empowerment.
- Fostering trust through enhanced clinician–patient interaction and mutually respectful relationships.
- Gaining confidence in progress toward goals from the positive emotional climate of the training process, which translates into better clinician morale and improved outcomes.
- Managing one's illness and being a responsible consumer of mental health services.
- Reducing negative symptoms.
- Employing pleasant conversation, empathy, and normal social etiquette to gain acquaintances and friends and thereby extending one's social network and inclusion, strengthening social support, and overcoming loneliness and depression.
- Meaningfully structuring one's daily routines so as to achieve optimal social stimulation, reintegration into community life, less stress, and shared problem-solving for work, school, and recreation.
- Reality-testing one's goals, pacing one's recovery, and gaining insight.
- Improving family relations and thereby reducing family stress, tension, emotional over-involvement, and burden.
- Coping with daily life hassles, disappointments, and major life events and thereby developing resilience in the face of stress.
- Pursuing advocacy relevant to one's needs for resources, benefits, and entitlements; access to treatment; and antistigma efforts.
- Achieving a wide variety of affiliative and instrumental role skills that are facilitated by the reliance of social skills training on procedural learning and memory that are intact in persons with serious mental disorders.

Note. The benefits of learning social and independent living skills are directly translated into empowerment, personal responsibility, hope, self-esteem, and other recovery-oriented processes.

There are manifold reasons why social skills training has relevance for persons with serious mental disorders. Many of these are listed in Table 5.5. The deficits in social and living skills have been well documented among persons with psychiatric disabilities: poor eye contact, inappropriate facial expression, constricted vocal intonation, low voice volume, abnormalities in the timing or synchrony of responses in conversations, and very low rates of spontaneous social interaction. Patients with schizophrenia suffer from very small social networks that are densely confined to family members, even before the onset of their psychosis. Those individuals with a small number of social contacts have more psychotic symptoms and worse social adjustment. There is evidence that psychosocial interventions can broaden patients' social networks.

Given the enduring psychobiological and neurocognitive vulnerability to relapse and poor social functioning among most patients with severe mental disorders, it becomes a priority to offer treatments that can fortify resistance to stress, attenuate vulnerability, and reduce stressors. Social skills training has been used in various forms and intensities to improve patients' conflict resolution skills, recruit social support, learn strategies for coping with stress, improve problem-solving skills, and diminish the stressful effects of overheated emotional climates in patients' living environments. When needs go unmet because of deficits in social communication, quality of life is diminished. Patients lacking social skills are thereby shut off from satisfying relationships with others and feel stifled, lonely, frustrated, depressed, and isolated. Because social skills training has been documented as an evidence-based service to help mentally disabled persons to function better and attain their personal goals, it has staked out an important place in the pantheon of rehabilitation services.

Many studies have found that premorbid social competence is a predictor of outcome in major mental disorders—as well as in medical disorders in general. This makes sense because social competence is important for persons to negotiate and obtain appropriate psychiatric and medical care, to rally social support for coping with a disorder, and to have the interpersonal skills and persistence to follow through with treatment and its many complications. If pre-illness social competence influences individuals' ability to meet successfully their many post-illness challenges in mental health services and community adjustment, it stands to reason that social skills training would raise their level of personal effectiveness for meeting their needs and coping with stressors.

Given the learning disabilities experienced by many mentally disabled persons, how can one justify teaching social skills, given the needed investment in scarce mental health personnel? The answer to this important question comes from an understanding of the mechanisms underlying disability. Although there is an emerging consensus that cognitive deficits are barriers to functional adjustment in the community, cognition only accounts for a modest portion of the variance to explain this. Identifying mediators that interface between cognitive problems and the performance of skills in the natural environment may help to identify treatments that are cost-effective. Knowledge and skills that are learned by patients during social skills training have been shown to mediate the relationship between cognitive functioning and social functioning in the community (Brown et al. 2006). In other words, the behavioral learning principles used in social skills training can compensate for cognitive deficits and empower patients to choose and attain their personal goals.

As was pointed out in Chapter 2 ("Principles and Practice of Psychiatric Rehabilitation"), there is a fundamental, inextricable interdependence among physiology, emotions, thoughts, and behavioral actions. When social skills training succeeds in teaching patients the *behavioral elements* of social-emotional expressiveness, all levels of their human experience—physiology, feelings, and thoughts—are favorably affected. In a similar manner, this interactional process is illustrated by the effects of behavioral interventions on the multiple dimensions of anxiety disorders. When patients respond to behavior therapy of anxiety disorders through behavioral exposure to the feared situations through imagery or real-life proximity, a normalization occurs in subjective reports of *emotion* reflected by fear and trepidation and *cognitions* of catastrophizing and thoughts of losing control, as well as in *behavioral observations* of worried facial expression, pacing, hand wringing, and muscle contraction.

▌ Research Examples

When social skills training results in improved social competence, a cascade of favorable subjective experiences ensues. Many research studies attest to the primacy of social effectiveness in self-esteem and quality of life. In a study of 600 adults, data from 1-hour interviews were elicited for each individual's self-reported happiness and social participation with friends, neighbors, and other people in organizations such as church, work, fraternal clubs, and civic groups. Results indicated that happiness was most highly correlated with social participation, both for psychiatrically healthy respondents and for respondents with mental disorders (Phillips 1967).

Neurobiological studies have pointed to social skills and social participation in the initiation of a chain of reactions in the central and peripheral nervous systems responsible for basic feeling states. When individuals smile—even a prompted, "forced" smile—changes are detected in the amygdala, where emotional experiences are processed, then rapidly transformed into more positive mood. We do not tremble because we feel afraid; rather, we feel afraid because we tremble. We gain confidence and self-esteem not by the power of positive thinking, but rather through successful person-to-person transactions, conversations, shared experiences, and positive reinforcement for social competence. Subjective life satisfaction reported by persons with long-term schizophrenia was most highly correlated with being able to create and maintain close interpersonal relationships, having close friends and confidantes, social effectiveness, and social support in living with others (Salokangas et al. 2006).

It must be understood that social skills training is not a "stand-alone" treatment for persons with serious mental disorders. As has been repeatedly pointed out in earlier chapters, the pervasive symptomatic and functional problems of patients with mental disabilities require the mobilization of *comprehensive, coordinated,* and *continuous* services, including social skills training, to accelerate the symptomatic and functional improvement of patients with mental disabilities. In fact, as we shall see later in this chapter,

LEARNING EXERCISE

Reflect for a moment and think of a patient of yours, past or present, who suffers from a persistent mental disorder and who might benefit from social skills training. On a piece of paper, or in conversation with a colleague, answer the following questions as you formulate a skills-training plan for that patient.

- As specifically as possible, what is the current level of social skills that the patient possesses in both instrumental and affiliative domains of life? For example, can the patient initiate conversations with strangers? Make a positive request of an agency worker? Go through a job interview? Give appropriate levels of self-disclosure?

- What behavioral goals or targets for training could be established in preparation for social skills training for this patient? Again, be as specific and operational as possible in pinpointing what the patient might be able to do, with whom, where, and when.

- If you had the requisite competencies, would you be willing to engage this patient in social skills training?

social skills training has become a key fixture in a number of comprehensive, evidence-based treatments.

The case vignette below illustrates the utility of social skills training when it is provided in the context of a comprehensive rehabilitation program. Do you have any patients under your care who have problems similar to those of this patient?

Social skills training empowers individuals with mental disorders to achieve their personally relevant goals in life. Insofar as empowerment is a motivating

CLINICAL EXAMPLE

Steve was a 20-year-old junior college student who had suffered a psychotic episode while on summer maneuvers with the National Guard. He heard voices deriding him and felt that his thoughts and actions were being controlled by his father. He was a religiously scrupulous young man who held very high expectations for himself. Steve received an array of services from his local mental health center, including medication and case management, psychoeducation for him and his family, and social skills training. After antipsychotic medication brought his psychotic symptoms into remission, Steve and his therapist used social skills training that could strengthen his recovery.

One problem that he faced was feeling awkward at work when his supervisor praised his efforts. Steve always felt he should be doing even better. His goal, then, was to practice in sessions how to verbally accept a compliment and then to apply this at work. A corollary to this was learning how to say to his supervisor, "I'm not quite getting this new procedure. Can you go over it again with me, please?" In this manner, he was able to reduce the stress he experienced at work. Also, he role-played asking a woman out for a date and then, upon getting the date, practiced asking open-ended questions and reflecting back interest and empathy to sustain conversations.

After 6 months of social skills training and antipsychotic drug maintenance therapy, Steve was able to attend a college away from home. To ensure his successful transition to college, he obtained tutoring and other supported education services from the university's office of disabled students. He also registered at a local mental health center, where he received psychiatric services. Steve participated actively with his new psychiatrist in regular medication management and in a weekly peer-run social support group. He wrote to his therapist a month after starting his junior year at college, "My ability to meet people and socialize is good. I've made lots of friends. I have a really swell roommate, and we get along well."

● **TABLE 5.6**

Relationship between empowerment and social skills training

Empowerment	Social skills training
Making choices and decisions	Setting specific long- and short-term goals
Participating actively in treatment	Role-playing and rehearsing social encounters
Knowing what it takes	Social modeling by peers
Gaining self-esteem	Positive reinforcement for achievement
Developing mastery and confidence	Repetition and cumulative real-life successes
Participating in society	Homework assignments for affiliation
Developing informed responsibility for oneself	Applying skills to everyday life situations

force in recovery from mental disabilities, social skills training plays a major role in the recovery process. The connections between how empowerment is gained through social skills training are delineated in Table 5.6.

▶ Basic Social Skills Training

TECHNIQUES TO HELP PATIENTS REACH THEIR PERSONAL GOALS

Social skills training is highly structured. The process follows a prescribed set of steps, each of which is based on social learning principles. The following guidelines set out the training steps that are used in helping patients to acquire social skills, which will be the building blocks for progressing toward recovery and a fuller and more satisfying participation in daily life. It is important to recognize that the structure involved in the training procedure actually frees the therapist or trainer to instill his/her own personal style into the interactions with the patients. In this manner, the systematic nature of the training procedure promotes spontaneity and liveliness in the therapist–patient relationship and ensures cohesion and active participation in the group.

Getting good results with social skills training requires individualizing training procedures to meet the needs of individuals with varying diagnoses, symptom severity, cognitive impairments, personal goals, social and family histories, extant social supports, and cultural values and norms. The pace and outcome of developing skills will vary greatly, but most individuals who participate in social skills training show personally significant improvement.

1. *Establish a reinforcing therapeutic alliance.* The initial task of the therapist, treatment team, or trainer is to engage the patient and family in a warm, accepting, and mutually respectful relationship.

   - Develop rapport by showing genuine interest and concern, expressing empathy, and using appropriate self-disclosure so the patient gets to know you at a human level.

   - Encourage the patient to be an active participant in treatment by saying, "You are the expert in building social skills because you know your personal goals and are aware of your strengths and limitations. I'm your consultant because I have the technical and human relations know-how to help you reach your personal goals."

   - Prior to the first session of skills training, provide an orientation to the patient for inculcating favorable yet realistic therapeutic expectations. Brochures that can be used for this purpose are available from the appendices of two definitive treatment manuals on social skills training (Liberman et al. 1989; Bellack et al. 2004). Make certain that directions for finding the location of the social skills training are clear—send a map if necessary, and inform the patient about public transport and parking. Provide transportation if needed.

   - At the first session, greet the patient warmly and check to find out how the patient prefers to be addressed—by first or last name. Take special care to describe details of the treatment contract and plan.

   - At the time of the initial skills training session, once again, provide the patient with a cogent, down-to-earth, and practical orientation to the purpose, aims, and format of the training procedures. Figure 5.3 shows a poster that is placed prominently in the room where skills training is done. The trainer asks "veteran" patients to go through the procedures, briefly describing what happens in the training process to orient new group members. Point out why the prescribed treatment or training is distinctive, and give a rationale for its value and utility.

PERSONAL EFFECTIVENESS for SUCCESSFUL LIVING

THE PATHWAY of PERSONAL EFFECTIVENESS to SUCCESSFUL LIVING

Identify your personal goal ··············· *How do you want your life to be different and better than now?*

Select a situation involving ··············· *Choose WHAT you want to attain, WITH WHOM you need to communicate, WHERE and WHEN you will be trying to take this step.*
another person that will be a SMALL STEP toward reaching your personal goal.

Watch a DEMONSTRATION ··············· *Learn by WATCHING the skills being used in the role-play.*
of the situation with another person taking your role.

Practice the skills for ··············· *Learn by DOING the skills in behavioral rehearsal with coaching and positive feedback.*
achieving your needs in a role-play, using good VERBAL & NONVERBAL COMMUNICATION.

Give and get POSITIVE ··············· *Positive REINFORCEMENT strengthens your skills and know-how.*
FEEDBACK for what you have done effectively.

Complete a HOMEWORK ··············· *Using your PERSONAL EFFECTIVENESS to make your life more successful and satisfying is where the rubber hits the road.*
assignment that enables you to use your skills in everyday life.

FIGURE 5.3 Poster placed prominently in the room where skills training is done. The trainer asks "veteran" patients to go through the procedures, briefly describing what happens in the training process to orient new group members.

- When the patient leaves the clinic, always say, "Goodbye. . . . Have a nice week. . . . I'll see you next time." In addition, remember birthdays and other special events to bring a personal touch into the relationship.

2. *Conduct a behavioral assessment at the start of treatment and continue it thereafter as a means of monitoring progress and areas in need of continuing training.* Identify the patient's strengths and

capabilities in various social relations and community situations in which affiliative or instrumental skills are needed. This is the behavioral assessment that can be drawn from the personal and social history provided by the patient and family as well as during cumulative observations in social skills training sessions.

- Does the person know how to meet people?
- Has the person maintained a friendship for a period of months or years?
- Can the person sustain a conversation by using appropriate levels of self-disclosure and asking open-ended questions?
- When needing something from someone else, can the person make a positive request?
- What skills are lacking that impede social competence and achievement of the person's life goals?

CLINICAL EXAMPLE

Desmond, although suffering from frequent hallucinations that caused him anguish, was able to engage in conversations that were rational and coherent for 15–20 minutes at a time. During conversations, he showed good active listening skills and appeared to comprehend the information being conveyed to him. His grooming and personal hygiene, however, were in need of improvement, and the therapist employed role-plays with other group members in which they received positive reinforcement for improving their dress, grooming, and personal hygiene. Desmond got the message through vicarious learning.

3. *Specify the interpersonal problem and its corollary, the long- and short-term goals, and then establish an interpersonal scenario that will enable the patient to reduce the problem and achieve the goal through communicating with one or more other people.* An interpersonal problem is an obstacle in successfully communicating to another person that is interfering with the patient attaining his/her personal goals. Setting short-term, weekly, or monthly goals is the most challenging step in conducting social skills training. Remember, there is no single "right" or "correct" scene and goal. Repeated practice is the soul of learning, so it is not "fatal" to select a situation that may not be the "best" one for this patient at "that time."

- At the beginning of the training session, the patient formulates, with the help of the counselor or trainer, the goals and scenes to be used in the training process.
- Patients, and their relatives or caretakers, are encouraged to participate actively in choosing their behavioral goals for the session.
- Some patients need much guidance and direction in the selection of appropriate goals, particularly in the early stages of training. The counselor, therapist, or trainer should not shrink from sharing the responsibility for goal setting and choosing scenes. Ethical precepts and knowledge of developmental milestones and age- and culturally appropriate goals and values can guide the therapist in this responsibility.
- When helping the patient decide on training goals, the therapist should make use of all information that he/she has on that person, including mental status, psychiatric and social history, behavioral assessments, family reports, and current assessment of assets and deficits.
- Practice scenes usually recapitulate the features of the real-life situation that holds a goal for a patient. These situations are almost always used for homework assignments that are subsequently given to the patient at the end of the training session.
- Some patients, especially those with significant cognitive impairments, need much guidance and direction in the selection of appropriate goals, particularly in the early stages of training. The therapist or trainer should not shrink from sharing the responsibility for goal setting and choosing scenes but should always check out the relevance and appropriateness of the interpersonal goal and scene for the patient before proceeding with it.
- Some scenes and goals are better than others. Help the patient identify short-term, weekly or biweekly, interpersonal goals by asking:

  » How do your symptoms and social disability interfere with the normative, personally relevant goals that you have for improving your life?
  » What needs, feelings, and initiatives related to attaining your personal goals are being blocked because you have problems expressing or communicating to others?
  » What social and living situations are causing problems or challenges?

> Be SMART in setting goals for social skills training:
>
> **S**pecific
> **M**easurable
> **A**ttainable
> **R**ealistic
> **T**ime-limited

» What daily life situations, relationships, and interactions would be desirable to manage and master in efforts to reach your personal goals?

» With whom do you want to establish social contact, improve a relationship, or obtain real-life needs in the community?

» Where and when does the problem situation occur?

CLINICAL EXAMPLE

Jenny was often involved in self-destructive and humiliating sexual relationships with men because she lacked the ability to perceive and identify characteristics of exploitative men, the assertiveness to say "no" to men who would use her for sex, and the knowledge and skills to develop relationships based on companionship. She was at a loss to determine how she might proceed to form relationships that were mutually respectful and marked by shared interests, values, and personal goals. After Jenny joined a social skills training group, the trainer asked her a number of questions to ensure that making friendships before getting romantically involved was a genuine goal of value to her. Then he asked her, "What places in the city can you go where you might meet someone with whom you share common interests?" Jenny replied, "Well, I enjoy dancing, playing tennis, and I do a lot of reading. I really enjoy nineteenth-century novels, but I read almost everything. Maybe I can meet someone at the library or in the parks and recreation district."

The trainer or leader then solicited other ideas from the group members, who came up with suggestions such as 1) asking the staff at the recreation center to add her name to the list of people seeking tennis partners with a proviso that she prefers playing with men; 2) inquiring about group lessons in dancing, tennis, racquet ball, and other sports; 3) joining book clubs that meet in the library and bookstores; and 4) looking into singles groups that sponsor sporting events, go to the theater, or meet in a church of Jenny's religious persuasion. Jenny decided to practice in the group asking a staff member at her local recreation district about registering for group lessons in one or another sport.

4. *Setting a goal for the skills training session.* It's important to move quickly from the patient's problems to formulating positive goals to be sought in the social skills training sessions. Undue focus on problems

can inadvertently reinforce them. Setting specific and concrete interpersonal goals is perhaps the most challenging step in social skills training. Formulate a scene that simulates or recapitulates the features of the real-life problem situation, but convert situations in which problems have occurred in the past into situations in which the patient can practice using improved communication skills.

Table 5.7 lists some of the important criteria used in helping patients to select their personally relevant goals. Extracting and developing functional and attainable goals with an interpersonal framework from rather vague or general problems that are described by patients is one of the most challenging steps in conducting social skills training. The guidelines and criteria that are used in designating goals, listed in Table 5.7, can be effectively used in social skills training.

5. *Select a person who can serve as a model for the patient.* Most patients with serious mental disorders are markedly deficient in social skills, and it would be counterproductive to have them engage in a "dry run" or initial behavioral rehearsal of the goal-oriented, interpersonal situation that is the focus of the training. Why have them practice ineffective behaviors and experience awkwardness and embarrassment? Practicing ineffective social behaviors is like continuing to push on the gas pedal when a car wheel is stuck in a rut; the more you push down, the more deeply the wheel digs itself into the rut. Therefore, the therapist selects another patient in the group, a coleader of the group, or himself/herself to serve as the model.

- Ask the patient to select someone in the group who can take the part of the other person who will be the focus of the interpersonal encounter and homework assignment. The person selected is usually someone who resembles physically or personality-wise the individual with whom the patient will be interacting.
- Arrange for a model to demonstrate more adaptive alternatives and prompt the patient to again give a rationale for the chosen alternative.
- Give the person who will serve as the model some clues on what to emphasize in the verbal and nonverbal communication that is likely to make the encounter a successful one.
- Ask the patient to give the individual role-playing the recipient of the communication some clues regarding the personal style of that person with whom the patient will be interacting. Providing such clues will make the behavioral rehearsal more realistic.

● TABLE 5.7

Guidelines and criteria for setting goals in social skills training

Goal setting is the most difficult and most important step in social skills training. Considerable experience enables trainers to elicit long-term, broadly defined, and personally relevant goals and even more clinical savvy to collaborate with patients in choosing a short-term goal that can be accomplished during the days or week before the next skills training session. Having goals that are attainable and relevant to the patient is where the "rubber hits the road" for social skills training.

Background information on the patient's relationships and living, learning, and working arrangements should be utilized in setting goals. Information derives from direct experiences and contacts with the patient, other mental health professionals who have known and treated the patient, psychiatric interview, mental status exam, behavioral assessments, family reports, and current day's assessment of the patient's cognitive capacities, symptoms, activation and motivation, and communication assets and deficits.

There is no absolute "best" interpersonal situation to practice in skills training. Repetition and multiple choices of situations will be employed during the course of any one patient's participation in social skills training; thus, the therapists or trainers should not be afraid of setting up a scene that may not carry much relevance for the patient. Practicing good communication skills by itself will be a boon for the patient, regardless of situational relevance of the scene being used in the role-play.

1. Engage individuals in a process leading to specification of one or more personally relevant, recovery-oriented goals that will improve quality of life outside the treatment program in the community. Involvement in setting their own goals empowers patients by according them choices, encourages a collaborative partnership in treatment, and enlivens self-control and self-direction in the management of their disorder.

2. Link long-term, broadly conceived goals with weekly, short-term goals. Short-term goals that have a high likelihood of achievement serve as stepping-stones to reaching the long-term goal that is motivating the patient's participation in skills training.

3. Set goals that are consistent with clinical imperatives. The clinical responsibility of the trainer is to ensure that goals are compatible with social and cultural norms, ethical standards, developmental and age-appropriate functioning, and patients' long-term, personally relevant aims.

4. Make goals that are specific, operational, and measurable. If behavioral goals used in the rehearsed scenes are general and vague, it will be difficult for the patient to implement them in real life and even more difficult for the trainer to know whether or not the goal was attained. It is helpful to join with the patient in describing specifically what he/she will have done and accomplished in fulfilling the goal.

5. Focus on positive and constructive behaviors as goals rather than decreasing the frequency of some unwanted behavior or interaction. Adaptive behaviors, when achieved, displace symptoms and problems; when patients achieve positive goals, their momentum toward personal, long-term goals is increased and they receive immediate reinforcement.

● **TABLE 5.7** (*cont'd.*)

6. Prefer functional behaviors as goals rather than "convenience" behaviors. Functional refers to those skills that, if acquired, would provide maximum payoff to the patient in his/her real-life situations. For example, practicing how to negotiate treatment arrangements with a social worker in a community agency where the patient will receive postdischarge, continuing care is preferable to negotiating over a conflict with a nurse in the hospital. Functional goals lead to improved functioning in the natural environment.

7. Set realistically attainable goals, which are more likely to meet with success in real-life settings. Focusing on more readily attainable goals will confer positive reinforcement and stronger motivation for patients to continue to pursue their longer-term goals. Goals need to challenge one's skills and abilities without discouraging effort, performance, and success.

8. Choose frequently occurring, interpersonal situations for goals over those that occur only occasionally, since the former provide more opportunities to achieve. For example, when there is strain in a marriage, it is preferable to have the spouses learn how to greet each other affectionately every day rather than practice exchanging affection on their wedding anniversary. Frequently occurring situations strengthen learning through repeated practice.

9. Use interpersonal situations and scenes that are practiced in the training session as those in homework assignments. Putting into effect what was learned in the skills training session within a week will promote generalization of skills into the real world and improved social functioning.

10. Debrief patients at the end of each session to explore possible roadblocks that they might anticipate in doing their homework. Ask each patient to identify any obstacles that might interfere with a timely completion of the weekly goal and, if necessary, engage the patient in problem-solving to try to remove the obstacle.

11. Promote support for patient's homework assignments by contacting family members, case managers, and other members of the patient's treatment team. Getting encouragement and positive reinforcement for homework completion from others with whom the patient relates can only increase the chances for goal attainment.

12. Always start a skills training session by inquiring about the patients' completion of homework assignments. If the trainer fails to convey self-responsibility to patients in regard to completing their real-life accomplishments, they will lose some of the motivation to transfer skills from the training location to real-life settings.

13. Reinforce tiny accomplishments, partly completed goals, and even effort for unsuccessful homework. Give spontaneous positive feedback when patients report completing their homework. You can never be too enthusiastic as long as it is genuinely felt. You can't "spoil" a patient with too much positive reinforcement if you are reinforcing adaptive behavior.

(continued)

● **TABLE 5.7** (*cont'd.*)

14. When, as is occasionally inevitable, patients return to the next session reporting that they were unable to complete their assignment, be positive and flexible and launch into a problem-solving mode. There are many reasons why homework is not completed and the trainer can consider:
    - » The interpersonal behavior of the assignment was too difficult and needs to be reduced in degree of difficulty
    - » Opportunities or encouragement was insufficient
    - » Opportunity for the interaction was lacking—the other person wasn't available
    - » Priority for achieving the short-term goal was downgraded with other problems intervening during the week
    - » Priority for achieving the longer-term, overall goal receded

15. Set goals that yield personally relevant and valued rewards. When goals are achieved, needs are met, relationships are established or sustained, and self-confidence and self-efficacy are strengthened.

- While the model is demonstrating appropriate communication, stand near the patient who is observing the process as it unfolds and annotate and highlight what the model is demonstrating so as to enhance learning by observation.

6. *Engage the patient in behavioral rehearsal.* A crucially important element in social skills training is having patients practice improved communication in situations that closely simulate their real-life situations where they must apply the skills. Role-playing real persons in the patient's life involves other patients in the group and the therapist as well. If possible, the therapist and/or cotherapist "shadow" the patients as they role-play, observing for assets and deficits and improvements that will be used for positive and corrective feedback.

   - Engage the patient in role-playing the scene, offering instructions and prompts as needed to initiate action and remind the patient of behaviors for remediation.
   - Provide on-line support, prompts, and positive feedback in coaching the patient to improve performance during the rerun of the scene.
   - Give generous praise to reinforce progress or acknowledge effort after the patient rehearses repeatedly. When giving positive reinforcement, focus on all dimensions of social competence in social skills training, including:

» Topical content and semantic choice of words and phrases
» Nonverbal components of expression
» Timing and reciprocity
» Appropriateness of context, cues, and expectations
» Receiving (social perception) and processing of skills
» Social problem solving

Figures 5.4 and 5.5 demonstrate the active mode of teaching used in social skills training. In these photos, the therapists are close to the patients, prompting, coaching, and reinforcing them "on-line" as the role-playing proceeds. This level of involvement makes more likely a positive learning experience that, in turn, is more likely to be generalizable to the natural environment.

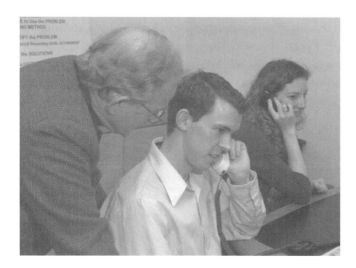

FIGURE 5.4 The patient is role playing a phone conversation that he has selected as his personal goal for the coming week. A trainer is taking the part of the person who will be the recipient of the phone call in the patient's real life. Dr. Liberman is closely observing the patient's social skills, ready to give positive or corrective feedback to improve the patient's performance.

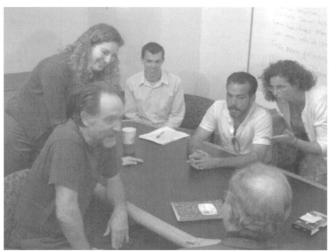

FIGURE 5.5 Social skills training is being carried out by a trainer or therapist who is prompting and giving "on-line" feedback and encouragement to a patient who is practicing conversational skills. The therapist takes an active and directive role in training and observes the interaction as it unfolds to determine interventions to use. While one patient is role-playing designated skills, another patient is being cued by a second therapist to observe the components of effective communication being demonstrated so that he can learn the skills through social modeling.

7. *Identify the assets, deficits, and excesses in the patient's performance during the role-play by focusing on receiving, processing, and sending skills.* Ask the patient the following questions:

- Who spoke with you in that situation? What did the other person say?
- How was the other person feeling?
- Did you get your short-term and long-term goals met?
- What are alternative ways you might have handled the situation?
- For each alternative, would your short-term and long-term goals have been met?
- Which alternative would be the most reasonable and most likely to lead to your meeting your goals? Why?

8. *Give positive feedback for specific elements of skills that were well done or correctly expressed.* Positive feedback should be given for specific verbal and nonverbal skills that were demonstrated in the patient's role-play or behavioral rehearsal. When positive reinforcement is given specifically focused on the behavior and immediately after the patient's rehearsal, skills are learned and strengthened.

- Give constructive and corrective feedback, not criticism, for deficits and problems with judgment, perception, and grasp of social norms. Solicit positive feedback from the group members or family members (depending upon whether the training is taking place in a group or family setting). Frame the feedback so it will not be critical and demoralizing by saying to another in the group or family, for example, "Tell Jane what she did well with her eye contact and voice tone . . . and would she make her point better if she spoke more slowly and clearly?"
- Ask the patient who has completed the role-play to repeat what and how he/she has communicated in the role-play and whether the intended communication would be successfully achieved if carried out in real life.
- Video feedback is particularly effective with persons who have deficits in verbal learning. In Figure 5.6 a social skills training role-play is being videotaped for subsequent playback for positive and corrective feedback.

9. *If necessary, repeat steps 5, 6, 7, and 8 until the patient's performance is reasonably competent and likely to meet the communicative requirements of the situation,* resulting in success when the patient employs the learned skills in real life.

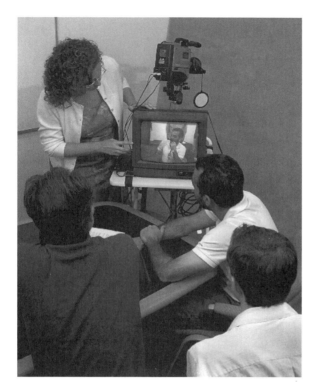

FIGURE 5.6 Videotaping as a means of providing feedback is a powerful technology for promoting improvement in social skills. The videotaped feedback is offered selectively to highlight the segments of the role-play when the patient was using good social skills.

10. *Shape behavioral changes in small increments, starting with where the patient has assets and without expecting much improvement at any one time.*

11. *When the patient has demonstrated in role-play form a reasonable degree of skill, instigate implementation and follow-through of social problem-solving by giving a homework assignment that the patient can carry out in the natural, community and home environment.* Involve the patient in the nuances of the homework assignment—for example, where, when, and how the patient can approach the other person, set the stage for a successful interaction, and eliminate distractions.

- Encourage the patient to give positive feedback to himself/herself even for making an effort, as the world does not always respond favorably to even the best social skills.
- Write down the assignment on an index or similar-size card, which can be specially printed for this purpose. An example of an assignment card is depicted in Figure 5.7. Homework assignment cards are as useful in mental health settings as they are in schools or as reminders of upcoming medical or dental appointments. In short,

homework assignment cards aid and encourage patients' compliance with homework. Having a card personally filled out and signed by their therapist or trainer boosts patients' morale and serves as a bridge between training sessions. Patients typically carry the card with them in their pocket, wallet, or purse.

12. *Ensure that the patient comprehends the problem, the short- and long-term goals, and the plan of action for the next week's homework assignment by reviewing these systematically at the end of the training session.* Inquire of the patient to make sure that he/she is reasonably confident that the homework assignment can be carried out during the coming week. Ask if he/she anticipates any problems that might interfere with the assignment being completed. If there are some problems, engage the patient in problem solving or suggest a different assignment.

**Personal Effectiveness
Assignment Report Card**

Name_____

Date assignment given _____

PE Assignment _____

_____

_____

Date assignment due _____ (_____)

_____

Cues for Personal Effectiveness

1. Maintain **Eye Contact**
2. Use your **Hands**
3. **Lean Toward** the other person
4. Maintain pleasant **Facial Expression**
5. Speak with **Intonation** and **Fluent** pace
6. Communicate your request, feelings, or needs **Clearly** and **Directly**

FIGURE 5.7 Example of a personal effectiveness assignment report card (front [top] and back [bottom]) to instigate completion of homework given to transfer the skills learned in the treatment venue to the patient's real life.

13. *Generalize improvements in social skills into real-life settings and strengthen durability over time through repeated practice and learning.*

- Implementing specific, attainable, and functional homework assignments
- Encouraging natural supporters (e.g., family, friends) or case manager to create opportunities and give encouragement and positive reinforcement to the patient for completing his/her homework
- Using positive feedback for successful transfer of skills to real life after each successful homework assignment
- Training in use of self-instructions, self-evaluation, and self-reinforcement
- Involving significant others in the training and implementation
- Fading the structure and frequency of the training

A step-by-step protocol for using basic social skills training is graphically displayed in the flow chart of Figure 5.8.

To exemplify the goal-setting process wherein short-term weekly goals are set and accomplished in real life en route to the patient's long-term overall goal, a case vignette is described in the following example. Cumulative experience with hundreds of patients over many years has revealed that approximately 75% of short-term goals are actually achieved through homework assignments. This has been confirmed by observational studies in which patients have been observed unobtrusively in the community completing their assignments.

EXAMPLE

Long-term, personally relevant goal: to improve relations with parents after years of alienation.

Sequence of short-term goals completed en route to attaining the overall goal:

- Ask case manager to help in obtaining parents' phone number.
- Make phone call to parents and describe improvements that you've made in treatment.
- Call parents and tell them how much you miss them and would like to see them after so many years; invite them to Los Angeles for a visit.
- Practice for upcoming visit; use open-ended questions to elicit information about your parents' life during the past few years and

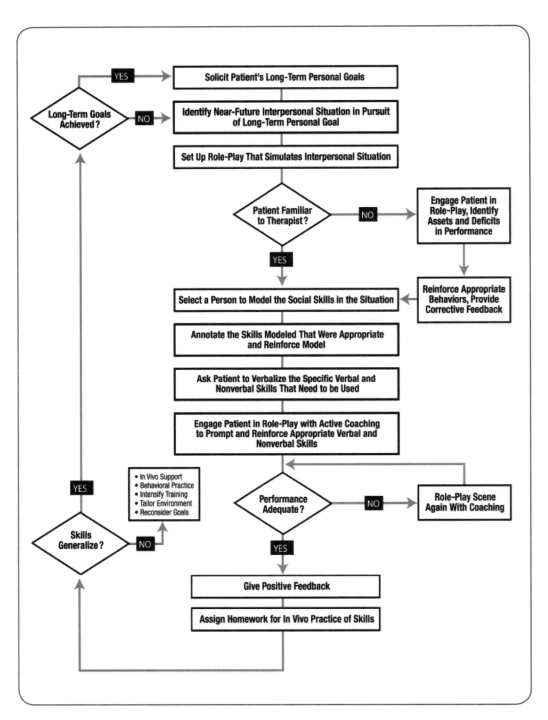

FIGURE 5.8 Flow chart for conducting the basic form of social skills training from soliciting goals to completing homework assignments. Generalization can occur if the person's social environment provides opportunities, encouragement, and reinforcement for using the skills in everyday life.

> reflect back to parents your interest and pleasure in talking with them.
>
> • During visit with parents, be sensitive to their or your discomfort and politely and affectionately terminate the conversation, saying something like, "It's been great talking with you and getting caught up with our doings. I'm kinda tired and would like to take a little nap at my apartment. Let's plan to meet later for dinner."

GUIDELINES FOR GENERALIZING SKILLS FROM TRAINING SETTINGS TO REAL LIFE

Transferring knowledge and skills from whatever classroom or simulation center, whether learning to fly an airplane, conducting surgical procedures, or selling merchandise, requires application in real-life situations where the knowledge and skills can be put to use. This is no different for using social skills that were learned in a clinic, community support program, or private office. To expect generalization to occur spontaneously goes against common sense as well as what we know about how people use what they learn in training. So what can be done to enable persons with mental disabilities to put their skills to use with those who await them in the natural settings of the community? The clinic-based forms of skills training attempt to do this by making the clinic-based training as close to the real situations outside the clinic as possible; for example, telephones and furniture arrangements are used as props, and group members do their very best imitating those people who are the real targets for intervention with the patients undergoing the role-play.

One possibility is to shift the learning into the natural environment where the skills would be used. For example, the *teaching interaction,* which is described in a later section of this chapter, consists of ad hoc training by nursing staff of social skills for hospitalized patients as interpersonal problems arise on the ward. Although in vivo training in the community would be more cumbersome, it is certainly possible for clinical case managers or rehab therapists to demonstrate specific interactions for patients and then observe and reinforce the patients as they engage in consumer behavior in stores, deal with employees of public agencies, and interact with psychiatrists regarding medication problems.

Whether it would be more cost-effective doing in vivo training in the community than in the classroom has not been tested; after all, it would require mobility and one-to-one tutoring, with the clinician modeling the skills, instructing the patient on what is to be done and how to do it, coaching the patient as the latter tries it out, and giving positive and corrective feedback for the performance. It might also require the clinical case manager to speak with the target person in the community in advance to get that person's cooperation in the training process.

Certainly, it would be desirable for case managers and other members of assertive community treatment teams to master the competencies of a social skills trainer and use some of their time teaching patients to function more independently in the community. In a study using *in vivo amplified skills training* as a supplement to a classroom-based training of social skills (Glynn et al. 2002), outpatients with schizophrenia were randomly assigned to 1) skills training in a clinic classroom or 2) classroom training plus having "booster" sessions in the community whereby a case manager strove to:

- Create opportunities in the community for patients to use the skills learned in the classroom.
- Encourage patients to take advantage of these opportunities.
- Reinforce patients' success in using their skills or in making an attempt to do so.

Patients in both treatment conditions showed significant improvements in their module-based skills and in overall community adjustment and quality of life. As seen in Figure 5.9, the patients who received the in vivo ampli-

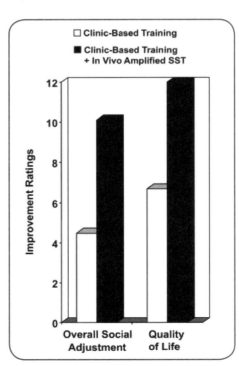

FIGURE 5.9 Greater improvements on social adjustment and quality of life at 60 weeks after start of training when case manager amplifies social skills training (SST) by providing opportunities, encouragement, and reinforcement to patients who are completing community-based assignments compared with patients who receive clinic-based SST alone. *Source.* Adapted from Glynn et al. 2002.

fied skills training plus clinic-based training achieved higher levels of social adjustment and quality of life in the community than their counterparts who participated in classroom learning only (Glynn et al. 2002). Improved generalization from in vivo amplified skills training has been replicated with three case managers in another controlled clinical trial, as well as when the community-based amplification was conducted by natural, nonprofessional supporters (friends, relatives, staff from residential care homes) nominated by the patients (Liberman et al. 1998; Tauber et al. 2000).

While basic training of social skills can be conducted very effectively in the context of individual or family therapy, there are decided advantages to using the procedures in group therapy. Groups can comprise from 3 to 12 (or more) participants, depending upon the patients' level of functioning, speed of learning, and availability of a second and third practitioner to serve as co-trainers. The advantages of conducting skills training in groups are delineated in Table 5.8.

▶ Attributes and Competencies of Social Skills Trainers

One of the limitations of many mental health treatments is their needing to be delivered by highly trained and licensed mental health professionals. In contrast, social skills can be taught by a wide array of mental health workers who do not need advanced, professional degrees. This is most important for service delivery, since the majority of clinical personnel at most mental health agencies have a college degree or less. There is a subset of competencies that are critical to the effective use of social skills training:

- Warmth, spontaneity, and genuinely expressed interpersonal skills
- Ability to teach specific skills with lively interactions with patients while following a structured program or manual
- Several years of working with mentally disabled persons and familiarity with their varied lifestyles
- Empathic understanding of the life experience of mentally disabled persons

When clinicians teach social and independent living skills, they are *teachers* and should be endowed with the skills that facilitate learning in any student—young or old, fast- or slow-learning, bright or cognitively impaired. Some attributes of effective teachers are similar to the characteristics of good therapists: empathic, capable of forming a therapeutic alliance, attuned to the individual needs of each student, positively reinforcing, clear

● **TABLE 5.8**

Advantages of conducting skills training in groups

- Offers naturalistic and spontaneous opportunities for trying out skills with members of the group—augmenting the practice of skills being learned in formal rehearsal
- Provides an arena for ongoing assessment of informally exhibited, peer-related social skills (the trainer is able to observe progress as well as note any problems and can use this information to inform future goal setting)
- Is more efficient and cost-effective than individual training, as 3–12 patients (or more) can be led by a single therapist, with the assistance of a co-therapist as required by the composition and size of the group
- Enables patients who have successfully completed social skills training to be empowered to serve as teaching assistants and even develop sufficient competence to be hired as skills trainers
- Makes it possible for patients to identify with other patients demonstrating the skills to be learned and hence social modeling becomes more credible and generalizable
- Amplifies positive feedback for incremental improvements in skill development beyond the single voice of the therapist
- Sets up role-plays with a variety of individuals who serve as surrogates from the real-life situation (role-plays are more like the real-life situation where the skills must be ultimately used; thus, generalization is enhanced)
- Multiplies modeling options for learning interpersonal skills, thereby making them more credible and easier to adopt when multiple peers are serving as models
- Develops cohesion in the group that magnifies the positive influence on symptomatic relief and the reinforcement value of feedback from peers and trainer
- Promotes more vitality in a group, more humor, and the ability for one or more people to serve as co-leaders, thereby enhancing empowerment (this often leads to a paid position in the agency as a consumer advocate or a personal support specialist)
- Forms and enhances cohesion in a group, which can be enhanced by shaping to bring more rapid symptomatic improvement and engagement in the community
- Creates opportunities for the participant to expand his/her social support network and develop friendly relationships outside of the group
- Assists participants in completing homework assignments through the use of a buddy system, in which participants provide encouragement and reinforcement to each other for applying their skills in the community
- Increases generalization of skills to real-life situations by allowing the participant to interact with a number of peers with different interpersonal styles
- Motivates the participant to persist in training through interactions with more "veteran" clients who can demonstrate their having achieved personal goals through participation in the group
- Enables peers, as well as therapists, to provide orientation and favorable expectations for the training

and specific in communicating, and genuinely interested in each student. In addition, trainers of social and independent living skills should have familiarity with behavior therapy principles, enthusiasm for working with severely disabled people, capacity both to follow detailed procedures and to adapt them to situational constraints, and ability to monitor patients' progress using worksheets and data.

Social skills training is a very active and directive therapy. The therapist or trainer must prepare for the sessions in advance and be able to quickly determine relevant interpersonal goals and scenes to use in the training. Goal setting can be accomplished prior to the social skills training session—for example, in a "problems and goals meeting" or through consultation with a patient's psychiatrist, personal support specialist, or primary therapist. Alternatively, goals and scenes can be set through focused interviewing of the patient at the start of the skills training session. The process of training requires movement and activity on the part of the therapist. The clinicians who are leading the training process, as shown in Figures 5.4 and 5.5, are out of their seats, in a coaching stance, and ready to whisper prompts, positive and corrective verbal feedback, and encouragement to the patient as the interaction unfolds.

Trainers must learn the basic elements used in teaching social skills: modeling, behavior rehearsal, prompting, feedback, reinforcement, and homework assignments. If clinicians do not adhere faithfully to these competency criteria, it is unlikely that they will obtain the favorable results that would otherwise be expected. As seen with other evidence-based treatments, when practitioners depart too far from the procedures that make an intervention effective, desired outcomes are not achieved.

For example, in one effectiveness study of modules conducted by our UCLA research center, a variety of patient populations and facilities were studied (Wallace et al. 1992). Notably, the only group of patients that did not significantly improve in their skills comprised residents at a board-and-care home where the home's director volunteered to do the training. Unfortunately, she took a short-cut in the training and failed to involve her group in the role-play learning activity. *No role-play practice, no skill acquisition.* Other staff members from other board-and-care homes achieved excellent results because they carefully followed all the learning activities for each skill area in the module.

An agency adopting skills training modules must also provide administrative and organizational support to meet the requirements of this unique modality—for example, decisions to set aside time for skills training, to supplant other activities with training sessions to subscribe to an educational and rehabilitative ideology, and to incorporate resources such as video recorders and monitors. Table 5.9 lists generic competencies for social skills trainers, as well as a sample of specific competencies for those leading modules in the UCLA Social and Independent Living Skills Program. When these competencies are fulfilled, the training process is likely to be of high fidelity and almost always leads to favorable outcomes.

The professional disciplines that are capable of teaching social skills are not as relevant to using this modality effectively as the specific competencies described in Table 5.9. However, it is noteworthy that these competencies are in a broad sense requirements for successful use of most of the evidence-based psychosocial treatments for the mentally disabled. If professional preparation and training of mental health professionals do not include competencies in the use of the interventions described in this book, those professionals will become somewhat redundant. Already, it has been well documented that psychiatrists are not prepared clinically to use or supervise evidence-based practices such as social skills training.

> "As most of the care of patients with schizophrenia and other severe mental disorders takes place in community-based settings, their treatment must include much more than psychopharmacology. Most psychiatrists with whom I've talked agree in principle with the psychosocial approaches for which there is an evidence base, but few use them or prescribe their use. For psychiatry, the bio-psychosocial model has become the 'bio-bio-bio model.'"
>
> STEVEN SHARFSTEIN, M.D.
> PRESIDENT, AMERICAN PSYCHIATRIC ASSOCIATION,
> 2005–06, *PSYCHIATRIC NEWS*, MARCH 3, 2006

▶ Training Social Problem-Solving Skills

Because it's not possible to teach patients how to deal with every interpersonal situation and problem that may arise to confound their recovery and quality of life, a procedure for training social problem-solving skills has been devised. In training social problem-solving skills, patients are assisted through a series of steps from identifying the nature of the problem to brainstorming alternative solutions to the problem, weighing the pros and cons of each of the alternatives, selecting from among alternative interactions one or more that might solve the problem, and then finally implementing the interaction. The advantage of this approach to social skills training is its broad generality and utility for almost any problem situation that crops up to block individuals' efforts to reach their personal goals.

Poor problem-solving skills are a major obstacle to recovery, in large measure because patients lose power, hope, and control over their lives when their efforts to reach their personal goals fail. Repeating the past is not a prescription for successful coping, adaptation, and reconstruction of the self. Integration into community life and active participation as a citizen

● TABLE 5.9

Generic competencies for social skills trainers and a sample of trainer competencies specifically linked to the modules in the UCLA Social and Independent Living Skills Program

Generic competencies
- Actively help the patient in setting functional, specific, and attainable goals.
- Assist the patient in building possible scenes in terms of "What emotion or communication?"; "Who is the interpersonal target?"; and "Where and when?"
- Instruct the patient about rationale and procedure, to promote favorable expectations and orientation before role-playing begins.
- Structure patient role-playing by setting the scene and assigning roles to the patient and surrogates.
- Engage the patient in behavioral rehearsal, getting the patient to role-play with others.
- Model more appropriate alternatives for the patient.
- Prompt and cue the patient during the role-playing.
- Coach or "shadow" the patient—being out of your seat and closely supporting the patient.
- Give patient corrective feedback for specific behaviors.
- Ignore or suppress mildly disruptive behavior.
- Get physically within one foot of the patient during role-play.
- Touch the patient, if appropriate, for support and positive feedback.
- Suggest an alternative behavior for a problem situation that can be used and practiced during the behavioral rehearsal or role-play.
- Give specific homework assignment.

Specific competencies for leading skills training modules (see pp. 246–259)
- Introduce each skill area by giving the benefits that accrue to participants who learn the skills of the module.
- Ask each member of the group to describe, in his/her own words, the benefits of participating in any particular skill area.
- Get participants to connect the benefits of the skill area and module as a whole with their own personal goals (motivational interviewing).
- Effectively elicit and sustain eye contact and attentiveness of all group members and demonstrate good verbal and nonverbal communication skills.
- Elicit correct responses to questions in Video Q and A learning activity from each participant, using prompting, fading, and modeling as needed.
- Engage each participant in role-playing, and repeat role-plays until interpersonal skills are within the normal range.
- Give specific, contingent positive feedback for improvements shown during role-playing, and solicit specific positive feedback from other group members.
- Get each participant to engage in problem-solving steps for resource management and problem-solving learning activities.
- When giving homework assignments, obtain accurate description of assignment from each participant and determine any obstacles to completion of assignment.

require the ability to solve problems as they arise in social and family relations, recreation, work, school, and spiritual and religious contexts. Also salient for problem solving is learning to manage one's illness and make decisions about treatment in collaboration with one's psychiatrist. To be human is to face and solve problems.

> "It's a troublesome world
> All the people who're in it
> Are troubled with troubles
> Almost every minute"
>
> DR. SEUSS

Solving the everyday problems of life almost always involves one or more other people, whether the others are part of the problem or are sought for assistance in solving the problem. Because of the pervasive, interpersonal nature of problems, teaching patients *social problem-solving skills* is an important rehabilitation modality. Fortunately, the same behavioral principles and teaching techniques used in the basic model of skills training can be used for inculcating social problem-solving. As in the basic training model, interpersonal scenes are specified, and the obstacles that are interfering with the patient's reaching a goal are clearly identified.

Modeling is used, as is brainstorming for problem-solving ideas from the other group members if the training is done in groups. The brainstorming focuses on generating potential solutions to removing the obstacles and attaining the goal. Once one or more alternative solutions are identified as feasible and potentially effective, the patient is engaged in a role-play. If

EXAMPLE

Problems can arise in any instrumental or affiliative relationship or situation. Having an appointment to meet with one's psychiatrist for a medication prescription is a goal that can be transformed into a problem when obstacles intrude on completing the appointment with the needed concerns about medication resolved. Some problems that may conspire against seeing one's psychiatrist are 1) transportation is not available, 2) the patient gets the flu and can't leave home, and 3) when arriving at the clinic, the patient discovers that the doctor has gone to a medical meeting that day. In solving problems, alternative measures need to be generated and evaluated, then tried in some sequence of feasibility until the obstacles are removed and the goal is achieved. In the case of problems associated with getting to see a psychiatrist, alternative approaches to reach that goal might be to consider a variety of transportation options, including asking a friend or relative for a ride, setting up a telephone appointment, requesting a meeting with another psychiatrist, or simply making a new appointment.

video equipment is available, a videotape of the role-play is made for review and positive feedback. For individuals with cognitive impairments, information from watching oneself on a video is much more readily assimilated for learning purposes than strictly verbal feedback.

A sequence of skills for training social problem solving is shown in Table 5.10. Because mentally disabled persons often lack the flexibility required for producing alternative ways of removing or taking a circuitous route around the obstacle, training in social problem-solving skills emphasizes the ability to consider options for dealing with challenges to obtaining one's needs. The mainstay of this approach is teaching patients how to identify the specific problem in a situation and then come up with alternative solutions to the problem and consider each alternative's relative efficacy. It is useful to view the training of social problem-solving skills as equipping patients with a "social prosthesis" to function more effectively and independently in everyday life. Much as artificial limbs, crutches, and wheelchairs are prostheses for the physically disabled, utilization of the problem-solving skills sequence is a prosthesis for the cognitive deficits that hobble the mentally disabled.

● **TABLE 5.10**

Sequential steps of training social problem-solving skills annotated by the use of Socratic questioning with patients that helps to induce their learning the skills

Identify and think of ways you could solve the problem.

Use a step-by-step method that helps you to identify the problem and then to develop ways to deal with it so you can obtain your goal.

Determine the nature of the problem.

Identify some situation, often involving another person, that is interfering with your immediate goal.

— How does this situation relate to your long-term personal goals?

— What is your short-term goal in the situation as a step toward your broader personal goals?

— What obstacles or situation do you have to remove or go around to be able to achieve your immediate goal at this time?

Identify all the different ways that the problem can be solved.

How many alternatives can you think of that might remove or circumvent the problem?

Don't be concerned about how realistic each alternative might be at this point in your problem solving.

(continued)

● **TABLE 5.10** *(cont'd.)*

Weigh the consequences of each alternative.

— What are the advantages, disadvantages, and feasibility of each alternative?

— What alternative or combination of alternatives could you use to achieve your goal in the immediate situation—alternatives that could help you remove, overcome, or avoid the obstacle between you and your goal?

How feasible is each alternative, and how likely is it that the alternative will enable you to reach your goal?

Determine which alternative or combination of alternatives you would select.

Would the chosen alternative help you achieve your immediate goal?

Determine how you would implement the alternative or combination of alternatives.

How would you use the chosen alternative(s) or option(s) for an effective social response, integrating both verbal and nonverbal skills?

Where, when, and how would you put your chosen alternative into effect?

Determine what resources you would need to be successful in using your chosen solution to the problem.

Who could help you with the solution?

Would you need money, transportation, or anything else to improve your chances of success?

If any one alternative doesn't work, try another.

If none of the alternatives are effective, consider altering your goal.

LEARNING EXERCISE

Now you should be ready to take the plunge and try to employ some of the social skills training techniques with one of your patients. Plan your strategy in advance of a therapy session, which might more easily be an individual session for your initiation into the fraternity of social skills trainers. Consider all the steps required for training an interpersonal skill and be modest in the goal or scene you select in conjunction with the patient. The guidelines for selecting goals for social skills training listed in Table 5.7, and the flow chart of the sequential training steps in Figure 5.8, can be helpful cues to you as you prepare for the session and then go through the steps.

❱ Variants of Social Skills Training: Different Strokes for Different Folks

Tailoring the goals, procedures, and format of social skills training is essential to meeting the needs of the full spectrum of patients who may benefit from improving their interpersonal competence. Individuals have differing diagnostic syndromes, personalities, comorbidities, and socioenvironmental supports and resources. Prospective patients for social skills training present with different constellations of social abilities, deficiencies, and learning rates. For such a varied population to acquire social skills and enjoy greater success in meeting their functional goals in everyday life, flexibility is required in the type of skills training and how that training is integrated into comprehensive treatment programs. Several training models, as well as variations on each model, are available to the clinician who wishes to adapt the basic training model into a broader array of populations and programs.

Given the important role of impaired psychosocial functioning in the criteria listed in the *Diagnostic and Statistical Manual of Mental Disorders*, most patients with schizophrenia, mood disorders, severe and persistent anxiety disorders, and personality disorders who seek treatment suffer from varying deficits in social skills. Table 5.11 lists a number of ways in which social skills training can be utilitarian for this broad array of patients. When integrated with other treatment interventions, social skills training complements the insight achieved cognitively with the action orientation that is the linchpin of behavior change. The emphasis on behavior as a mediator of changes in emotion and cognition is summarized by the adage "Action is the proper fruit of the tree of knowledge" (Thomas Fuller, *Gnomologia: Adages and Proverbs,* 1732).

ASSERTIVENESS TRAINING

Being able to appropriately and effectively express one's feelings and needs in situations where others may seem to be intimidating, dominating, or exploitative has been long a special focus of social skills training. Individuals are often caught in the trap of responding to such situations with two different types of responses, neither of which results in achieving their goals. The two maladaptive responses are passivity and aggressiveness. Recognizing the differences between these two inappropriate and counterproductive responses is the first step to learning more adaptive ways of self-assertion. Assertiveness generates positive reinforcement

● TABLE 5.11

Types of social skills training for varied types of patients

PATIENT POPULATION	SOCIAL SKILLS TRAINING APPROACH
Schizophrenia	*Personal therapy:* Uses social skills training to teach patients how to reach their personal goals and improve their relationships with family members. Patients also learn how to become more accurate in perceiving stressful situations and to take assertive or other actions to reduce experiential stress.
	Cognitive enhancement therapy: Uses social skills training groups to teach patients to practice and use their newly learned cognitive skills (e.g., social attention, social perception, decision making, problem solving) in their everyday lives.
	Neurocognitive enhancement therapy: Uses computerized training of sustained attention, verbal learning and memory, and executive functions followed by social skills training groups for patients to learn ways to use their cognitive skills in their work.
Bipolar disorder	Focuses on social judgment, empathy, family relations, and work.
Major depression	Increases behavioral activation and positive reinforcement. Practicing assignments, to be completed in vivo, are given in the context of cognitive-behavioral, interpersonal, and social rhythm therapies.
Somatoform disorder	Diverts attention from self-concerns and impairments to small, incremental interpersonal goals that can lead to success and positive reinforcement.
Obsessive-compulsive disorder	Provides training to help the patient to engage in social interactions, starting with easily attainable yet functional goals that can begin to displace preoccupation with obsessions and compulsions. Patients learn to request assistance from family members in complying with exposure and response prevention assignments from cognitive-behavioral therapy.
Posttraumatic stress disorder (PTSD)	Provides training for improving skills in a variety of relationships that have been "stretched" and in which the other persons have become "burned out" and alienated.
	Training includes giving positive feedback and compliments, thanking people for their assistance, expressing a desire to maintain one's job with one's supervisor, and improving

● **TABLE 5.11** *(cont'd.)*

PATIENT POPULATION	SOCIAL SKILLS TRAINING APPROACH
	communication skills with family members and with mental health professionals working in the PTSD programs of the Department of Veterans Affairs.
Social phobia	Provides training in assertiveness, making eye contact, and speaking clearly, slowly, and with appropriate intonation. Practicing conversing with others in a gradually increasing variety of venues and topics and with a number of conversants.
Asperger's disorder	Helps participants develop verbal and nonverbal conversation skills and provides training in problem solving in a variety of vocational and social situations.
Borderline personality disorder	Improves relationships and mood regulation as a principal component of dialectical behavior therapy (DBT).
Marital and family distress	Focuses on interpersonal communication and problem solving, mutual acceptance, and behavioral activation in behavioral marital therapy, family-focused therapy for bipolar disorder, behavioral family therapy, and psychoeducational approaches for relatives of the severely mentally ill.
Conduct disorder and delinquency	Uses a teaching interaction with a here-and-now, on-the-spot format to provide training in problem solving for remediating interpersonal friction and conflict between peers and peers and adults.
Older adults	Combines skills training and health care self-management to enhance the social functioning and independent living skills of elders; cognitive-behavioral social skills training improves coping skills, social functioning, and reality contact.

from others because one's needs are more likely to be met; thus empowerment, self-esteem, self-responsibility, dignity, and respect are acquired by an assertive person.

It is unfortunate that many people equate assertiveness with aggressiveness. Definitions that highlight the differences in traits among persons who are passive, assertive, and aggressive are given in Table 5.12. The first step in assertiveness training is learning the norms of society and accurate social perception of the incoming verbal and nonverbal messages from the person with whom you are speaking. Often, nonverbal and paralinguistic cues are as important for conveying the meaning of a message that lies along the passive–assertive–aggressive continuum as the words themselves.

12

how assertiveness differs from passivity and aggressiveness on behavioral dimensions

PASSIVE PERSON	ASSERTIVE PERSON	AGGRESSIVE PERSON
Has rights violated; is taken advantage of	Protects own rights and respects the rights of others	Violates rights; takes advantage of others
Does not achieve goals	Achieves goals without hurting others	May achieve goals at expense of others
Feels frustrated, unhappy, hurt, and anxious	Feels good about self; has appropriate confidence in self	Defensive, belligerent; humiliates and depreciates others
Inhibited and withdrawn	Socially and emotionally expressive	Explosive; unpredictably hostile and angry
Allows others to choose for him/her	Chooses for self	Intrudes on others' choices

Knowing the nuances of cultural variations in norms and expectancies can be critical in determining an appropriate composite of behaviors to orchestrate in teaching a person personally effective assertiveness. The case example on p. 243 shows how a small miscue by a culturally naïve skills trainer led to an adverse result.

PERSONAL THERAPY

To reconcile social skills training with the need to adapt it for the phase of a person's disorder, a personal therapy was devised (Hogarty et al. 1997). The importance of yoking a form of treatment with the requirements of acute, stabilizing, stable, and recovery phases of schizophrenia and other severe mental illnesses was underlined in Chapter 3 ("Illness Management"). Personal therapy is applied twice a month over a 3-year period in three graduated stages that take into account the sensitivity of persons with severe mental disorders to excessively intense treatment and cognitive deficits. Goals for training include addressing affective, cognitive, and physiological experiences of stress, including teaching patients to recognize stressors and cope with them. Thus, the training that is used in personal therapy has

CLINICAL EXAMPLE

Juan had made a rapid recovery from his first episode of psychosis and wanted to persuade his parents to extend his hours of unaccompanied hanging around with his friends. His parents had been somewhat over-protective of him after the traumatic experience of his psychotic break and wanted to observe him at all times. In Juan's social skills training class at the day treatment center, his therapist inquired about how Juan might effectively deliver his request for longer hours before a curfew. Juan indicated that this was a request that he would have to address to his father, as his family was unacculturated and from a rural part of Mexico where the father's patriarchal role was ascendant. Juan practiced making a positive request, using good eye contact, with wording like, "Dad, I feel a lot better. I'm taking my medication and have been told by my doctor that I'm ready to spend more time with my friends. It's really important for me to get your permission for staying out a few more hours each night."

Juan returned the next day to the mental health center with a black eye and considerably chastened by his efforts to apply assertiveness at home. It became evident that, while his verbal request was culturally acceptable, making eye contact with the family's authority figure during a request for more autonomy was perceived by his father as aggressive. This anecdote illustrates the importance of cultural competence for trainers of social skills. Soon thereafter, the mental health center hired a Chicana who was well versed in Latino culture and was able to consult with Anglo staff members to increase their sensitivity to the role of culture in communication.

greater breadth and depth in goals as well as teaching patients to monitor and use interpersonal and other skills for self-regulation of affective disturbances. The skills training sessions are provided individually in the context of a supportive relationship that offers psychoeducation for patients, empathy, reassurance, reinforcement of health-promoting initiatives, and reliance on the therapist for advocacy and problem solving in times of crisis.

To advance to the next higher stage of therapy, patients have to demonstrate that they can apply selected social skills strategies and their symptoms have stabilized with effective doses of maintenance medication. In the advanced stage, which usually begins late in the first year of treatment, training focuses on vocational situations, relapse prevention, and accurate perception of the effect of one's behavior on others. Consistent with the growing consensus regarding the time scale for improvement from psychosocial treatments, the benefits of personal therapy are greatest after three full years of treatment. Compared with supportive therapy, personal therapy yields significantly better outcomes for negative symptoms, social relationships outside the home, normalization of behavior and adjustment, enhanced work performance (with 43% working part-time or full-time), and an improvement in leisure pursuits (Hogarty 2002).

HOME-BASED SOCIAL SKILLS TRAINING

Assertive community treatment is the best known among a variety of intensive case management programs to maximize comprehensive, coordinated, collaborative, consumer-oriented, and consistent care for persons with disabling mental disorders. With an increasing number of mental health agencies adopting this outreach form of providing psychiatric services, social skills training can be performed when the treatment team makes contacts with patients in their homes and other locales in the community rather than in a mental health clinic or facility.

In one such program, two to three mental health professionals made an initial home visit to acquaint the patient and family with the purpose and benefits of social skills training. A detailed orientation was given with the aim of establishing positive therapeutic expectations and an active, participatory role for the patient. The patients selected goals that were individualized by personal preference. While most of the goals related to the patient's relationships with friends and acquaintances in the community, family involvement was mobilized with an explanation of the importance of helping the patient use the skills taught during the sessions by providing opportunities, encouragement, and reinforcement for any constructive efforts. Training was given twice weekly, with each visit lasting 90 minutes. A portable video camera was utilized to give the patient and family members positive, graphic feedback of role-played interactions.

After 6 months, results revealed significantly greater improvement in symptoms in the patients participating in the home-based skills training as compared with a matched control group of patients who participated in a psychosocial club. Both groups received similar types of medications and bimonthly visits with a psychiatrist. There were several advantages of furnishing skills training in the home: 1) because the training included relapse prevention, family members were able to alert the visiting staff when prodromal signs of relapse arose; 2) communication and problem-solving skills improved, leading to reductions in family conflicts; and 3) families were noted to give encouragement and reinforcement to their mentally ill relatives' use of skills for friendships and activities outside the home, which translated into greater autonomy (Moriana et al. 2006).

THE TEACHING INTERACTION

The *teaching interaction* is a variation of the social skills training model, useful for spontaneous teaching of skills to patients right in the very settings where interpersonal problems arise. This variant of training inculcates constructive modes of communication under tense and stressful conditions in settings where skills need to be learned "on the spot." These settings include supported living residences, family homes, group homes, ordinary places and situations in the community, psychosocial rehabilitation clubs, partial and inpatient hospital units, and board-and-care homes.

The teaching interaction is a sequence of training steps (Table 5.13) that is especially helpful for patients needing to learn how to interact and communicate more effectively in novel or provocative situations. For example, the teaching interaction is particularly useful in situations where irritation, confusion, frustration, and anger might erupt into disruptive or aggressive behaviors. This variant of social skills training supplants counterproductive, emotionally impulsive, and inappropriate behaviors by inculcating more

● **TABLE 5.13**

Ten steps for developing new communication skills using the teaching interaction for remediating disruptive or aggressive behavior

1. Express positive affect to the offending patient using a smile, a special greeting, or warm physical contact.
2. Praise what the patient has been able to accomplish in the recent past or some positive progress or recent adaptive behavior.
3. Describe the inappropriate and disruptive behavior that was just exhibited.
4. Describe the appropriate alternative behaviors that could be used instead in a similar situation.
5. Give a rationale to the patient for using the appropriate behavior.
6. Describe the consequences that must be imposed for the inappropriate behavior.
7. Ask the patient to acknowledge what has happened.
8. Practice the situation that was conflict laden, using more appropriate alternatives to threats and violence.
9. Give feedback to the patient during the time he/she is practicing alternative behaviors, offering both praise and corrective feedback.
10. Reward the new and more appropriate behavior with praise and tangible reinforcers.

constructive interpersonal skills (Fixsen et al. 1973). The learning of more appropriate interactions results in empathy, problem solving, and reconciliation in tense interactions while strengthening relationships between patients or patients and staff members. The 10 steps of the teaching interaction are listed in Table 5.13.

Skills training effectively increases social participation for a wide range of psychiatric patients with moderate to severe disabilities, including those from various walks of life, from minority cultures, and with little education or few verbal skills. Even individuals with autism and moderate degrees of retardation have been successfully taught communication and problem-solving skills and, as a result, have been able to function more independently in regular jobs and live in ordinary homes and apartments. Figure 5.10 illustrates the efficacy of the teaching interaction when used in a group home with disruptive and aggressive adolescents who have serious mental disorders combined with conduct disorder.

In summary, effectiveness of social skills training with the full spectrum of cognitively impaired persons with mental disabilities requires individualized assessment and goal setting, systematic use of behavioral assessment, precision teaching, and principles of human learning. Skills learned in a classroom-type setting are much more generalizable to community life when patients are given opportunities, encouragement, and reinforcement for using their skills outside the classroom.

▶ Modules for Training Social and Independent Living Skills

An innovation in social skills training has been the design of structured, topical, and prescribed "modules" for the development of know-how and skills for achieving social success and independent living. This variant of skills training has utility for almost all mentally disabled patients across the entire range of functioning because patients can be matched with those modules that fit their particular needs and personal goals. The modules can be readily used in all mental health settings, from private practice offices to community support programs, psychosocial rehabilitation clubs, intensive case management, outpatient clinics, and psychiatric hospitals and day programs.

An advantage of a modular approach to skills training is its "user-friendliness," which enhances its exportability to practitioners of all disciplines who work in settings with varied resources. As depicted in Figure 5.11, each module is self-contained, with a trainer's manual, a participant's

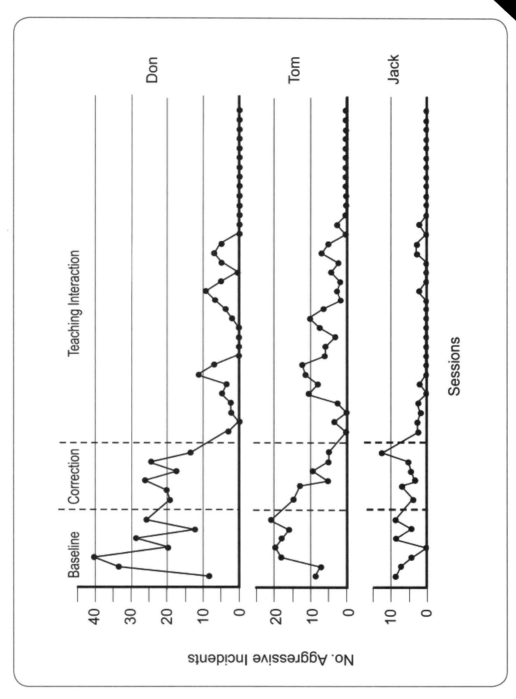

FIGURE 5.10 Improvements in the social behavior of three adolescents with combined conduct disorder and serious mental disorders as a function of the introduction of the *teaching interaction*, a variant of social skills training. Counselors were trained to use the teaching interaction in a group home whenever verbal or physical aggression occurred or was threatened.

FIGURE 5.11
Examples of a trainer's manual, participant's workbook, DVD or videocassette, and a video playback system for a skills training module.

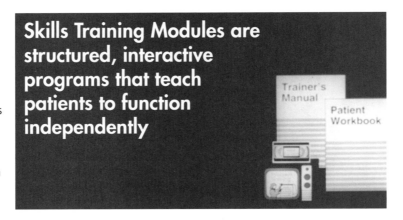

Skills Training Modules are structured, interactive programs that teach patients to function independently

Trainer's Manual

Patient Workbook

workbook, a user's guide, and a DVD or videocassette that serves to demonstrate the skills for the respective module. With a highly prescriptive trainer's manual, mental health workers who are experienced in working with their mentally disabled patients can lead skills training groups without substantial in-service training or external consultation.

What does make a difference, however, are trainers who have natural teaching skills; that is, spontaneity, enthusiasm, and a desire to reach out and individualize the training to patients in the group. Module trainers can be activity and occupational therapists, mental health associates, social workers, nurses, nursing assistants, rehabilitation technicians, psychiatrists, or psychologists. Even patients who have graduated from one or more modules and are good communicators have effectively served as module leaders.

Because many mentally disabled patients share a common spectrum of skills deficits for independent living, why not "package" a generic set of training materials to remediate these areas of disability? Think of mentally disabled persons as needing to attend a school for community integration. Some higher-functioning patients may need to take only one course or module, say in substance abuse management (Roberts et al. 1999). Others who had poor premorbid functioning and developed their illness before having had opportunities to learn life skills may sign up for four modules, two in the morning and two in the afternoon, 4 days per week. The bottom line is that participation in modules is individualized—one suit does not fit all. Table 5.14 lists the modules that are currently available through Psychiatric Rehabilitation Consultants (P.O. Box 2867, Camarillo, CA 93011-2867; 805-484-5663; www.psychrehab.com).

One advantage to generic packaging of skills training in modules comes from the standardization of the training protocol from one module to another. The skills being taught are vastly different, but for the wide

● **TABLE 5.14**

Modules of the UCLA Social and Independent Living Skills Program

Medication Management	Symptom Management	Substance Abuse Management
Community Re-entry	Basic Conversation Skills	Friendship and Intimacy
Recreation for Leisure	Workplace Fundamentals	Involving Families in Services

diversity of mental health and rehabilitation professionals and paraprofessionals who use them, familiarity breeds contentment, competence, and consistency. Because the modules' training manuals provide detailed, step-by-step instructions, the modules can be used with minimal orientation and education for the practitioner. Clinicians can obtain direct exposure to module procedures by using a self-paced DVD or videocassette training program that features multidisciplinary practitioners demonstrating each of the learning activities with real patients. In these training videos, annotation by the narrator of each learning activity offers the neophyte trainer further information and pointers for conducting social skills training. For the practitioner, modules offer a structured protocol for teaching skills to patients that allows rapid and faithful delivery of the essential training while still permitting leeway for the personality and individual, interpersonal style of the trainer.

For the patient, the module format mandates active and increasing degrees of participation in the therapeutic process, with the goal of enhanced ability to use the functional area of each module independently. The trainer or therapist teaches the skills using a combination of video demonstrations, focused instructions, specialized role-plays, social and video feedback, and practice in the "real world." Each module consists of a set of sequential learning activities that:

- Introduce the patients to the purpose and rationale for the module and heighten their motivation to participate.
- Train patients in the skills required to fulfill their needs in the subject area of the module.
- Teach the patients how to gather the resources they will require to put their skills to use.

- Teach patients how to anticipate and solve problems that might be encountered as they try to employ their skills.
- Arrange for practice of the skills in the "real world," followed by autonomously completed homework assignments.

SKILL AREAS AND LEARNING ACTIVITIES

The organizational content of each module, as shown in Table 5.15, comprises a number of skill areas that, when integrated and cumulatively learned, provide the abilities and knowledge to cope with and surmount the challenges presented by that segment of life in the community. Each module is divided into separate skill areas, with each area having specific, target behaviors for training. Thus, the skill areas composing the *Basic Conversation Skills Module* enable patients to acquire the skills required for starting, maintaining, and terminating conversations with others in their natural environments.

The specific behavioral criteria required for patients to learn in the skill area "Keeping a Friendly Conversation Going," included in the Basic Conversation Skills Module, are shown diagrammatically in Figure 5.12. In the first skill area of this module, "Starting a Friendly Conversation," patients learn "conversational openers" such as:

- Choosing a topic from something in the immediate situation (e.g., book, picture, activity, time of day, weather).
- Talking about something that you and the other person are doing (e.g., waiting in line, purchasing a commodity, watching a game or event).
- Complimenting the other person for his/her appearance or behavior.
- Asking a question about what the other person is doing.
- Asking for or giving information or an opinion.
- Saying "hello" or "hi" and introducing yourself.

The modules are designed to teach patients two types of competencies: 1) the ability to perform skills necessary for successful community adjustment and 2) the ability to solve problems that arise as obstacles to the use of these skills. The skills taught in each module have been identified as important for functioning by mental health and rehabilitation professionals, patients themselves, and family members.

The skills in each module are taught through seven highly prescribed learning activities (as shown in Figure 5.13), which are repeated in each

● TABLE 5.15

Skill areas of a subset of the modules for training social skills

● **Medication Management**
  » Understanding benefits of psychotropic medications: therapeutic and prophylactic
  » Learning self-administration of medication and self-monitoring of its effects
  » Identifying minor and serious side effects of medication
  » Negotiating medication issues with a psychiatrist or other health care provider
  » Learning benefits of long-acting injectable medication

● **Symptom Management**
  » Identifying warning signs of relapse
  » Monitoring warning signs and developing a relapse prevention plan
  » Coping with persisting symptoms
  » Understanding the hazards of alcohol and illicit drugs of abuse

● **Substance Abuse Management**
  » Receiving basic training in damage control, an emergency card, habits and control of craving, high-risk situations, warning signs, healthy pleasures, and healthy habits
  » Quitting after a slip
  » Reporting and self-disclosing a slip
  » Refusing drugs offered by a dealer
  » Refusing drugs offered by a friend or relative
  » Getting a support person
  » Asking someone to join you in a healthy pleasure
  » Negotiating money management with a representative payee

● **Basic Conversation Skills**
  » Developing verbal and nonverbal communication skills: "go" and "no go" signals for conversations
  » Starting a friendly conversation
  » Keeping a friendly conversation going
  » Ending a conversation pleasantly
  » Putting all the skills together

● **Recreation for Leisure**
  » Identifying benefits of recreational activities
  » Getting information about recreational activities
  » Finding out what's needed for a recreational activity
  » Starting, evaluating, and maintaining a recreational activity

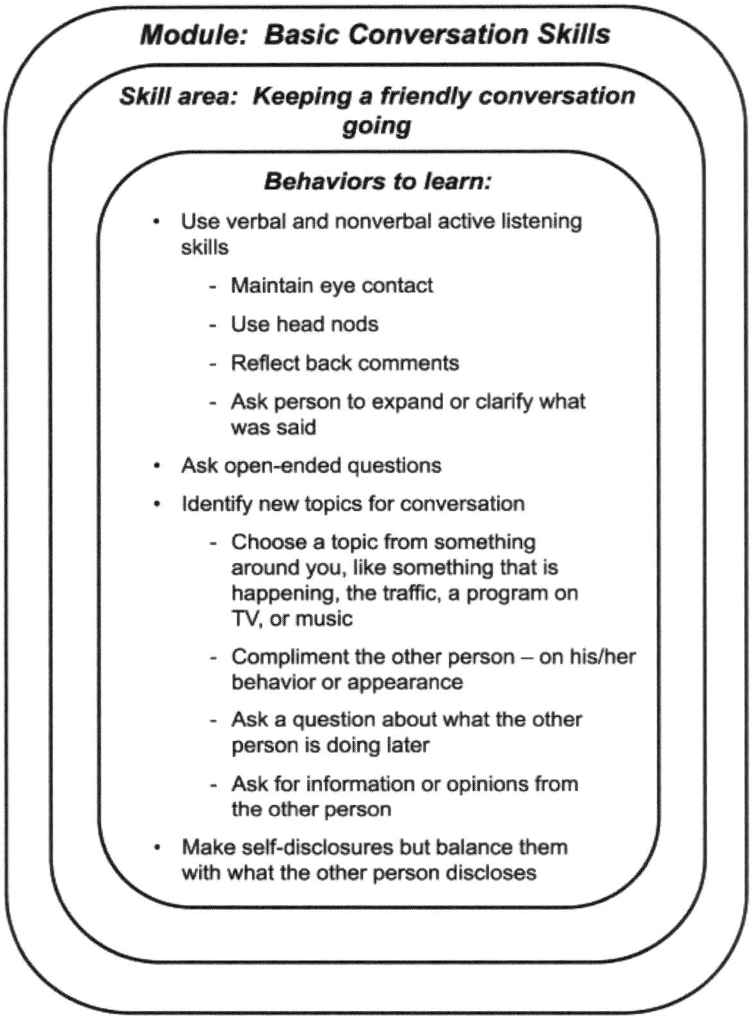

FIGURE 5.12 Educational or specific behavioral objectives in the skill area "Starting a Friendly Conversation" in the Basic Conversation Skills Module.

skill area. The learning activities are infused with principles of learning that facilitate patients' acquiring the know-how and behavioral skills of the module. One might view the learning activities of a module as tantamount to special education for the mentally disabled.

To guide trainers through the complexities of the seven learning activities, each activity is preceded by explicit directions to the clinician regarding the outline of the educational objectives of each learning activity, a list of resources and materials needed (e.g., videocassette, flip chart or whiteboard, handouts for the participants), and a summary of the steps to follow in leading the participants in the learning activity.

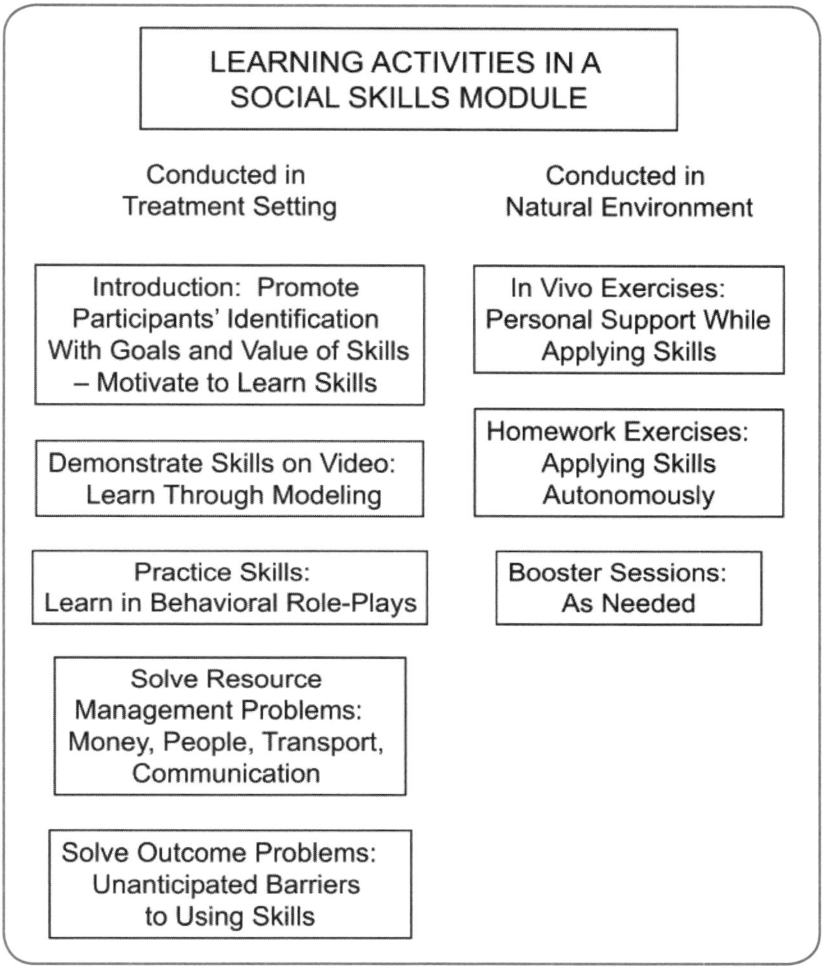

LEARNING ACTIVITIES IN A
SOCIAL SKILLS MODULE

Conducted in
Treatment Setting

Conducted in
Natural Environment

Introduction: Promote
Participants' Identification
With Goals and Value of Skills
– Motivate to Learn Skills

In Vivo Exercises:
Personal Support While
Applying Skills

Demonstrate Skills on Video:
Learn Through Modeling

Homework Exercises:
Applying Skills
Autonomously

Practice Skills:
Learn in Behavioral Role-Plays

Booster Sessions:
As Needed

Solve Resource
Management Problems:
Money, People, Transport,
Communication

Solve Outcome Problems:
Unanticipated Barriers
to Using Skills

FIGURE 5.13 Learning activities used to teach the educational or behavioral objectives for each skill area in each module.

Introduction to the Skill Area

In the introduction, patients are encouraged to identify the goals of the module and of each skill area, the steps necessary to achieve the goals, and the benefits that will accrue if the goals are achieved. The aim here is to connect patients' participation in the learning activities of each module's skill area with their own, individualized personal goals. This process is termed *motivational interviewing* because it strengthens patients' determination to participate in the module. In addition, the exchange of questions and answers in this exercise introduces patients to the terminology used in various aspects of the training.

EXAMPLE

The following dialogue from the Introductory Learning Activity of the second skill area of the Basic Conversation Skills Module, "Starting a Friendly Conversation," is repeated with each participant in attendance until all members have shown that they understand the purpose and value of the module for themselves.

TRAINER: What will you learn in this skill area?

DON: I'll learn to find places where there are people to talk to, people who are willing to talk with me, and topics for starting friendly conversations.

TRAINER: That's right. How will learning these skills benefit you? For example, how will the skills help you reach your own particular goals?

DON: I'll know how to start conversations with people and that will give me a chance to get out to places for recreation, make friends, and spend time with other people instead of being so lonely and bored at my care home.

TRAINER: You've got it! I can see that you understand how this class will be useful to you and your personal goals. What will you learn during the entire module?

DON: I'll learn how to start conversations, keep them going, and end them without feeling embarrassed.

TRAINER: Very good! That's as good a summary as I've heard of what you'll be learning and why it's worthwhile.

Videotape and Questions and Answers

In the second learning activity, patients view videotaped demonstrations of correct performance of the skills. The tape or DVD is stopped periodically to allow the trainer to ask questions that assess and sustain the patient's attentiveness and comprehension.

If there are incorrect answers, feedback is provided and the videotape or DVD is replayed. Presenting the information until it is understood allows patients to proceed at their own pace, thereby individualizing the training even though it is offered in a group.

Role-Playing

In the third learning activity, patients are asked to role-play or practice the skills they have just viewed. Videotaping this performance for subsequent review is recommended. When reviewing the role-play, the trainer and

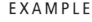

EXAMPLE

The video has shown four young adults talking about their learning experiences in a conversation skills class they are taking. The trainer checks for participants' learning the skills by using a question-and-answer protocol.

TRAINER: Name three types of places that the people on the video said were good for meeting people.

JOE: Places where people get together, like parks, and places where you go frequently, like coffee shops.

TRAINER: Right on, Joe. There's one other type of place where you can find people to have brief but friendly chats. Marie, can you help out with this third type of place?

MARIE: Yes, they're places where you'd be standing around or waiting in line for a while—like a bus stop, a supermarket checkout counter, or a concert or ball game.

TRAINER: Exactly. You've hit it right on the nose, Marie. OK, we've got all three types of places. Now, I'm going to ask each of you in the group to tell me what types of places they are. Remember: places where people get together, where you go often, and where you'll be hanging around or waiting in line for a while with others.

---

other patients evaluate the performance for the presence of such behavior as good eye contact, alert posture, and audible voice volume—in other words, good communication skills. Feedback is presented in a positive light, with the destructive consequences of criticism minimized. Role-plays are repeated as many times as needed for patients to demonstrate the knowledge and skills depicted in the videotape.

Videotaping of the role-play can be used for reinforcing the adaptive elements of the patient's behavioral repertoire demonstrated during the rehearsal. As shown in Figure 5.14, video feedback is provided after the role-play, and the patient, other members of the group, and the trainer focus on the positive elements in the patient's performance. Positive feedback is solicited and, because it is contingent on the positive skills shown by the patient, has a profound effect on the patient's learning and subsequent implementation of the skills of each learning activity.

Resource Management

After each skill has been correctly role-played, patients are taught how to obtain and manage the resources required to use that particular skill. Resources must be gathered for patients to implement a particular com-

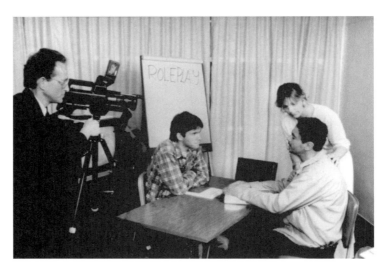

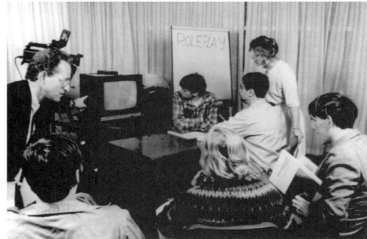

FIGURE 5.14 Video feedback is used to provide "self as model" and to reinforce the patient's verbal and nonverbal behaviors in the role-play learning activity of a module.

munity living skill. For example, even if an individual has the skills to perform competently during a job interview, he/she needs money, clothes, a typed résumé, and transportation to attend the interview. The training methods consist of role-played exercises and interactions designed to assess the patient's ability to process the various alternatives open for effective resource management. The trainer describes the skill and then asks a series of questions designed to have patients actively consider the resources they might need to perform the skill. Resources usually fall into the categories of *time, money, people, places, materials, transportation, telephone, Internet,* and *clothing.* For each resource mentioned, patients discuss how they could go about obtaining it. Patients then evaluate each resource by deciding what the advantages and disadvantages might be.

EXAMPLE

In the Resource Management learning activity of the Basic Conversation Skills Module, the trainer solicits ideas from participants about resources for getting to a park for a concert where there will be people who have similar interests with whom to start conversations.

TRAINER: What resources will you need to be able to use your skills of starting friendly conversations at a concert in the park?

BRITNEY: We won't need money because the concert is free. But it would be good to bring a cushion or blanket to sit on and something to drink during the concert. And we'd need to have transportation to the park, and there's no bus line that goes there.

TRAINER: What other ways could you get there besides by bus?

MIKE: We could walk or take a taxi. But taxis are expensive."

HAL: Or hitchhike.

PAT: I don't think it's safe to hitchhike if you're by yourself. But I could ask my brother to drive me over there.

After exhausting most alternatives for transportation, the trainer and participants consider the feasibility of each one, leading each person to make a judgment that fits his/her own situation, preferences, and potential resources.

Outcome Problems

After patients have been trained to marshal the necessary resources, they are taught to solve the problems presented when the environment fails to respond as expected and unanticipated barriers to effective use of knowledge and skills must be overcome. Inevitably, patients will encounter unexpected obstacles to obtaining their goals, despite their best presentation of skills.

For example, the trainer might open this learning activity by saying, "Pretend you're at a party and see a person you'd like to start a conversation with across the room. He's alone, but as you walk toward him to introduce yourself, two other guys start talking with him. What do you do in that situation?" Each of the participants in the module is asked for his/her ideas, first without considering their feasibility. The brainstorming generates a lot of ideas, some of them humorous, which adds some pizzazz to the learning process. Each idea is then evaluated for feasibility, advantages, and disadvantages. In the case of the party, some alternatives are to 1) wait until there's a break in the conversation; 2) find another person to start a conversation with; and 3) go to a small group of people who are conversing, listen to their conversation, and then wait for a pause to join in.

Without training in problem solving, many patients will respond to such baffling and frustrating experiences with social withdrawal, demoralization, anger, hostility, passivity, or stereotyped symptoms. By teaching the patient a variety of alternative response modes, the patient becomes more resilient and better able to clear obstacles out of the way of goals. Here, as for resource management, problem-solving skills are systematically applied.

The trainer begins by reading a description of an attempt to use the skill and the obstacle posed by the environment. The trainer then asks the patients questions designed to have them consider a variety of alternatives that might remove the obstacle. The entire problem-solving process is aided by the use of a form listing seven steps for problem solving. The stepwise approach to problem solving was described earlier in this chapter (see "Training Social Problem-Solving Skills"), and the form used for learning the steps is shown in Figure 6.7 in Chapter 6 ("Involving Families in Treatment and Rehabilitation"). Again, there are no predetermined answers. The use of the systematic problem-solving process for each skill area helps the patient to internalize this process for use in everyday life.

In Vivo Exercises

It is imperative that patients have the opportunity to practice in the natural environment the skills they have learned. In vivo exercises take the patients out of the training group—but not too far out. Patients perform the skills in their world, with the trainer along to observe their performance as well as to provide prompting, encouragement, and positive feedback. An example of an in vivo exercise for a person in the Basic Conversation Skills Module would be to start a conversation with the receptionist at the mental health center after establishing a few questions about that person's background and interest in her job that are appropriate for interacting with a relative stranger.

Homework Assignments

Finally, patients are given the opportunity to perform independently the skills they have learned. Since it is the goal of the program to teach them to function independently, this represents the ultimate step in training. Wherever possible, patients' performances are evaluated by examining tangible evidence or permanent products of their efforts. For example, if the assignment is to obtain information about medication from a community pharmacist, the patient can report the information to the therapist and bring back the pharmacist's business card.

A central task for the trainer of skills in modules or other formats, which carries the greatest importance for generating and maintaining motivation to learn, is to give frequent, enthusiastic, and genuine positive reinforcement *contingent upon the specific behavioral responses and examples of learning of the participants in the group.* Because teaching even the most disabled individuals yields progress when clinicians use the full array of behavioral learning principles, there are few more rewarding enterprises in psychiatric practice than training social skills.

LEARNING EXERCISE

Now that you have been exposed to the various models for conducting systematic and structured social skills training, it's time to evaluate your own skills in using this modality with your patients. Respond to these decision-making requests to help you actually use what you have learned from this chapter.

List four individuals for whom social skills training would be appropriate. These can be either patients whom you have primary clinical responsibility for or patients whom you have clinical contact with during the week. Of these four patients, which one do you think you would be most likely to be successful with in using the social skills treatment methods?

What general problem area (e.g., obtaining employment, meeting new friends, talking with a family member) would you choose to work on with this patient? Describe the specific scene and task that you would create to give the patient a chance to practice this new behavior. At what specific place and at what specific time would you be doing this social skills training? What behavior(s) could you or someone else model for the patient that he/she could learn from? What realistic, "outside the therapy session" assignment could you give the patient based on his/her performance?

Review the checklist of therapist generic competencies shown in Table 5.9 before and after applying the methods of social skills training to one or more of your patients. Then check off those skills that you feel you've gotten under your belt.

▶ Effectiveness of Social Skills Training

Social skills training has found a place in the treatment of numerous psychiatric disorders and problems. Evidence supports its efficacy in schizophrenia, depression, bipolar disorder, social anxiety, borderline personality disorder, somatoform disorders, marital discord, conduct disorder, and developmental disorders. While considering the amassed evidence supporting the effectiveness of social skills training in schizophrenia and other disabling mental disorders, we must keep in mind that, like medications or other single treatments, this technique is never used as a stand-alone modality. Recovery is not achieved by skills alone. Even the most socially competent individuals without mental disorders will encounter stressors and problems that will not be readily surmounted. Social skills training is one therapeutic component, along with the many others described in this manual, that when carefully combined can raise a patient's prospects for recovery.

ASSESSMENT OF EFFECTIVENESS OF SOCIAL SKILLS TRAINING

Any evaluation of the efficacy of social skills training requires methods for determining the impact and outcomes of training. Outcomes can be viewed on a continuum of time and space. At the most proximal level, measurement of the acquisition of skills that was the mainspring of the training is a logical point of departure. Greater weight can be given to the impact of training when skills that were similar to, but not the same as, the ones trained show significant improvement. The most challenging outcomes are those distal to the focus of training—for example, when skills related to social judgment are learned and these, in turn, enable the individual to make sound and realistic decisions regarding money management and choice of friends.

In evaluating skills training, it is essential to understand what this modality can be expected to accomplish for individual patients and what outcomes are simply out of the question. For example, it is certainly reasonable to forecast the impact of training on the completion of homework assignments. There is a reasonable expectation that the skills practiced in a clinic session will be used in real life, since the skills rehearsed at the training site were those chosen by the patient to put into real-life action. However, to fairly weigh the completion of homework assignments as indicative of putting skills to use in one's everyday life, it's necessary for clinicians to give realistic and attainable homework assignments. Generalization of skills into patients' natural environments also requires trainers to promote accountability by inquiring at the start of each session about the results of each person's homework assignment. Further, abundant positive reinforcement must be proffered for any approximation to the completion of the homework.

From another angle, for skills to be durable and to transfer to patients' natural environments, training must be of sufficient duration, intensity, and extensiveness. Many studies of social skills training conducted during the 1970s and 1980s were relatively brief and delimited in focus, so it's not surprising that the outcomes were modest. Training frequency of twice or more per week for durations of up to 18 months has become more the rule than the exception in studies of the past 15 years.

Also, skills training programs are increasingly incorporating methods for providing opportunities, encouragement, and reinforcement for patients using the skills in their everyday lives. As would be expected, these more recent studies have shown greater efficacy, effectiveness, durability, and generalizability. The reasonable next step would be to design social skills training for indefinite, long-term use in customary clinical settings, not unlike the time-unlimited, continuous, and flexible availability of medication management, supportive case management, supported employment, and supported housing.

Given the cognitive deficits of many persons with mental disabilities plus the erosion of skills that are insufficiently practiced or reinforced, continuation therapy is simply essential if the full range of social and independent living skills is to be sustained and strengthened.

> "A key component of community integration of the seriously mentally ill is an active approach to the analysis and modification of social systems, including engineering natural environments that maximize adaptation. This social and community approach leaves open the possibility that many adverse outcomes can be averted by effective consultation with families, neighbors, clubs, employers, schools and social organizations."
>
> R.P. LIBERMAN, L.W. KING, AND W.J. DERISI (1976)

Recovery requires that long-term environmental supports and contingencies of reinforcement buttress skills that were learned in mental health settings. Natural rather than professional supports can be harnessed to transform skills into higher levels of social functioning for community life (Liberman et al. 1976; Tauber et al. 2000; Tharp and Wetzel 1969).

LEARNING AND RETENTION OF SOCIAL SKILLS

Because of schizophrenia patients' psychotic symptoms and cognitive deficits, many clinicians may question the cost-effectiveness of investing in skills training services. But these learning disabilities are the main reason for offering social skills training to persons with schizophrenia. Social skills training capitalizes on the implicit or procedural learning and memory capacities of individuals with schizophrenia that are not compromised by this neurodevelopmental disorder. The techniques inherent in social skills training tap implicit learning processes that facilitate the acquisition of targeted behaviors: repetition, role-playing and behavioral rehearsal, social modeling, and shaping of skills through reinforcement of successive approximations.

There is no question that social skills training, when competently carried out, results in predictable learning among persons with schizophrenia.

Attesting to its efficacy are more than 100 research studies, backed up by numerous meta-analyses, reviews of the literature, catalogues of best practices, and endorsement by practice guidelines such as those of the American Psychiatric Association. The types of skills that have been learned range from basic conversation to job maintenance and from communication with family members to assertiveness with social agencies.

Examples of the learning of four types of skills relevant to the recovery of persons with mental disabilities are depicted in Figure 5.15: medication self-management, symptom self-management, basic conversation, and recreation for leisure. Patients with schizophrenia and other disabling mental disorders were randomly assigned to receive 6 months of training in these skills, to participate in expressive arts and crafts, or to receive treatment as usual. Patients in both types of psychosocial services also received treat-

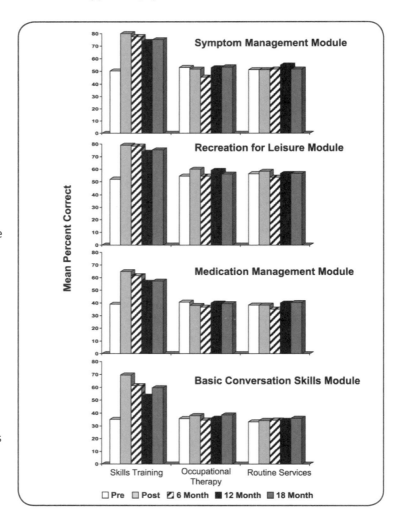

FIGURE 5.15 Evidence for the specific effects of social skills training on the learning of targeted skills in several areas of community functioning for patients at a community mental health center. Patients with serious mental disorders who received social skills training exhibited large-scale increases in the skills taught, whereas individuals who received other forms of treatment showed no improvement in these skills.

ment as usual that included case management and medication management. Not only was there significantly greater acquisition of skills when specific training was used, but the skills remained at a high level for 2 years after the start of training (Wallace et al. 2001). The specific efficacy of skills training was demonstrated by the lack of skills acquisition in the two comparison groups.

GENERALIZATION OF SOCIAL SKILLS TRAINING TO COMMUNITY LIFE

Do social skills that are improved in training have a broader or more generalized impact on novel situations, community functioning, and other measures of well-being? There are several ways to promote generalization of social skills to the natural environment. Adhering to the following guidelines can improve the likelihood that skills get used in real-life situations:

- Help patients to select frequently occurring, realistic, attainable interpersonal interactions that are related to their personal long-term goals.
- Always give specific homework assignments and positive reinforcement for their successful completion and even for effort.
- Anticipate obstacles that may interfere with application of the skills by engaging the patient in a problem-solving process.
- View social skills training as a transformational, gradual, long-term process that may take years for patients to achieve their personal goals.
- Be persistent and persevere, giving opportunities, encouragement, and positive reinforcement for efforts to put skills into everyday use.
- Be generous with positive feedback, for even small steps can make a difference in giving hope to patients for continued progress.

When patients with schizophrenia are given opportunities, encouragement, and positive reinforcement for using skills in novel community settings that have been learned in a hospital, clinic, or office, generalization usually takes place.

Often, the use of homework assignments is a sufficient spur to generalization, since such exercises embody opportunities, encouragement, and then positive reinforcement when the assignment is successfully completed. A socially isolated young woman with schizophrenia attending a weekly social skills training group set numerous goals during the training sessions. She reported success in implementing the skills required for those goals more than 70% of the time. Her principal goal was to develop friendships. She practiced stepwise skills involving social communication and interpersonal relationships in the group, which were then further developed as homework assignments to implement in her everyday life. Results are shown in Table 5.16, reflecting her progress toward dating and friendships.

As documented by a 2-year study of social skills training with 80 outpatients with schizophrenia, when provisions are made to encourage utilization of the skills learned in a clinic to patients' everyday lives, generalization is clearly seen in patients' community functioning. Patients were randomly assigned to expressive and insight-oriented occupational therapy or training in social and independent living skills. The skills training consisted of a curriculum using Basic Conversation Skills, Recreation for Leisure, Medication Management, and Symptom Management Modules (Liberman et al. 1998).

● **TABLE 5.16**

Sequential homework assignments given to a young woman with long-term schizophrenia whose personal goals were to expand her social network by making new friends and eventually dating

- *Invite parents to attend church with you and provide encouragement for you to ask the minister about joining the young adults' social group.*
- *Phone coordinator of the social group and obtain information about date, time, place, and number and gender of participants.*
- *Attend a session of the social group and introduce yourself to other members.*
- Find out three things about one of the group members and share three facts about yourself.
- *Repeated assignment above and achieved it.*
- *Tell group facilitator how much you enjoy and value the group.*
- Invite Terry to join you for coffee after the group.
- *Offer to give a ride home to Terry so she doesn't have to take the bus.*
- *Invite Terry to join you for coffee after the social group.*
- *Ask Terry to choose from among three popular movies and go with her, offering to purchase the popcorn.*
- Ask Terry if it's okay to invite another group member to join you both for coffee after the group.
- *Repeated assignment and achieved it.*
- *Find out about the computer dating service used by Terry.*
- *Invite Josephine to join you and Terry for coffee after the social group.*
- *Ask Terry to accompany you to a speed dating service.*

Note. The assignments that she completed in her community activities are shown in italics.

Treatment consisted of 15 hours of training per week for the first 6 months, with the frequency declining over the next 18 months. Clinical case management was also provided to assist participants in realizing their personal goals. Medications were stabilized and prescribed on an optimal, "doctor's choice" basis. The aim of this study was to determine whether intensive skills training would result in changes in patients' self-esteem, subjective distress, and involvement in community activities. In this study of patients with persistent symptoms, as shown in Figure 5.16, the participants who received the skills training had significantly better social functioning, improved self-esteem, less distress, and a more satisfactory quality of life over the 2-year period.

Conducting treatment research in ordinary clinical settings with unselected patients having comorbidities and with the treatments delivered by the actual staff of the customary facilities—as opposed to research staff—is referred to as *effectiveness research*. Because effectiveness research has

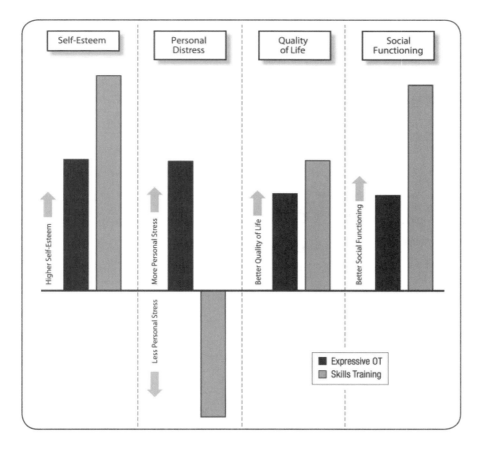

FIGURE 5.16 Generalization of social skills training to overall functioning in the community and quality of life. OT = occupational therapy.

greater generality to the field as a whole, the results of skills training with patients living in state hospitals and community care homes are of interest. In Figure 5.17, results of training in social skills with the UCLA modules in these facilities show clearly that learning does take place. As expected, the long-stay patients in the state hospitals had much lower initial skills than their counterparts living in the community. After training, the patients in the state hospital did not reach the same level of skills achieved by patients living in community residences, but *patients in both types of settings showed significant evidence of learning* (Wallace et al. 1992). In fact, their acquisition of recreation for leisure, conversation, and medication management skills was nearly double that exhibited at the start of training. Patients randomly assigned to treatment as usual showed no apparent increase in skills. *If you want patients to learn skills, you must teach them.*

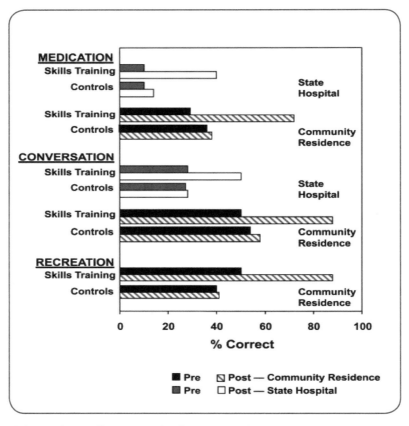

FIGURE 5.17 Effectiveness of skills training modules in customary treatment settings: state hospitals and community residences. Nursing staff members in psychiatric inpatient units and operators of residential care facilities were trained to use modules on a twice-weekly basis with their residents. Consultation was provided by experts in social skills training.

OVERVIEW OF EFFECTIVENESS OF
SOCIAL SKILLS TRAINING

Notwithstanding the evidence in support of the effectiveness of social skills training, there are some individuals with mental disabilities who are less likely to respond to training. Rehabilitation practitioners should never give up on a patient, as even the most challenging and refractory individual has some assets and sources of motivation that can be tapped as a starting point for eventual recovery. Readiness for rehabilitation or social skills training is not decided by an "open" versus "closed" door. The benefit derived from any form of rehabilitation is relative and marked by continua of time, phase of disorder, and amount and rapidity of responsiveness.

So the question is not "Can this person respond to social skills training?" but rather "How can we adapt and apply principles of learning to enable the individual to participate and succeed in social skills training?" For some small proportion of individuals, despite the efforts of the most creative and experienced skills trainers, the training process is slow, arduous, and time-consuming, with progress toward goals measured in tiny increments. Some of the factors that appear to constrain the efficacy of social skills training include:

- Thought disorder with incoherence, derailment, and loose associations
- Frequent distractibility and severe cognitive deficits such as poor attentiveness and memory
- Deficit syndrome or enduring, primary negative symptoms
- High levels of social or performance anxiety, especially when social skills training is conducted in groups
- Difficulties in identifying personally relevant goals that can be used as long-term motivators for the week-by-week interpersonal objectives that are stepping-stones to one's overall goals
- Negativism toward participating in skills training or rehabilitation of any form

Fortunately, methods are being developed and tested that are able to compensate for some of these limitations of learning capacity. For example, research is accumulating that cognitive impairments can be remediated, often with computer-aided instruction, which is described in Chapter 10 ("New Developments for Rehabilitation and Recovery"). Another promising finding is the improvement in cognitive functioning that ensues when training in social skills is used on a daily basis in a milieu permeated by positive reinforcement for adaptive behavior (Spaulding et al. 1999). When patients and trainers engaging in social skills training become discouraged with the pace of progress toward recovery, they should answer two questions before giving up on their efforts:

- Are the personally relevant goals of the patient being carefully parsed so that the training endeavor is functional, attainable, and rewarding?
- Is the trainer adhering to the fidelity competencies required by effective social skills training?

Beyond the characteristics of the individual patient delineated above, ability to benefit from social skills training is influenced by the social environment: interactions and comfort level with the social skills trainer, motivation provided by family members and others close to the patient, and incentives to participate that may be identified from the *reinforcement survey* and *functional assessment* described in Chapter 4 ("Functional Assessment"). Successful participation in social skills training more than any other factor depends on the spontaneity, genuine friendliness, and enthusiasm of the trainer. Learning of social skills is hampered by stilted leadership styles, verbosity, and efforts to explain *why* patients feel or behave the way they do instead of *how, what, when, where,* and *with whom* they may be able to reach their own personal goals.

The general, overall utility of social skills training can be estimated by a statistical technique called *meta-analysis.* Meta-analysis of treatment research includes all studies that have been scientifically designed and carried out, with proper control groups and well-defined patient populations, characteristics of the treatment, and measures of outcome. This statistical approach permits direct comparisons of results across all published studies. A meta-analysis of 22 studies of social skills training for 1,521 persons with schizophrenia found significant efficacy for this modality in:

- Acquiring the skills that were taught in the training sessions.
- Performing social and daily living skills in natural settings.
- Improved community functioning.
- Reduction of negative symptoms.
- A broad array of clinical facilities such as psychiatric hospitals, community mental health centers, day treatment programs, residential care homes, community support programs, assertive community treatment, and psychosocial rehabilitation centers.

The analysis found only small benefits of social skills training on positive psychotic symptoms and relapse (Kurtz and Mueser, in press). The results provide strong evidence for the value of social skills training in elevating the psychosocial adaptation of individuals with schizophrenia. Lest we err

in conflating evidence-based practice with our success using social sk
training with any particular patient, we must not forget that we are trea
ing individuals, not statistical means and levels of significance. After mor
than three decades of research and development, the prospects for recovery
from mental disabilities are boosted by *practice-based evidence* as well as
evidence-based support for social skills training as an element in a comprehensive approach to rehabilitation.

▶ Cross-Cultural Applicability of Social Skills Training

A stern test of the robustness and external validity of a treatment is whether
or not the treatment can be effectively adapted to meet the needs of patients
in different countries with varied ethnic and cultural values and systems of
mental health services. The modules in the UCLA Social and Independent
Living Skills Program have been translated into 23 languages and implemented in countries located in Asia, Africa, Europe, South America, Australia, and North America. Figure 5.18 depicts a map of the world with the
countries darkened that have translated and adopted the modules for clinical
use. In many of these countries, controlled research has been conducted to
document the efficacy of the skills training (Liberman 2007).

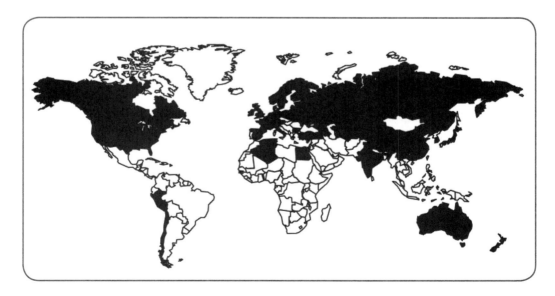

FIGURE 5.18 Countries of the world where social skills training has been implemented using the modules
of the UCLA Social and Independent Living Skills Program.

As an example of the cross-cultural efficacy of social skills training: The largest psychiatric hospital in Tokyo adapted the Community Reentry Module, using 16 sessions of training, for developing a relapse prevention plan and teaching patients how to manage medications independently, how to cope with stress in the community, and how to connect with aftercare services following discharge. The 32 inpatients in this evaluation averaged 47 years of age and had been hospitalized for over 4 years. They had little or no insight into their illnesses and were still experiencing psychotic symptoms. Sixteen patients were randomly assigned to participate in the skills training module, while the same number of patients in a comparison group were randomly assigned to receive 16 sessions of the hospital's standard milieu treatment including occupational therapy. The occupational therapy included participating in prevocational activities and expressing their feelings and concerns through arts and crafts.

Patients who participated in the skills training, but not in the occupational therapy, showed substantial increases in their knowledge and in the skills taught in the module, demonstrated higher levels of functioning, and were more than three times as likely to be discharged from hospital. Superior outcomes for skills training over comparison treatments have been demonstrated in cross-national, controlled studies using the modules of the UCLA Social and Independent Living Skills Program in Poland, Bulgaria, Finland, the Netherlands, Germany, Switzerland, Sweden, Norway, Denmark, France, Turkey, Mexico, Canada (Quebec), Korea, Hong Kong, and China.

▶ Summary

Participation in community life through pursuit of one's desired goals in life requires interpersonal and social skills. Psychotropic medications alone cannot teach any of the skills needed for everyday life. Just as medications and other biological treatments are designed for control of symptoms, social skills training is designed to convey the knowledge and skills for personal effectiveness and successful living. From the vantage point of the vulnerability-stress-protective factors model of major mental disorders, social skills training can be appreciated as one of the major factors protecting against stress-induced relapse and behavioral disabilities. Recovery from mental disabilities is achieved when persons acquire the skills and supports for empowerment, self-responsibility, and a life with dignity, satisfaction, and personal meaning. Many persons whose efforts put them on track for recovery can use their skills and supports to transform their hope for a better future into reality, shedding their mental disabilities and moving closer to a fulfilling life as a normally functioning citizen.

A variety of specific skills are involved in any successful social encounter. These include initiating conversations; giving and asking for information, opinions, and assistance; expressing feelings; making and complying with requests; giving and accepting affection and compliments; and negotiating and resolving differences and conflicts. Cultural norms also play a part in determining the appropriateness of social communication. Because skills must be demonstrated in a large variety of interpersonal contexts, the individual must be attuned to the norms and expectations, the rights and responsibilities, and the needs and goals of himself/herself and others.

Social skills training focuses on affiliative and instrumental skills. The former are needed to develop and sustain social relationships among family and friends. Instrumental interactions function to provide food, shelter, income, and other tangible needs for life. Training social skills requires clinicians to be spontaneous yet systematic, enthusiastic yet analytic and knowledgeable in the use of basic principles of human learning. These principles include specification and operationalization of goals that are relevant to the individual with a mental disorder, motivational enhancement, instructions, cueing, prompting, coaching, positive reinforcement, behavioral rehearsal, generalization programming, and precision teaching.

A large reservoir of empirical studies attests to the effectiveness of social skills training in enabling mentally disabled persons to learn a wide range of skills, retain the skills for lengthy periods of time, and use the skills in their everyday lives. Social validation of skills training is supported by its successful adaptation by mental health professionals in countries throughout the world. In many of these countries, controlled studies have replicated the effectiveness of social skills training that has been found in the United States.

While the technology for social skills training has matured and the empirical validation for its efficacy has grown over the past two decades, its use is still limited to a relatively small number of behaviorally oriented practitioners. Many institutions and clinics offer socialization groups and experiences for the chronically mentally ill, but very few offer structured and systematic social skills training. If a recovery orientation to clinical services is to be more than a shibboleth, teaching skills to patients with cognitive impairments should employ techniques that can overcome their learning abilities. This requires translating basic principles of learning into the educational process. Using conventional, verbally mediated lecture and discussion groups will produce a lot of words but very little action in promoting empowerment, shared decision making, self-directed responsibility, and attainment of personally relevant goals. A major challenge in the field is to promote wider dissemination and faithful use of social skills training. Psychiatric rehabilitation requires *comprehensive* biobehavioral treatments. Therefore, patients with schizophrenia or other disabling mental disorders have their chances of recovery enhanced by social skills training only if they are concurrently receiving antipsychotic medication; illness management; continuing care with supportive, mutually respectful, and reliable therapeutic relationships; intensive case management; supported housing; vocational rehabilitation; financial entitlements; peer support; and family education.

▶ Key Points

- If recovery from a serious mental disorder signifies that a person is participating as a member of the community in meaningful and satisfying ways, social and independent living skills are the "membership dues."
- Social skills are the means for communicating and obtaining needs for instrumental and affiliative roles. Verbal, paralinguistic, and nonverbal behaviors are the currency with which individuals demonstrate their social skills.
- Social competence is the desired outcome of interpersonal interactions wherein mentally disabled persons obtain their immediate and longer-term personal goals by communicating to others with their social skills. A skilled communicator gains social competence only as instrumental and affiliative needs are cumulatively achieved. Social skills are the bridge that enables the mentally ill to cross over from the "near shore" of disability to the "far shore" of competence, social participation, personal responsibility, empowerment, and hope for recovery.
- An information-processing model of social interaction defines the means by which social skills and social competence are acquired. There are three steps in this model:
  » "Receiving skills," or accurate social perception

> » "Cognitive processing skills," or social problem solving
> » "Sending skills," or communication behaviors that enable individuals to obtain their needs and reach their goals

- Acquiring skills empowers individuals for functional, self-directed achievement of their desired roles as worker, student, family member, advocate, and friend. Because of the cognitive and symptomatic impairments inherent in serious mental disorders, "special education" must be used to ensure that skills are learned and then used in everyday life.

- Methods by which human beings learn skills include motivational enhancement, social modeling, behavioral rehearsal, contingent positive reinforcement, shaping and chaining behaviors, prompts and cues, repetition, and homework assignments. Generalization occurs when individuals use the skills learned during training in their everyday lives.

- Mentally disabled persons require supplemental assistance from family and other natural supporters, as well as from practitioners, for opportunities, encouragement, and positive reinforcement to use their social skills in ordinary community settings.

- Internationally, widespread use of social skills training has been facilitated by the development and dissemination of user-friendly, highly structured modules for providing training for a broad spectrum of social and independent living skills: medication and symptom self-management, substance abuse management, basic conversation, recreation for leisure, community re-entry, workplace fundamentals, and friendship and intimacy.

- Social skills training is thoroughly validated as an effective, evidence-based treatment for the seriously mentally ill. When the training incorporates social learning principles, is given in an adequate amount, and is linked to opportunities, encouragement, and reinforcement for using skills, patients with schizophrenia and other mental disabilities can learn and retain social skills and use them to achieve their goals in the community.

▶ Selected Readings

D'Zurilla TJ, Nezu AM: Problem-Solving Therapy: A Social Competence Approach to Clinical Intervention, 2nd Edition. New York, Springer, 1999

Heinssen RK, Liberman RP, Kopelowicz A: Psychosocial skills training for schizophrenia. Schizophr Bull 26:21–46, 2000

Hogarty GE, Anderson CM, Reiss D, et al: Family psychoeducation, social skills training, and maintenance chemotherapy in the after-care treatment of schizophrenia. Arch Gen Psychiatry 43:633–642, 1986

Hollin CR, Trower P (eds): Handbook of Social Skills Training, Vols 1 and 2. Oxford, UK, Pergamon Press, 1986

Kopelowicz A, Liberman RP, Zarate R: Recent advances in social skills training. Schizophr Bull 32 (suppl 1):S12–S23, 2006

Liberman RP, Wallace CJ, Blackwell G, et al: Skills training vs psychosocial occupational therapy for persons with persistent schizophrenia. Am J Psychiatry 155:1087–1091, 1998

Liberman RP, Eckman TA, Marder SR: Training in social problem-solving among persons with schizophrenia. Psychiatr Serv 52:31–33, 2001

Liberman RP, Glynn SM, Blair KE, et al: In vivo amplified skills training: promoting generalization of independent living skills for clients with schizophrenia. Psychiatry 65:137–155, 2002

Linehan MM: Skills Training Manual for Treating Borderline Personality Disorder. New York, Guilford, 1993

▶ References

Bellack AS, Mueser KT, Gingerich S, et al: Social Skills Training for Schizophrenia, 2nd Edition. New York, Guilford, 2004

Brown CE, Rempfer MV, Hamera E, et al: Knowledge of grocery shopping skills as a mediator of cognition and performance. Psychiatr Serv 57:573–575, 2006

Curran JP, Monti PM (eds): Social Skills Training: A Practical Handbook for Assessment and Treatment. New York, Guilford, 1982

Fixsen DL, Phillips EL, Wolf MM: Achievement Place: experiments in self-government with pre-delinquents. J Appl Behav Anal 6:31–48, 1973

Glynn SM, Marder SR, Liberman RP, et al: Supplementing clinic-based skills training with manual-based community support sessions: effects on social adjustment of patients with schizoprenia. Am J Psychiatry 159:829–837, 2002

Hogarty GE: Personal Therapy for Schizophrenia and Related Disorders. New York, Guilford, 2002

Hogarty GE, Kornblith SJ, Greenwald D, et al: Three-year trials of personal therapy among schizophrenic patients living with or independent of family. Am J Psychiatry 154:1504–1513, 1997

Kurtz M, Mueser KT: A meta-analysis of controlled research on social skills training for schizophrenia. J Consult Clin Psychol (in press)

Liberman RP: A behavioral approach to group dynamics: reinforcement and prompting of cohesiveness in group therapy. Behav Ther 1:141–175, 1970

Liberman RP: Reinforcement of social interaction in a group of chronic schizophrenics, in Advances in Behavior Therapy, Vol 3. Edited by Rubin R, Franks C, Fensterheim H, et al. New York, Academic Press, 1972, pp 151–159

Liberman RP, DeRisi WJ, Mueser KT: Social Skills Training for Psychiatric Patients. New York, Pergamon, 1989 (available from Psychiatric Rehabilitation Consultants; www.psychrehab.com)

Liberman RP, DeRisi WJ, King L, et al: Behavioral measurement in a community mental health center, in Evaluating Behavioral Programs in Community, Residential and Educational Settings. Edited by Davidson P, Clark F, Hammerlynck L. Champaign, IL, Research Press, 1974, pp 103–139

Liberman RP, McCann M, Wallace CJ: Generalization of behaviour therapy with psychotics. Br J Psychiatry 129:490–496, 1976

Liberman RP, Wallace CJ, Blackwell G, et al: Skills training versus psychosocial occupational therapy for persons with persistent schizophrenia. Am J Psychiatry 155:1087–1091, 1998

Liberman RP: Dissemination and adoption of social skills training: social validation of an evidence-based treatment for the mentally disabled. Journal of Mental Health 16:553-572, 2007

Moriana JA, Alarcón E, Herruzo J: In-home psychosocial skills training for patients with schizophrenia. Psychiatr Serv 57:260–262, 2006

Phillips DL: Mental health status, social participation and happiness. J Health Soc Behav 8:285–292, 1967

Roberts L, Shaner A, Eckman TA: Overcoming Addictions: Skills Training for People With Schizophrenia. New York, WW Norton, 1999

Salokangas RKR, Honkonen T, Stengard E, et al: Subjective life satisfaction and living situations of persons in Finland with long-term schizophrenia. Psychiatr Serv 57:373–381, 2006

Spaulding WD, Fleming S, Reed D, et al: Cognitive functioning in schizophrenia: implications for psychiatric rehabilitation. Schizophr Bull 25:657–676, 1999

Tauber R, Wallace CJ, LeComte T: Enlisting indigenous community supporters in skills training programs for persons with severe mental illness. Psychiatr Serv 51:1428–1432, 2000

Tharp RG, Wetzel FJ: Behavior Modification in the Natural Environment. New York, Academic Press, 1969

Wallace CJ, Liberman RP, MacKain SJ, et al: Effectiveness and replicability of modules for teaching social and instrumental skills to the severely mentally ill. Am J Psychiatry 149:654–658, 1992

Wallace CJ, Liberman RP, Kopelowicz A, et al: Psychiatric rehabilitation, in Treatments of Psychiatric Disorders, 3rd Edition. Edited by Gabbard GO. Washington, DC, American Psychiatric Publishing, 2001, pp 1093–1112

Involving Families in Treatment and Rehabilitation

Involving Families in Treatment and Rehabilitation

Relatives must learn not to be consumed by their family member's illness. But this is easier said than done because living with schizophrenia is like living on the edge of a volcano.

DONALD RICHARDSON, PAST PRESIDENT,
NATIONAL ALLIANCE FOR THE MENTALLY ILL

NUMEROUS FACTORS have converged during the past three decades to facilitate the development and refinement of evidence-based approaches for strengthening families that are coping with serious mental disorders. The merging of these social and professional movements has led to the germination of therapeutic and educational services for families. Consumed and overwhelmed by the responsibilities for the daily management of relatives with serious psychiatric disabilities, families need and deserve professional assistance (Dixon et al. 2001a; Fadden et al. 1987; Hatfield and Lefley 1987; Tessler and Gamache 2000). Factors that have contributed to a focus on the family include:

1. Deinstitutionalization, which has produced a mass exodus from mental hospitals, reduced accessibility to hospitals for even floridly ill psychotic patients, and increased responsibilities for care and support of the mentally ill by their relatives.
2. Realization that families are not responsible for causing serious mental disorders and deserve the respect, support, attention, and education that they need to participate constructively in the management and treatment of their mentally ill relatives.
3. Empirical studies that have shown how families can serve to protect their ill relatives from relapse and dysfunctional lives if they are prepared to cope with the enormous challenges posed by the illnesses in their midst. In a contrary fashion, patients experience high rates of relapse when living or interacting with relatives who lack the skills and resources to constructively collaborate in the treatment enterprise.
4. Stress and burden experienced by families who are ill equipped to

manage their mentally ill relatives at home. Families have become assertive in requesting information and training to deal with stress that can result in anxiety, depression, and demoralization.

5. Recognition that the stress-induced dysfunctions in communication and problem solving within families are a consequence, not a cause, of mental disorders.

6. Growth of a vital advocacy and self-help movement by relatives of mentally ill persons that has organized nationally and spawned hundreds of local chapters with hundreds of thousands of members.

7. Disenchantment with reliance solely on maintenance antipsychotic medications, with their noxious side effects, for the treatment of schizophrenia. This change in perspective has been accompanied by the realization that while pharmacotherapy can reduce or eliminate symptoms, stress-related relapse and functional decompensation require psychosocial services, including the mobilization of families as a factor in achieving recovery.

8. Development of behavioral, cognitive, and educational methods for clinical problems in psychiatry that offer practical help for patients and families of all social classes and that supersede less applicable psychodynamic and insight therapies.

9. Reduction of stigma of mental illness and increased public awareness about and acceptance of mental disorders as bona fide illnesses that deserve treatment. Reduced stigma has led to families "coming out of the closet" to seek professional assistance to become educated about their relatives' mental disorders, and to advocate for their relatives' treatment and rehabilitative needs.

10. Availability of well-designed and evidence-based practices that can reliably strengthen the coping, communication, and problem-solving skills of the entire family unit, including patients and their relatives.

EXAMPLE

Families of persons with schizophrenia and other disabling disorders usually pass through 10 phases as they try to adjust to living with the uncertain prospects and life-changing challenges of a mentally ill relative. These phases are not always linear but can recur in cycles depending upon the stability of their ill relative and the assistance they receive from psychiatrists, other mental health professionals, and self-help organizations. Having the competence and emotional resilience to assist families as they move through these phases is a major responsibility for clinicians caring for the ill relative. Bearing with the family through the phases requires continuity of collaborative care—too little in evidence in present-day mental health services. The 10 phases are as follows:

1. Initial awareness that a problem exists—early signs of symptoms and abnormal behavior "must be just a phase he/she is going through"
2. Denial of a mental illness—attributing the symptoms to a temporary aberration, stress, or illicit drugs
3. Searching for a cure—"give me my son/daughter back again"
4. Accepting the existence of a mental illness but frustrated by its inadequate, limited treatments
5. Demoralization, depression, anxiety, worry, anger—"it's like losing a loved one, but there's no death and the person is still there but not the same person"
6. Becoming educated and knowledgeable about the illness
7. Advocating for better treatment and rehabilitative services for the ill relative
8. Cycles of optimism and pessimism as new treatments appear promising then fail to deliver sustained improvement or prevent relapses
9. Cumulative know-how in coping with the illness—navigating with increasing confidence through the stormy seas of the inevitable ups and downs of the illness and facilitating access to services
10. Participating in self-help groups, advocating for better services, becoming active in fighting stigma—helping others through the phases of adaptation to long-term illness and disability

---

The new and effective family interventions do not stigmatize families as being "sick" or in need of therapy to "straighten them out." Rather, congruent with the vulnerability-stress-protective factors concept of serious mental disorder (see Chapter 2, "Principles and Practice of Psychiatric Rehabilitation"), family interventions are viewed as conferring added therapeutic protection to the patient and relatives. These interventions have in common practices that are structured, planned, and systematic for teaching coping skills to all members of the family in which a mentally ill member resides. When provided know-how and skills in collaborating with practitioners for managing mental illness, families face fewer stress-induced relapses in their relatives who are vulnerable to psychosis.

Most interventions offer services for all members of the family, including the relative in the family who suffers from a psychiatric disability. Effective family procedures can be conducted by a wide variety of mental health professionals with experience in treating serious mental illness. Competencies in delivering the techniques of family programs, as shown in Table 6.1, are more important than the discipline to which a practitioner belongs. The new and effective interventions vary in small ways, one from another, and have been entitled *behavioral family management, behavioral family therapy, multiple-family therapy, family psychoeducation,* and *family support.* However, the specific names for these similar and overlapping practices of family assistance are largely irrelevant, as they all have survived validation studies over the years.

Educational and supportive programs for families have brought a new optimism to the management of disorders that previously carried a poor prognosis. The optimism is not generated by faddish attachment to an ideology or philosophy of treatment, but rather by availability of pragmatic, well-replicated empirical studies that have documented considerable reductions in relapse rates in patients living in countries worldwide—from China to

● **TABLE 6.1**

Common elements in interventions that provide education, skills, and support to families containing a seriously mentally ill person

- Show empathy and concern and provide opportunities for catharsis and ventilation of stress and helplessness.
- Provide education on the nature of mental illness; its causes, course, and prognosis; resources available in the community for treatment, rehabilitation, and self-help and peer support programs; and social and financial benefits and housing.
- Give practical advice on coping with a mental disorder, including mitigating symptoms, cognitive impairments, and functional disabilities.
- Encourage families to obtain or sustain their own life trajectories, healthy pleasures, relationships, and personal goals.
- Teach family members to acquire appropriate and effective communication skills and use these to reduce stress and improve their relationships in everyday life.
- Teach family members to use their newly learned communication skills in dealing constructively with frequent, daily problems that can include interpersonal friction, disagreements, disappointments, finances, privacy, and independence.
- Assist family members in using modes of stress management and assertiveness in advocating for needed services and resources in the community.

England and from India to the United States. Replicated findings are scarce in psychiatry, so when clinical researchers report upward of 50% reduction in relapse during the 9–24 months following a hospitalization, mental health and rehabilitation practitioners take notice (Dixon et al. 2001a; Lehman et al. 2004; McFarlane et al. 2003; Pitschel-Walz et al. 2001).

▶ Effectiveness of Family Interventions

Clinical, social, family, and economic benefits are achieved by adding psychosocial family interventions to a comprehensive array of services required by persons with mental disabilities. It should be understood that family interventions are not stand-alone modalities; rather, they are coordinated with pharmacotherapy, illness management, crisis intervention, clinical case management, skills training, and supportive services (vocational, educational, housing) that help patients to achieve their personal goals. More than 25 controlled studies of family interventions with favorable outcomes have been published for schizophrenia alone, with many more focusing on disabling forms of depression, bipolar disorder, obsessive-compulsive disorder, and eating disorders (Falloon et al. 1999). Because many of the studies were carried out in different countries, cross-cultural validation adds to their evidence base for efficacy.

When weekly interventions last 6 months or longer—a minimum threshold of sessions for efficacy—significantly greater benefits can be documented for procedures that include structured and educational forms of family intervention compared with services that do not.

The empirically validated benefits of the more substantial, methodical, and well-organized family treatments include:

- Fewer psychotic or affective episodes of exacerbation or relapse by the patient
- Increased self-worth and quality of life by patient and family members
- Enhanced collaborative relationships with psychiatrist and other members of the treatment team and stronger therapeutic alliance
- Markedly reduced hospitalizations
- Improved family morale and less emotional burden
- Better adherence to medication and psychosocial treatments by the patient
- Enhanced social functioning of the patient
- Fewer deaths and suicides
- Better cost-effectiveness

Involving families in services for the seriously mentally ill should be viewed as affording primary and direct benefits to the relatives of the mentally ill person—not just indirect benefits to the patient. Even when patients are no longer living with their families, family members' stress levels are just as high as those in family members whose ill relatives do live at home; moreover, upward of 25% of family members report symptoms that are tantamount to stress-induced psychological disorders.

FAMILY EDUCATION AS A PARADIGM SHIFT IN THE TREATMENT OF SEVERE MENTAL DISORDERS

For more than two centuries prior to 1970, families were either excluded from the treatment of the seriously mentally ill or stigmatized for bearing some of the responsibility for the onset and chronicity of these disorders. During the 150 years of institutional care, patients were effectively exiled from their families to live in closed communities comprising the large, state psychiatric hospitals. The psychoanalytic movement and its derivatives, such as systemic family therapy, spotlighted "family pathology" as having a role in the genesis of schizophrenia and other major mental disorders. These pejorative views of families as sources of psychopathology penetrated the therapeutic ideology of mainstream American psychiatry from the 1920s to the 1970s.

As a psychiatric resident in the 1960s, the author soon became dissatisfied with the refractoriness of his patients with schizophrenia to psychodynamic therapy. He was disenchanted with the indifference of his academic teachers to the evident failures of their theoretically imposing but therapeutically bankrupt psychoanalytic approaches. Seeking alternatives to help his patients improve their functioning so they could resume their long-lost lives in the community, he recognized the practical value of hitching behavioral learning principles to an educational framework for involving families in the treatment of his mentally disabled patients. Family members were seen as positive sources of therapeutic influence for their mentally ill relatives while at the same time in need of knowledge, coping skills, supportiveness, and collaboration with professional caregivers.

The prototype for involving family members as active partners in treatment and rehabilitation is called *behavioral family management* or *behavioral family therapy*. Other, more recent treatments for families are derivatives of the conceptual foundations, goals, and format of this approach.

Drawing from his direct clinical experiences, the author designed and evaluated *behavioral family therapy* in the late 1960s and early 1970s to meet the needs of patients and their family members for coping with serious mental disorders (Liberman 1970, 1972; Liberman et al. 1973, 1980). The term *behavioral family management* was coined because behavioral learning principles and educational techniques were used to help families cope with and *manage* the stress, challenges, and symptoms of interacting with a mentally ill relative. While this approach was certainly "therapeutic" in intent and practical use, the term *therapy* was minimized in the interest of protecting families from the stigma associated with "treatment" and the implicit pathology, sick role, and blame that accompanied the use of this term. With the passage of time, families have assumed a strong and positive role in the treatment of severe mental disorders; hence, the term *therapy* is no longer viewed as pejorative and alienating. Thus, in this book, the terms *behavioral family management* and *behavioral family therapy* will be used interchangeably.

Behavioral family management incorporates methods derived from social learning theory, encompassing structured and directive behavioral techniques such as goal setting, modeling, behavioral rehearsal, coaching, reinforcement, and homework assignments. Patients and their relatives, in joint sessions, learn about schizophrenia and its treatments and practice adaptive communication and problem-solving skills. In 1975, while working in London as an NIH International Research Fellow, the author recruited a young psychiatric resident, Ian Falloon, to test behavioral family management with schizophrenia patients hospitalized at the Maudsley Hospital (Liberman et al. 1984a). The further evolution of this approach included adapting behavioral family management for multiple family groups (Liberman et al. 1984b) and for use as a home-based service (Falloon et al. 1985).

In the first controlled clinical trial of behavioral family management, Falloon studied 36 young adults with schizophrenia who were living at home in stressful relationships with parents. The patients were randomly assigned to in-home behavioral family management or clinic-based supportive, individual therapy. All patients received antipsychotic medication, case management, and other services as needed. Before entering therapy, all patients had had their psychotic symptoms stabilized with at least 1 month of antipsychotic drug treatment. Regardless of treatment condition, all patients followed the same treatment schedule: weekly visits during the first 3 months, biweekly visits for the next 6 months, and monthly visits thereafter for a total of 2 years. In addition to receiving behavioral family management or individual therapy—which was conducted by mental health professionals—all patients were seen monthly at the clinic by a psychiatrist responsible for prescribing optimal doses of neuroleptic drugs. The psychiatrist, as well as other service providers, was blind to the type of psychosocial therapy (Falloon et al. 1985).

The comparative effectiveness of the behavioral family management and individual therapy was assessed by a battery of outcome instruments, including ratings of psychotic symptoms, community tenure, social functioning, family burden, and cost-effectiveness. Statistically significant advantages of behavioral family management were noted in each of the outcome dimensions. The results for clinical outcome are depicted in Figure 6.1. Whereas only 6% of the patients receiving behavioral family management experienced a relapse or exacerbation of their schizophrenic symptoms during the first 9 months of treatment, 44% of those receiving individual therapy did so. The 44% relapse rate actually compares favorably with the approximately 55% relapse rate over a 9-month period in patients returning to live in households marked by stress. Even more promising than the very low relapse rate (6%) among behavioral family management patients is the high rate (56%) of full remission of schizophrenic symptoms at the 9-month point among these individuals, many of whom were functioning relatively normally in social and vocational roles.

Two years after treatment began, at the point when the behavioral family management entered a "maintenance" stage, the relapse rates for the two treatment conditions were 11% for behavioral family management and 83% for those in individual therapy. For patients hospitalized during the 2-year

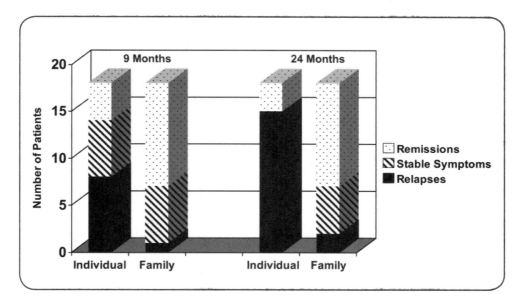

FIGURE 6.1 Comparison of outcomes of schizophrenia patients randomly assigned to behavioral family management or individual supportive therapy (*N*=18 in each group) for 9 and 24 months after entry into the respective treatment programs. By the end of 24 months, 66% of behavioral family management–treated patients had experienced full remission of their psychotic symptoms, compared with only 17% of the individually treated patients. *Source.* Adapted from Falloon et al. 1985.

period, the average number of days spent in the hospital for the behavioral family management patients was 1.8 days per year versus 11.3 days per year for those receiving individual therapy. Since symptoms are only one dimension of outcome, how did behavioral family management affect patients' social adjustment? Whether one evaluated overall social adjustment, leisure activities, family life, self-neglect, work, or friendships outside the family, the patients receiving behavioral family management had significantly better outcomes. Family burden was vastly reduced for the relatives receiving behavioral family management but little changed for relatives of patients getting individual therapy. Even though the costs for time and transportation of therapists to the behavioral family management home sessions were higher than those of the clinic-based program, the much lower rates of rehospitalization and other clinical services for the behavioral family management patients yielded a much better cost-effectiveness than the individual therapy (Falloon 1986).

At first glance, the results of this research study suggest a major breakthrough in the treatment of schizophrenia. Another interpretation might be, however, that behavioral family management merely improved the medication compliance of patients, which in turn resulted in lower rates of relapse. Data from many other studies of treatment of schizophrenia, however, controvert this interpretation, since approximately 30%–40% of patients relapse in a year even when reliable antipsychotic medication use is assured. Moreover, in this controlled study, the amount of medication prescribed for patients in behavioral family management was about 100 mg/day less, in chlorpromazine equivalents, than that prescribed for their counterparts in individual therapy. Thus, the superior treatment outcomes for behavioral family management were obtained with patients requiring much less antipsychotic medication.

Don't rush to the conclusion, however, that medication is not important for patients participating in behavioral family management. That would be a false assumption. Almost all patients in behavioral family management did require continuation of their maintenance antipsychotic drug, albeit at a lower dose level. In fact, the only patient in the behavioral family management group who relapsed during the first 9 months was an individual who had failed to take his medication regularly. The important lesson from this study that can be carried back into our clinics and mental health centers is that a combination of optimal drug therapy and family management is a potent treatment for mentally disabled patients (Liberman and Liberman 2003; Mueser et al. 1994).

❱ Role of Family Coping Skills in Neutralizing Stress and Vulnerability

Let's try to understand how the remarkable results from Dr. Falloon's study relate to the stress-vulnerability-coping-competence model of mental disorder (see Chapter 2). Individuals with the neurobiological vulnerability to schizophrenia or other major mental disorders are extraordinarily sensitive to stressors. A wide variety of stressors can provoke an episode of illness or exacerbate existing levels of symptoms and cognitive impairments. Stressors may occur as time-limited life events—for example, loss of a job, termination with a valued therapist, death of a loved one, moving to another residence or city. Longer-lasting, ambient tensions in a person's day-to-day environment can also function as stressors. These usually affect everyone in the family and can include social withdrawal, feelings of helplessness, demoralization, subtle or overt interpersonal conflicts, and unpredictability in the home environment.

Stressors external to the family, such as when a patient is denied Social Security benefits or a family member becomes unemployed, can heighten the ambient stressors within the family because of financial pressures. Ongoing family stress, including disappointments that ensue from a patient's failure to meet community standards of behavior, may summate until it exceeds a threshold of vulnerability above which a relapse or exacerbation of florid symptoms may occur. Coping with stressors can be impeded by awkward and ineffective efforts at communication and problem solving among family members. Expressing ideas and feelings, making requests of each other, and breaking big problems into small steps are skills that few families have mastered. The ways in which effective and ineffective communicating and problem solving interact with stressors can increase or decrease the risk of relapse, as shown in Figure 6.2.

Behavioral family management aims to inculcate coping skills through teaching patients and their relatives better ways of communicating and solving daily problems. In fact, Falloon discovered that patients and their relatives did improve their coping and problem-solving skills as a result of being exposed to behavioral family management. Those families that displayed the greatest improvements in coping also had the best clinical outcomes. We might postulate, therefore, that the enhanced problem-solving capacity of patients and their relatives in the behavioral family management program blunted the pathogenic impact of stressors on the schizophrenic disorder.

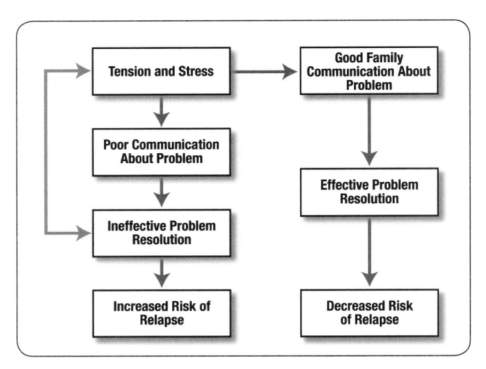

FIGURE 6.2 Constructive and positive communication skills are used for effective problem-solving that reduces tension and stress within the family, thereby decreasing the risk of relapse. Lack of communication skills yields ineffective problem solving and a reverberating cycle of increasing stress that increases the risk of relapse.

Moreover, improved coping and competence in these families enabled patients to remain out of the hospital with little in the way of schizophrenic symptoms and with less need for the protective antipsychotic effects of medication.

In the stress-vulnerability-coping-competence model, psychobiological vulnerability is an enduring trait that changes slowly, if at all, in response to environmental, personal, or biological events. If vulnerability did not change significantly and yet medication needs were reduced, how then did behavioral family management–induced coping and competence promote such positive outcomes? As can be seen in Figure 6.3, the relapse threshold is more easily exceeded by patients living in households where tension and stress are at a high pitch. Given the unpredictable and unsettling experience of living with schizophrenia at home, most families understandably struggle with high levels of tension and stress. Behavioral family management, by providing patients and relatives alike with problem-solving skills, enables the family group to directly address sources of stress, such as finding ways to allow one another needed privacy or having more effectiveness in dealing

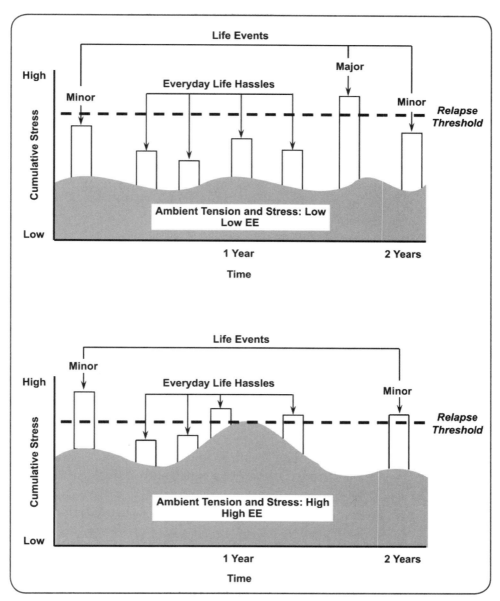

FIGURE 6.3 Ambient levels of tension and stress within the family of a person with schizophrenia are additive with intercurrent life events and daily hassles that may exceed the vulnerability threshold for relapse of the individual with schizophrenia. High expressed emotion (EE) consists of relatives whose stress from living with a family member with schizophrenia leads to maladaptive coping efforts that include emotional overinvolvement and/or excessively high expectations and criticism of that family member. Low EE consists of emotional attitudes of relatives who are tolerant, supportive, and realistically expectant of the family member who has schizophrenia, thereby providing protection against relapse. The probability of relapse of a person with schizophrenia is three to four times greater in a high EE versus a low EE household. The same stress-related relapses based on family EE are found in major depression, bipolar disorder, and other medical and psychiatric disorders.

with social agencies. Whether the sources of stress emanate from within or outside the family boundaries, they can be deflected by active coping and use of constructive alternatives. In this manner, both ambient levels of tension and external threats to the integrity of the family unit are defused, and the stress experienced by patients and relatives falls considerably below the relapse threshold.

▶ Family Burden of Mental Illness

With the deinstitutionalization of the severely mentally ill and the contraction of mental hospital beds throughout the United States, the burden of caring for the hundreds of thousands of patients with schizophrenic and affective disorders has shifted from hospitals to the family and other community-based agencies. Each year, an estimated one million families receive a mentally ill person back into the home after a psychiatric hospitalization. Approximately 65% of discharged mental patients return to their families, on either a full-time or a part-time, intermittent basis. Since long-term institutional care is becoming rarer, patients tend to spend more time in proximity to their relatives. For example, in the current era of brief, revolving-door hospitalizations for treatment of psychotic and other severe disorders, three times as many patients return to live with their relatives than do patients who are hospitalized for 6 months or longer.

Since the 1950s, psychiatric researchers have documented the emotional, physical, and financial strain imposed upon family members who have the responsibility of caring for a mentally ill person (Jungbauer and Angermeyer 2002). There are a number of elements to this strain, termed *family burden*. One source of family burden derives from the pervasiveness and severity of the symptoms of mental illness and the associated impairments in most spheres of life. Schizophrenia, for example, presents family members with immense challenges to understand, react to, contain, and cope with thought disturbances, delusions, hallucinations, and incoherence; in addition, the impairments in work, recreation, affects, habits, activities of daily living, and socializing create even more difficult dilemmas for caring relatives. How are family members to cope with inappropriate or bizarre behavior, tenaciously held false beliefs, extreme social withdrawal, unpredictable moodiness and irritability, and even violence?

Most American families would prefer to see their young adult children develop independence and competence for life on their own. In contrast to the prevailing cultural norms in the United States, some cultural and ethnic groups, such as Latino and Asian families, encourage closer and more enduring family ties and extended kin networks. But even in the case of cultural diversity, almost all parents enjoy the successful transition of their children away from the family home. Just at the time when independence is expected to occur, individuals who are biologically predisposed to serious mental illness can break down with schizophrenic or major affective disorders. The emergence into independent adulthood is halted and, in many cases, interrupted for long periods of time. The symptoms and associated social and occupational impairments of major mental disorders interfere with the maturational process. As a result, whether they were actively promoting a young person's move toward independence or not, parents find themselves having to care for their sick relative, provide food and room for extended periods, expedite the search for treatment and rehabilitation, and undertake a monetarily and emotionally draining commitment.

Another source of burden comes from the heightened economic responsibility that having a nonworking young adult in the household produces. Estimates of the annual costs to families for supporting their mentally ill relative are $13,891 for patients with mental disabilities versus $3,547 for young adult offspring of the same age but without a disability. It is increasingly difficult to obtain financial assistance and entitlements from federal, state, and local authorities. There are also costs and obstacles attached to even public mental health care in the current period of fiscal constraints on government budgets. For example, in Los Angeles County, individuals with private insurance are not accepted for services at county-run mental health centers; indigent patients must first obtain Medicaid to qualify for services, and undocumented immigrants are reluctant to seek services for fear of being returned to their home countries. As co-payments for increasingly expensive psychotropic drugs escalate, many patients discontinue their medication, relapse, and require costly hospitalizations. The huge numbers of patients needing psychiatric services mean that each psychiatrist working in county-affiliated mental health centers has clinical responsibility for 300–400 patients. This translates into visits of 10–15 minutes for medication reviews that are available less frequently than at monthly intervals. In the long run, however, these constraints on public mental health care have been unloaded onto the family, which is expected to pick up the tab and perform the effort required to connect a patient with a therapist, case manager, psychosocial rehabilitation, psychiatrist, and appropriate residential arrangements.

Sometimes, this labor of love leads parents to neglect other children who may be younger than the patient but who appear to require less attention and nurturance. The dependency foisted on families by major mental disorders also can lead spouses to neglect each other and can thus threaten the integrity and satisfaction of a marriage. Therefore, families need assistance in deciding how much they can invest, emotionally and economically, in the continued care and support of a chronically mentally ill relative. They need to sort out their tangled web of emotions and make realistic decisions about their future and the future of their sick relative. Some families will opt to engage in a major caretaking role for extended periods. Others will be able to engage in caretaking intermittently with periods of respite. Some will decide that support and caretaking are beyond their capacities and means and will benefit from professionals who can assist with making arrangements for public assistance funding, residential care facilities, and other social agency support.

However families ultimately decide on the degree of their involvement in caring for their sick relative, the fact is that scarce and limited resources, personnel, and facilities for mentally ill persons force the caregiving function on most families. According to various reports, approximately one-third of the one million severely chronically mentally ill persons in the United States live with their families, most often with their parents. Even when the mentally ill person is not continuously residing with parents or spouse, there is considerable involvement of the family in the form of phone contacts and home visits; transactions with professional caregivers; provision of food, money, clothing, and transportation; and offerings of temporary housing at home during times when fiscal constraints or interpersonal problems make alternative housing untenable.

With the unpredictability of major mental disorders, families assume responsibility for extensive monitoring and supervision of their ill relative.

LEARNING EXERCISE

Reflect for a moment on your own caseload. Which of your patients are living at home with relatives? Which patients plan to return home after a current period of hospitalization? Write down the names of at least two such patients and next to their names list the kind of problems that the relatives are likely to face in living with the patient. Finally, place a check mark next to the anticipated problems for which you, as a responsible mental health professional, could provide information and technical assistance, perhaps preventing tension and stress from occurring in the first place. Ask one of your colleagues to share his/her experiences in responding to the problems posed by family burden in the management of serious and persistent mental disorder.

Vacations go by the boards, and interruptions in nighttime sleep become commonplace. Patients tend to have reversals in their day and night routines, and many wander from the home and local community to become counted among the thousands of mentally ill homeless individuals. Little wonder, then, that many families coping with a mentally ill relative have their integrity threatened. As conflicts and differences in caregiving between spouses emerge, family separation and divorce may ensue.

Even for families that survive intact, the intrusive impact of harboring a severely and chronically mentally ill person is oppressive. There is a major price to pay beyond dollars and cents. Caregivers suffer from mental strain and feelings of utter defeat. Anxiety and tension, guilt, resentment, demoralization and depression, grief, and frustration exact great emotional costs on the family members and have inevitable repercussions on the clinical status of the ill relative as well. The stressful experiences reported by relatives of the mentally ill often include psychiatric and physical symptoms and illnesses; thus, caregiving is not only burdensome but also hazardous to the caregiver's health.

CLINICAL EXAMPLE

Mr. J and his wife had looked forward to his retirement as a chance to travel and enjoy their many hobbies. They didn't count on their 24-year-old son's developing schizophrenia and forcing them to give up most of their leisure in efforts to care for him. They took turns sleeping to make sure that their son's nocturnal prowling did not result in fires caused by his careless smoking habits. "Even when he's away from home, we're constantly worried and thinking about him. Is he OK? Will he find his way home all right? Will we get a phone call from the police?" This couple exhausted their financial and emotional resources in caring for their adult son. When seen by a psychiatrist in consultation for their son, Mrs. J was so depressed and anxious that she required treatment for herself.

STRESS, TENSION, AND GUILT

Surveys of family members living with a mentally ill relative have repeatedly revealed significant amounts of stress and tension in the households. It is natural and understandable that relatives living with the erratic and sometimes dangerous behavior of a mentally ill person should themselves experience personal tension and distress that often reaches symptomatic and dysfunctional levels. In one national survey carried out with a sample of 281 relatives of chronically mentally ill persons, over one-third reported such symptoms as sleep disturbances, excessive worry, fear, frustration, grief, depression, anxiety, and a sense of despair. Typically, siblings could not comprehend the patient's acting-out symptoms and tended to blame the patient for misbehaving and the parents for not controlling the behavior.

> "We always were on guard, constantly concerned about what would happen next. This produced mental and emotional exhaustion with little patience to cope."

> "Our lives have been unbearable at times, since our son became ill. It's been like having an emotional chain around our necks which ties us to feelings of utter defeat."

> "With our daughter's unpredictable outbursts and strange behavior, we feel like we're on a knife's edge."

A psychiatrist intoning the diagnosis of "schizophrenia" can evoke reactions as tragic as the news of an incurable, fatal disease; however, the mourning process that follows death and can bring psychological healing often escapes relatives of the mentally ill. Grief over the loss of a once-promising child who now seems like a stranger in the home recycles with the remissions and relapses that are often characteristic of schizophrenia and other major mental disorders. No sooner are hopes raised by improvements in symptoms and functioning of the ill family member than they are dashed by a relapse and rehospitalization. Prominent publicity given to new "breakthroughs" in treatment of schizophrenia, which tend to appear on a yearly basis, injects family members with false and unrealistic hopes for cures and sets them up for subsequent disappointment and despair when the prophecy fails.

Guilt is another emotional reaction shared by many family members. Upward of 50% of relatives experience guilt, usually stemming from their felt failure to recognize the early warning signals of the disorder, prevent its occurrence, better manage the illness, or influence the patient to seek and accept treatment. Guilt can be accentuated by the misguided views, and inadvertent comments by professionals about family dynamics can be easily misinterpreted by relatives who are predisposed to hear that they are responsible for their offspring's illness. On the other hand, guilt can be reduced by straightforward explanations by professionals of the unavoidable genetic and biological vulnerability to schizophrenia.

▶ Stress and Relapse

The uncertainty, unpredictability, and mystification that surround a family attempting to adjust and cope with a mentally ill relative all too readily yield a harvest of helplessness, powerlessness, frustration, and tension. Increased family tension can corrode the stability of families and bring normal-functioning relatives to the brink of psychiatric symptoms and role impairment. Stress-related disorders such as hypertension, headaches, insomnia, and depression have been reported by relatives. Some relatives react to ongoing and fluctuating stress by withdrawing from the situation or by outright rejection of the mentally ill member of the family.

LEARNING EXERCISE

Consider a meeting you could arrange with the relatives of a patient in your current caseload. Whether the patient's diagnosis falls within the schizophrenic, affective, or anxiety disorders, make a plan for eliciting and then reducing any guilt experienced by the relatives for the patient's disorder. How will you elicit their possible guilt feelings? You might start by saying, "Many relatives of persons with mental disorders have the impression that somehow they contributed to the person's illness. Have you ever had those thoughts about your son [or daughter]?" In reducing guilt, write an outline to organize your presenting to the relatives a rationale for the stress-vulnerability-coping-competence model of major mental disorders. How can you put into lay terms the idea that schizophrenia and other serious psychiatric disorders are stress-related, biomedical illnesses, not unlike those of rheumatoid arthritis, diabetes, and heart disease?

It should not be surprising that some relatives cope with a severe and unremitting mental disorder by attempting to compensate for their sick member's deficits by nurturing and providing solicitous responses. Wanting to minimize disability and overcome the ravages of symptoms on social functioning, well-intentioned parents or spouses can easily take over a patient's life and become emotionally overinvolved in attempts to motivate the patient to higher levels of performance. Overconcern about the patient's whereabouts, dress, grooming, and daily activities can produce an intrusive pattern that has unhappy consequences for patient and relative alike. Other relatives, baffled by the impairments in functioning without any noticeable physical disease, continue to hold previous expectations for performance that were appropriate during the premorbid period but that are translated into criticism and defeatism once an illness has begun. As family members become sensitized to the emergence of psychotic symptoms or disturbing behavior, quite naturally they attempt to suppress the patient's incoherence, strange thoughts, and hostility. Unfortunately, attempts to preempt an eruption of psychosis and unusual behavior tend to be laced with worry, stress, and tension. Communicated to the patient whose perception is often impaired, these emotional efforts to stave off an unpleasant situation tend to exacerbate the disturbance in the patient and make matters worse. In this fashion, a vicious cycle gets established in which symptoms of mental disorder and dysfunctional family relations have reciprocally negative effects.

Studies carried out in London, Los Angeles, Chicago, Spain, China, and India have documented the adverse impact of overheated family emotional atmospheres on the course of schizophrenia and depression (Butzlaff and Hooley 1998; Leff and Vaughn 1985). As can be seen in Table 6.2, patients returning to live with relatives whose homes are marked by high stress, and

● TABLE 6.2

Nine-month relapse rates among patients with schizophrenia in seven studies: comparison of high–expressed emotion (EE) families and low-EE families

| | % RELAPSE RATES | |
| | High-EE | Low-EE |
STUDY	Families	Families
London, 1972 (*N*=101)	58	16
London, 1976 (*N*=37)	48	16
Los Angeles, Anglo American families (*N*=54)	56	17
Los Angeles, Mexican American families (*N*=55)	52	25
Chicago, Caucasian and African American families (*N*=24)	91	31
Chandigarh, India (*N*=70)	30	9
Los Angeles, recent-onset cases (*N*=29)	37	0

Note. Relapse was conservatively defined by return or exacerbation of psychotic symptoms, not rehospitalization. *High expressed emotion* refers to families with excessively high a) expectations of their mentally ill family member, b) criticism of the mentally ill member's functioning and behavior, or c) emotional overinvolvement and overprotectiveness with the mentally ill family member. Low expressed emotion consists of emotional attitudes of relatives who are tolerant, supportive, and realistically expectant of the family member who has schizophrenia, thereby providing protection against relapse.

Source. Data from Leff and Vaughn 1985.

who express criticism and hostility toward or emotional overinvolvement with their ill family member, have a three to four times greater likelihood of relapsing in the 9 months following discharge from the hospital. In contrast, patients returning to live with relatives who have a better understanding of the illness, and consequently more realistic expectations for performance and a greater tolerance for their sick family member's deviance, have a better than expected outcome. Most studies show that approximately 40% of patients with schizophrenia will relapse during the first year after discharge from the hospital; yet, in the group of patients returning to live with more tolerant and accepting relatives, only 15% relapse. It appears that tolerance and acceptance of the illness actually confer protection against relapse to the sick family member.

When high levels of stress and cycles of negative emotionality are present in families, relapse becomes much more likely in a wide range of mental and physical disorders: eating disorders, mood disorders, obsessive-compulsive disorder, posttraumatic stress disorder, alcoholism, myocardial infarction, and ulcerative colitis (Butzlaff and Hooley 1998). This general pattern across so many disorders reflects the expected upsurge in distress and pressure in families contending with an emotionally burdensome illness. Fortunately, evidence-based family treatments have been shown to reduce levels of expressed emotion, with the consequence that relapse rates often decline. Among young persons with the recent onset of schizophrenia, expressed emotion levels have predicted occupational and school functioning as well as relapse. In seeking recovery from serious, stress-related disorders, it is reassuring for patients, family members, and professionals to know that the everyday interactions that combine to produce stress are modifiable and treatable.

EXAMPLE

There are cultural differences in the ways that families respond to a severe mental disorder. There are variations among ethnic groups in terms of their attitudes toward mental disorders, acceptance, and accommodation to the mentally ill patient within the family and reactance to the subculture's stigma toward the mentally ill. Research has shown how these cultural differences in attitudes and ways of coping may profoundly influence the course of illness among various cultural groups. When families experience high amounts of stress or "high expressed emotion," relapse rates are twice as high as when families learn to cope with the illness, accepting its realities and modulating their expectations of the patient.

In London, approximately 47% of the families experienced high stress with criticism and overinvolvement. In the western European countries of The Netherlands, Italy, and Spain, the rates of "high expressed emotion" were above 70%. In Los Angeles, Anglo Americans tended to more frequently respond with "high expressed emotion," with two-thirds of them expressing critical or emotionally overinvolved attitudes toward their mentally ill relative (Vaughn et al. 1984). On the other hand, mostly unacculturated Latinos in Los Angeles appeared to have lower expectations of their mentally ill adult children and greater acceptance of their having a real, medical illness. Only one-third of the Latino families were judged as having high expressed emotion, and the rate of relapse among the family members with schizophrenia was correspondingly lower.

At the other end of the developing world and cultural spectrum, in India, where the course of schizophrenia appears to be more benign than in the United States or western Europe, less than 10% of relatives were rated as critical or overinvolved. The marked differences in family emotional climates and coping patterns may help to explain why schizophrenia appears to run a smoother course in underdeveloped nations (Hooley 1998).

The most likely explanation for this strikingly replicated finding on expressed emotion and its impact on relapse is that families are overstressed by the demands of caring for a seriously mentally ill member. Not having a professional perspective on the nature of mental illness and lacking the skills to cope with a person who has mental illness, family members react with whatever they can muster as overburdened caregivers, including excessively high expectations for functioning, criticism, or overnurturance.

The same pattern of stress-linked relapse is found in residential care homes for the mentally ill. The day-to-day interactions are between patients who reside in these homes, and the staff of the homes who are largely lay-people without training in mental health. Given the nature of the residents' disorders and the ambient stress that is inevitably a concomitant of living in close quarters with little to occupy their time, it is not surprising that behavioral disturbances ensue from time to time. When residents of these homes are viewed by staff members as uncooperative, agitated, hostile, or impulsive, the employees tend to speak critically of them. This, in turn, elicits negative attitudes by those residents toward the staff. The vicious cycle proceeds and can eventuate in relapse or the extrusion of the resident from the home. On the other hand, those patients receiving positive comments and warm feelings from staff report high satisfaction with the quality of their life in the home, symptom stability, and greater levels of independence.

Thus, it is not just within the family that the emotional climate appears to generate stressful or protective effects on the course of a patient's illness. The stress level—based on the attitudes and interactions of individuals living with the person having an illness—is a relevant predictor of relapse or worsening of symptoms wherever patients may live and with whomever they interact. The generalized validity of the emotional climate as an indicator of stress-linked relapse is also found in many other mental and physical disorders: bipolar disorder, depression, agoraphobia, learning disabilities, obesity in women, eating disorders, posttraumatic stress disorder, alcoholism, bronchial asthma in children, diabetes, seizure disorders, breast cancer, and myocardial infarction. Most importantly, "expressed emotion" reflects an interactional process that is bidirectional in its effects. The disturbing and unpredictable behavior and the symptoms and disabilities of the patient cause stressful reactions in those with whom the patient associates, and those, in turn, feed back on the patient. From this reverberating circuit, two adverse effects sometime ensue: 1) a stress-related negative and worrisome mood in the caregivers, who may cope with the problems by overprotecting the individual, and 2) a stress-related relapse in the patient.

IMPORTANCE OF CONTACT AND COMMUNICATION WITH PROFESSIONALS

The stress and dysfunctional coping efforts of such a large number of American families are compounded by the indifference of many professionals to the needs of families. Too many professionals continue to ignore relatives, rather than involve them in obtaining information about the patient to improve the accuracy of diagnosis and effectiveness of treatment planning and evaluation. Too many practitioners pay obeisance to a misguided conception of privacy and confidentiality. There is no violation of confidentiality when a clinician *solicits information from family members.* Can anyone picture an internist or surgeon failing to invite a close family member to provide confirming and converging information regarding the patient as a key element in diagnosis and choice of treatment? Relatives are lucky if they get in to see the professional responsible for the patient's treatment, much less hear of the diagnosis and prognosis. Plainly speaking, relatives are ignored by mental health professionals.

Despite the indifference of professionals to the needs of family members for support and counseling, relatives still express a strong desire for contact and communication with professionals, especially the psychiatrist responsible for the patient's care. Because of the great stress and anxiety associated with living with a person suffering from schizophrenia or other severe mental illness, relatives regularly articulate a need for information and assistance from professional caregivers. Families report the following needs for professional help in coping with the mentally ill relative: 1) motivating the patient to accept medication and other treatments, 2) understanding appropriate expectations for the patient, 3) assisting in times of crisis, 4) comprehending the nature of mental illness, 5) accepting the illness, 6) locating housing and financial support resources, 7) obtaining Social Security benefits, 8) obtaining a conservatorship, 9) understanding use of medications and their side effects, and 10) gaining referral to self-help and advocacy organizations such as the National Alliance on Mental Illness.

Mental health professionals and family members have profoundly different "worldviews" of mental disorder—a situation that contributes to a harmful schism and to obstacles in developing therapeutic alliances. Practitioners see patients as their primary concern and will often try to "protect" the patient from putative, harmful family influences by withholding information from the family and hiding behind the cloak of confidentiality. There is a blind spot in the vision of many professionals, who forget that the family directly shares in the caregiving functions. In fact, except for time spent with a therapist, psychiatrist, case manager, or outpatient treatment and rehabilitation facility, the patient with a severe mental disorder receives the bulk of his/her caregiving from family members. The role of the family with outpatients is similar to the role held by nursing staff when patients are hospitalized. Since modern psychiatry has emphasized interdisciplinary teamwork among hospital and community mental health staff, including high levels of communication and sharing of responsibility, it is curious, hypocritical, and tragic that professionals have shut out families from active roles in the treatment and rehabilitation of a mentally disabled person.

Recovery from mental disabilities cannot occur solely with a cooperative relationship between the patient and psychiatrist; nor can recovery be expected if other treatment team members are added to the effort. Evidence-based medications and psychosocial treatments added to the mix will also fall short of recovery. The involvement of the family is the catalyst that can move the reactive process toward recovery. The family knows the patient best and has information to share with treaters that will enhance their efficacy. When the family is collaboratively involved as genuine members of the treatment team, they can lend their resources, observations, support, and influence cumulatively to all of the other protective factors for achieving:

- Optimal stabilization and remission of symptoms.
- Gradual improvement in social and vocational functioning.
- A better quality of life.

But how can a practitioner invite the family to join the team for sharing of information and treatment planning unless the patient gives permission?

EXAMPLE

What are the specific needs of relatives for information and contact with professionals? Relatives of the mentally disabled want to know:

- Can mental illness be cured? Can treatment restore the patient to normal?
- In the absence of a cure, what can be done to bring symptoms under control and facilitate better psychosocial functioning?
- How is the diagnosis made, and can brain imaging tell us what's wrong?
- What other treatments are effective in helping the patient to recover?
- What are the causes of mental illness and its effective treatments?
- What are the side effects of medication, and how serious are they?
- For how long does the patient have to continue taking medication?
- Is mental illness caused by genetics and inheritance? Should first-degree relatives have children? What are the earliest signs that mental illness may be starting?
- How can we manage difficult situations, respond to psychotic speech, and find practical ways to keep the home safe?
- How shall we cope with disturbing behavior, such as social withdrawal, aggression, mood swings, and poor daily living skills?
- What can be done in a crisis situation when irrational behavior threatens to escalate into anger and assault?
- Should the patient live at home or elsewhere?
- How can we ensure consistency and continuity of treatment?
- Where are the best services located to help our loved one?
- What can we reasonably expect from our mentally ill relative in terms of school, work, and maintaining self-care capabilities at home?
- What medications are available, and how do they work? How can we motivate our loved one to take them reliably?

Of course, most clinicians will be able to discriminate readily between information that should be kept confidential and information that can be shared openly with family members. Few patients will refuse to a continuing exchange of information with their family members. In over 40 years of clinical work, I've had only a handful of patients who have refused to involve the family. It may take some time to persuade patients of the importance of the family as integral members of the treatment effort—but eventually most will agree.

LEARNING EXERCISE

How can psychiatrists and other clinicians persuade their mentally disabled patients to agree to an open sharing of information with their family members about their illness and treatment? Have you been successful in bringing families into the treatment and rehabilitation enterprise? If so, how did you do it?

I've had success by presenting the benefits and value of family involvement for the patient. Then I elicit from the patient how an involved family, motivated to provide supports and resources, can promote the patient's progress toward achieving his/her personal goals and recovery. I say to my patients when explaining the importance of including their families on the treatment team:

"Without having your family members as active partners with you in the rehabilitation effort, it's like tying one therapeutic hand behind my back. We all need to work together on your behalf. Reading from the same treatment page will also help your family members to cope with their stress and feelings of helplessness—which will further reduce tension for you. However, if there is personal information that you don't want to share with your family—for example, your use of illicit drugs or an abortion—simply tell me and I will honor your confidentiality."

Given the central importance of the family in the care, course, and outcome of major mental disorder, it becomes essential to redress the grievances that relatives have regarding their lack of access and relating to professionals. The scope of these grievances has a basis in the gaps that have grown between professionals and relatives of the mentally ill. For example, one survey of relatives in England found that virtually none of the families had received any advice about the nature of the condition, how to supervise medication, the likely outcome of treatment, or how best to respond to disturbed behavior (Tarrier and Barrowclough 1986). In the United States, one survey of relatives found that over half felt that mental health professionals had "not very adequately at all" helped them to understand the psychiatric illness of their family members, most of whom had schizophrenia (Hatfield 1983). In the same survey, more than 60% still expressed desire for greater collaboration with practitioners serving the patient. Despite their frustration and bitterness toward professionals, families continue to see professionals as key resources in their times of need. They want more information, translated to their level of comprehension, so they can grasp the reality of their present and future situation with an ill relative. Until recently, professionals have not been prepared or trained for responding to these needs of families.

FAMILY SELF-HELP AND ADVOCACY GROUPS

Because of the centuries-long stigma toward mental illness, families and patients living with psychiatric disorders took much longer than other groups of medically disabled persons to organize into self-help and advocacy organizations. For decades, families of persons with mental retardation have sustained a vigorous advocacy and lobbying organization—the National Association for Retarded Citizens—that has met great success at the national and state levels for promoting services, research, and quality of care for developmentally disabled persons. It wasn't until 1979 that the National Alliance for the Mentally Ill (NAMI)—now the National Alliance on Mental Illness—was formed as an umbrella organization for an increasing number of consumer-oriented, advocacy, and self-help groups that had spontaneously developed throughout the United States. Similar, but smaller, advocacy and support groups exist for other disorders, including the Depression and Bipolar Support Alliance, the Anxiety Disorders Association of America, and the Obsessive Compulsive Foundation.

NAMI is by far the largest of these self-help organizations and has exerted an enormous positive effect on the delivery of services to mentally ill family members. NAMI rates states for the quality of their mental health services, has successfully lobbied the National Institute of Mental Health to support more treatment research for schizophrenia and other mental disorders, and has influenced state and local mental health programs to offer evidence-based services and better educational programs for family members. Several hundred local chapters now exist throughout the country, and the national office, located near Washington, D.C., has become one of the most effective lobbying groups on behalf of the needs of the mentally ill. More than 250,000 persons are members of NAMI, and the organization sponsors a large, education-oriented convention each year that brings the newest research findings to the attention of family members. The aims of NAMI are a) to engage in cooperative efforts and group action to become informed about mental disorders, b) to learn about the mental health delivery system and its resources, and c) to press for improvements in this system through consumer advocacy and legislative and judicial action. A commitment to grassroots action is a notable feature of local NAMI groups, some of which have already secured influential positions within the advisory bodies to public mental health agencies.

One important benefit of the NAMI groups is self-help and mutual support. Most of the local groups sponsor counseling activities carried out by peers and by professionals as well as support groups that meet on a weekly basis to share coping styles and problem-solving experiences. Although sound professional advice and easy accessibility to professional caregivers are important coping resources for the families of the mentally ill, referral to a local NAMI self-help and support group can also yield tangible reductions in stress and tension in the home, with resultant benefits for the relatives and patient alike. Thus, the mental health professional with a working relationship to the self-help family organizations in his/her locale can magnify the impact of educational and informational efforts.

The rapid growth and increasing popularity of NAMI groups in the past 5 years are both a cause and an effect of the reduction in stigma attached to mental illness. Wider public education and more sophisticated media coverage of mental illness have helped to demystify psychiatry and the victims of psychiatric disorders. More citizens view mental illness as a bona fide medical disorder, not dissimilar from diabetes, kidney disease, or neurological disorders. Moreover, the popular press and other media—as well as professional and advocacy organizations—have been effective in publicizing the treatability of serious mental disorders. Like cancer before it, mental illness is being gradually destigmatized as the public increasingly realizes that these disorders can be controlled, with many patients returning to a life trajectory of recovery. Especially important in this change of zeitgeist has been education about mental illness by NAMI and its many local affiliates. As a result, many relatives and patients "come out of the closet" and openly advocate for improved services for the mentally ill.

A scant 15 years ago, surveys revealed considerable social stigma among relatives of the mentally ill. However, in a recent survey of 125 families, the large majority of respondents said they did not experience social stigma. Three-fourths indicated that they continued socializing with friends in the presence of the ill relative and were able to speak to coworkers about the illness. Eighty percent said they did not avoid friends or relatives because of embarrassment or shame.

The acceptance of mental illnesses as stress-related biomedical disorders will lead to public support for more empirical research on causes and treatments of these illnesses. It will also serve as a launching pad for increased partnership in treatment and rehabilitation among patients, relatives, and professionals.

LEARNING EXERCISE

To help you, as a mental health professional having contact with relatives of psychiatric patients, improve the quality and amount of communication and information exchange, recently published books on the needs and views of families can serve as a key resource. These books can also be used as a medium of communication between you and the patient's relatives, since you can loan a copy to them and give them reading assignments, quiz them on what they have absorbed, elicit how their situations compare with those presented in the books, and use these discussions as points of departure for family education and management advice. Go to your library or local bookstore and obtain at least one of these volumes:

- *The Family Face of Schizophrenia: Practical Counsel From America's Leading Experts,* by Patricia Backler. New York, Jeremy Tarcher/Putnam, 1994

- *The Family Intervention Guide to Mental Illness,* by Bodie Morey and Kim T. Mueser. Oakland, CA, New Harbinger Publications, 2007

- *The Complete Family Guide to Schizophrenia: Helping Your Loved One Get the Most Out of Life,* by Kim T. Mueser and Susan Gingerich. New York, Guilford, 2006

- *Surviving Schizophrenia,* by E. Fuller Torrey. New York, Harper, 1995

- *Conquering Schizophrenia: A Father, His Son and a Medical Breakthrough,* by Peter Wyden. New York, Knopf, 1998

- *The Bipolar Disorder Survival Guide,* by David Miklowitz. New York, Guilford, 2002

- *Surviving Manic Depression: A Manual on Bipolar Disorder for Patients, Families and Providers,* by E. Fuller Torrey and Michael Knabe. New York, Basic Books, 2002

- *I Am Not Sick, I Don't Need Help! Helping the Seriously Mentally Ill Accept Treatment,* by Xavier Amador. New York, Vida, 2000

After you obtain one or more of these books, read through some of the material and select a chapter or excerpt that you could review with the family of a patient. Make a list of questions that could serve as a focal point for discussing the material after they read it and as a way for you to check on whether they have comprehended the information.

LEARNING EXERCISE

You can work synergistically with NAMI groups in your city, county, or state and thereby promote the coping efforts of relatives of your patients. But it is first necessary that you make contact with such groups and get acquainted with their current goals, advocacy issues, educational programs, leadership, and membership. Then you can find avenues for mutual assistance. NAMI members often know more about mental health, housing, and social services in the community than mental health practitioners. You can even make referrals of family members and patients to the excellent NAMI-sponsored *Family-to-Family* peer-led seminars and a similar seminar series for patients called *Peer-to-Peer.*

One concrete way to develop a working alliance with these groups is to offer to give a talk or lead an informal coping and support group in a discussion of mental illness. This exercise is a prompt for you to locate at least one NAMI group near your place of professional practice and expose yourself to its activities and members. To locate the nearest group, visit their Web site at www.nami.org or check your phone book under National Alliance on Mental Illness, or write or phone the national headquarters of NAMI at Colonial Place Three, 2107 Wilson Blvd. Suite 300, Arlington, VA 22201-3042. Tel. 1-800-950-NAMI.

▶ Evidence-Based Treatment Services for Families and Their Relatives With Mental Disabilities

Given the key role of supportive families in the recovery of their relatives with severe mental disorders, the importance of a wide array of services available for strengthening the family's coping capacities cannot be overstated. When families are knowledgeable about the mental illness of their relative, can adjust their expectations accordingly, are equipped with coping skills, and offer judicious support and advocacy to meet their relative's needs, the possibilities for recovery are amplified. In a parallel fashion, both the family and the patient have similar desires and aims for recovery. The patient wants to overcome the obstacles of an illness to enjoy independence, employment, education, friendships, recreation, and spiritual fulfillment. The family members of the patient want to surmount the burdens and stress of "living on the edge" with a disabled and symptomatic relative so they can feel liberated to study, work, attend church, engage in leisure activities, and socialize without feeling hindered by caregiving needs. Both healthy family members and their mentally ill member wish to have rewarding and low-stress relationships with each other. Hope for a better future, self-responsibility and autonomy, self-efficacy, and meaningful lives are aspirations for all persons in the family.

The common ground for mentally ill persons and their families is complicated by differences between what each views as desirable at any one point of time. For example, the well family members may have little tolerance for the mentally ill person, whose behavior may be undisciplined, bizarre, and disturbing. At such times, the family may feel impelled to assume responsibility for the mentally ill relative, even at the expense of antagonism over the latter's desire for autonomy and freedom. Interventions by the family may then be viewed by the mentally ill person as overly involved, intrusive, and controlling. In a reciprocal manner, patients may not recognize that their unpredictable, dangerous, and impulsive behavior provokes anxiety, stress, criticism, and helplessness in their family members. Studies have shown that when the family members are emotionally burdened, they try to compensate for the dysfunctions of their mentally ill relatives by closely monitoring and hovering over them. Emotional overinvolvement often paradoxically backfires as patients react negatively by failing to take their medications and relapsing (Perlick et al. 2004).

Achieving shared goals and fervently desired recovery depends upon interventions that take into account the respective needs and wishes of all members of the family and provide the wherewithal to reach them. Fortunately, a spectrum of family-oriented services is now available for persons with serious and persisting mental disorders. A wide variety of these services have been shown to be effective and helpful in evidence-based studies (Dixon et al. 2001a). Sadly, few mental health practitioners and agencies have gone the extra mile to become trained and proficient in offering these services; for example, it has been noted that fewer than 20% of mental health agencies offer any systematic, planned, and dedicated services to families of the mentally ill. The reasons for this deplorable void are listed in Table 6.3.

With continuing advocacy for family services, supports, and education by consumer organizations such as NAMI, we expect improvement in their availability in the coming years. There is every good reason to expect our field's adoption and provision of mental health services for families with a seriously disabled, mentally ill member. The entire field of medicine is being pressed to offer education to patients and their families, ensure that they are informed about their illnesses and available treatments, and invite their collaboration in decision making about treatments. This trend will be accelerated in the next decade or two as national health insurance emerges with an essential emphasis on prevention of relapses, hospitalizations, and

- **TABLE 6.3**

  Factors that have delayed the deployment of services for family education by practitioners and mental health agencies

  - All too often, mental health professionals consider the patient as the only relevant person needing services and ignore the family as being an intrusive bother.
  - It is often assumed that many adult patients have little or no contact with families, but even two-thirds of homeless, severely mentally ill individuals have regular contact with their families, who are eager to participate in treatment.
  - Clinicians have not had substantial training in doing structured, planned education with families of persons with schizophrenia and are uncomfortable in that situation.
  - Descriptions of the new evidence-based approaches have been published in books and journals and presented at conferences—none of which serve to provide competency-based training for clinicians.
  - Agencies and practitioners are not typically reimbursed for educational services.
  - Mental health agencies are buffeted by politically correct priorities with such rapid turnover that their administrative leadership promotes fashion over function. Thus, so-called wellness centers that offer drip-dried, consumer-led discussions and drop-in programs on the benefits of exercise, nutrition, and sundry other topics are funded, while evidence-based family education programs languish in the shadows.
  - It is administratively difficult to establish enduring and utilitarian programs of services for families because:
    » Engaging families at various points of contact within a community mental health agency—such as at the time of initial contact, at intake of the patient into inpatient services, or at the time of hospitalization—requires planning, initiative, and designation of staff responsibility.
    » Ensuring that the educational intervention is designed to meet the varied needs of families and patients within the context of a true collaboration among patient, family, and professional is still alien among mental health providers.
    » Integrating families with other services available to patients in a comprehensive and coordinated system of care is challenging even to the most experienced and enterprising mental health agencies.

disability. While greater resources should be invested in the provision of services to the families of the severely mentally ill, the effort should not be done piecemeal but rather in synchrony with the full range of rehabilitation programs that are evidence-based, continuous, consumer-oriented, and aimed at assisting patients to reach their maximum feasible independence along the road to recovery.

SPECTRUM OF FAMILY SERVICES AND TREATMENTS

A flexible approach to the provision of family services and treatments is consonant with the important principle of fitting the intervention to the patient and family. The needs, phase of illness, goals, interests, and choice of the patient and family are prepotent over the biases and preferences of practitioners. Thus, some families may be satisfied with their level of knowledge and coping ability regarding mental illness, preferring to meet with their mentally ill relative's primary therapist or psychiatrist on an "as needed" basis. Others may be more comfortable attending a peer-to-peer support and education group before becoming involved in a more intensive and effortful intervention like *behavioral family management*. Matching the particular educational and treatment modality to the specific needs and wishes of the family is aided by a "menu" of services that can be shared with the family at the time of orientation. An informed family that is accorded decision-making power by a practitioner who invites active participation and collaboration in the planning and implementation of services is already touching the bases of a recovery orientation. Differences among the various types of empirically validated family interventions include the dimensions and goals listed in Table 6.4.

The prototype for the panoply of family interventions and psychoeducation is *behavioral family management,* which is also called *behavioral family therapy* (Mueser and Glynn 1999). When behavioral family management is integrated with the requisite comprehensive services for the mentally disabled—including judicious types and doses of psychotropic medications,

---

● **TABLE 6.4**

Differences among the various types of empirically validated family interventions

- Frequency, length, and duration of sessions
- Participation by the family alone or the family together with the patient
- Priority given to the well-being, knowledge base, skills, and clinical improvement of the family alone or conjointly with the patient
- An emphasis on didactic education for knowledge and attitudinal change versus action-oriented, behavioral building of communication and problem-solving skills
- Single-family, multiple-family group, or mixed sessions (with some featuring a focus on single family and others a focus on multiple families)

training in illness management, social skills training, vocational rehabilitation, and continuous treatment teams—patients can expect to gain self-control in their lives, overcome the obstacles to their personal goals posed by their illnesses, experience fewer relapses and rehospitalizations, attain higher levels of social and occupational functioning, and enjoy a better quality of life. As co-participants, families can expect to achieve cognitive mastery over the heretofore baffling mental illnesses of their relatives and develop coping skills for dealing with the emotional and financial burdens as well as the everyday stressors and challenges of living with a mentally ill person. Behavioral family management can engender hope and confer empowerment to families that were mired in helplessness and despair.

The diverse offshoots of behavioral family management have appropriated various components of the parent program, adapted for practical use with families in designated situations. After describing behavioral family management, we will illustrate its variants, highlighting the importance of using flexible levels of intervention in our work with the mentally disabled. These approaches have been used successfully with families and patients representing many psychiatric disorders: schizophrenia, bipolar disorder, recurrent depression, obsessive-compulsive disorder, posttraumatic stress disorder, panic and agoraphobia, and autism spectrum disorders.

DIVIDING THE RESPONSIBILITIES FOR PERSONAL SUPPORT SERVICES

An overarching issue in the use of behavioral family management or any of its congeners is the extent to which family members should be accorded responsibility for meeting the considerable needs for activities of daily living, illness management, socialization, and advocacy for services. In a truly collaborative venture, there will be an open discussion of the proportion of the patient's personal support services that might be best managed by the mental health system—divided among the various members of a multidisciplinary team—or by the family. The goal, of course, is for the patient to assume more and more responsibility for self-management, initiative, and autonomy. Realistically, patients' taking greater and greater self-responsibility for the management of their illness and fulfilling their personal goals is a long-term process. Initially an "engine" is required to provide energy for the patient to move farther along the road to recovery. How much "horsepower" of that engine should be allotted to the family and how much to the mental health program?

In some situations, it may be necessary for the patient to leave the family home and receive treatment and rehabilitation in a residential or transitional rehabilitation center or in a supported living apartment. This is often desirable when the family is exhausted, feels utterly defeated, and has few personal and financial resources. We might view this approach as "constructive separation" between patient and family. The patient is necessarily involved in the planning and decision making and in fully comprehending the rationale for such a decision. Motivational interviewing is used by the responsible clinician to ensure that living separately serves the long-term personal goals of the family and patient.

It is totally unacceptable for a mental health professional to encourage the family to give the patient an ultimatum to "shape up or ship out." Patients and families are to be viewed as always "doing the best they can," given their knowledge, skills, personal and financial resources, treatment, and severity of illness. It is the responsibility of the responsible mental health clinician to work out a plan that enables the patient and family to take some initial steps toward their respective personal and family goals. Families in dire straits, whose members are emotionally drained, will often misinterpret recommendations for constructive separation as meaning they should use "tough love" and "kick the patient out of the home." If precipitous and unsupervised actions are taken to force the patient to leave home without making all necessary arrangements for continuing care and rehabilitation, the mental health system loses credibility and is teetering on a balance beam of unethical conduct.

CLINICAL EXAMPLE

For 3 years, John had resisted all efforts of his family to seek consultation for his extreme social isolation and paralysis of personal action. He spent all of his time in his room at home, which was decrepit and filthy. He never showered, shaved, or washed his clothes. He repeatedly accused his parents of trying to poison him and ate only late at night when his parents were sleeping, when he would grab items from the kitchen and consume them in the privacy of his room. After a home visit and motivational interviewing identified John's long-term goals of employment and living independently, medication was presented as a step that John could take to reduce his current unwanted feelings of helplessness and hopelessness.

During several months of slow improvement, John and his parents participated in learning how to manage his disability and symptoms by participating in the *Symptom Management and Medication Management Modules* (Psychiatric Rehabilitation Consultants 2007). As the family embarked on a systematic plan for psychiatric rehabilitation, discussions focused on how John might obtain his goals most expediently. By considering the various alternatives and what they had to offer John and his parents, everyone settled on a decision for John to enter a transitional rehabilitation center for a 3-year program leading to independent living. The family and John continued to meet on a weekly to monthly basis during the next 3 years, participating in behavioral family management with John's psychiatrist. The focus of the sessions was on improving their communication and problem-solving skills—especially how to give positive reinforcement, or "warm fuzzies," to each other as they became increasingly aware of the mutually helpful and considerate actions that were being taken by all three members of the family.

When it is determined that the family wants to assume the responsibilities for much of the patient's needs for case management or personal support, the mental health clinician can assume the role of supervisor or mentor to family members as they undertake the arduous task of fulfilling many rehabilitative responsibilities. Some of the responsibilities falling to the family's shoulders in this type of situation include assisting in the patient's linkages to and engagement with needed services, being aware of the comprehensive needs of the patient, monitoring the quality of the services being rendered, helping the patient with meeting daily living needs, being available in times of crisis, and engaging in advocacy efforts to enhance services.

Table 6.5 lists the kinds of assistance that can be provided by relatives and the things for relatives to avoid. Professional and family caregivers can work in partnership to optimize the quality of services provided to patients with chronic mental disorders. In this partnership, professionals must respect the needs and desires of family members for the type and amount of involvement in the care and management of the patient's illness.

Behavioral family management sessions have been conducted in the home, in the hospital, in clinics and mental health centers, and in storefronts in shopping malls. Multimedia aids are helpful in the teaching process: videotapes have been produced that convey educational material and highlight coping strategies, and flip-charts and blackboards are the constant companions of professionals plying the family management approach.

▶ Behavioral Family Management

The overall purpose of behavioral family management is to empower patients and their family members alike in a collaborative process with the knowledge,

● **TABLE 6.5**

Ways for family members to assist in the treatment and rehabilitation of a seriously mentally ill relative

FUNCTIONS TO SERVE	TRAPS TO AVOID
Assist in locating, linking, and sustaining treatment and rehabilitation services	Becoming overinvolved with ill relative and trying too hard to help and comfort
Encourage supportive use of medication	Nagging or using excessive criticism
Advocate for better services	Becoming isolated from family and friends
Maintain tolerant and low-key home atmosphere	Taking for granted small signs of progress
Reduce performance expectations to a realistic level	Expecting too much improvement too quickly
Encourage participation in treatment and low-stress activities	Depriving self and other family members of fun, recreation, vacations, and personal activities
Know how the mental healthcare system works	Not getting information from other families through NAMI affiliate
Participate in planning and implementing treatment as an active partner	Passivity and intimidation by psychiatrists and other mental health professionals
Keep an accurate, cumulative journal of the illness and treatments received	Failing to include relative benefits of past treatments and effectiveness versus side effects of medications
Educate professionals regarding the patient's functional assets and strengths	Considering only the patient's problems
Track early warning signs of relapse	Warning signs are noted by patient (subjective symptoms) as well as by family and mental health professionals (objective signs and symptoms)

skills, strategies, and attitudes that will facilitate patients achieving their personally relevant goals in life. Recovery from the disabilities associated with serious mental disorders is the optimal outcome of this process. Recovery is not tantamount to remission of symptoms or elimination of relapses. Our definition of recovery goes beyond symptoms, encompassing a person's being able to achieve his/her personal goals, enjoying a meaningful and reasonably normal life with personal satisfaction, autonomy, and responsibility. With the collective experience of evidence-based practice and practice-based evidence, behavioral family management is the model of family intervention that offers hope for recovery when combined with other essential services for comprehensive rehabilitation described in this manual.

In behavioral family management, participants are taught to understand the mental disorder they are living with as well as the treatments and rehabilitative services that have been demonstrated to be effective in helping to overcome the symptoms, cognitive impairments, and disabilities associated with the disorder. Patients and their family members learn how diagnoses are made; about the interactions of genetic, brain, and environmental influences in causing mental disorders; and the way in which stress, vulnerability, and protective factors determine progress toward recovery. The importance of forestalling relapses and the disabilities that are inevitable accompaniments is highlighted by teaching participants how to recognize the early warning signs or symptoms of relapse and to develop an emergency plan to prevent or attenuate it.

While acquiring information and understanding concepts relevant to severe mental disorders is a key element in behavioral family management, even more important is the systematic and active learning of ways to communicate emotions, needs, and information to each other. Unless family members can shift from focusing on the unpleasant and frustrating interactions that dominate everyday life to constructive communications, clinical progress is slowed. Patients learn how to be direct and positive in making requests of their family members, and the latter learn how to ignore arguing with their ill relative about delusions and instead encourage conversations about mundane but ever-present topics in the "here and now."

Effective communication is basic to all normal relationships—whether in families, at work, with friends, or in community situations. If our goal is the pursuit of recovery, what is a more important investment in the therapeutic enterprise than helping patients and their relatives to normalize their relationships through successful communication? When family members are capable of communicating effectively, they can work constructively together on solving the problems they face in meeting their needs and goals. Problems are ever present in all of our lives—even more so when family members are contending with a disabling mental disorder. Thus, putting together information, concepts, and know-how and fostering communication skills can empower patients and their family members to get on top of their problems instead of being crushed by them.

When successful, behavioral family management enables families to suffer less, acquire more self-control and self-efficacy, and, most importantly, experience the joys and simple pleasures that are available to everyone. Behavioral family management seeks to strengthen the capacities of the family so its members can remove the obstacles to their needs and goals using their own resources and abilities. Therefore, the underlying basic mechanism for this modality is the *teaching* inherent in all phases of behavioral family management. Clinicians who are competent in behavioral family management are teachers as much as they are therapists.

THE WHERE, HOW, AND BY WHOM OF BEHAVIORAL FAMILY MANAGEMENT

While behavioral family management requires special training—usually through workshops and supervised, on-the-job practice—a wide variety of mental health professionals, including psychiatrists, psychologists, social workers, nurses, and occupational therapists, have been indoctrinated into leadership roles. The particular disciplinary background is not as important as a directive and assertive style, openness, candid comfort in dispelling myths and mystifications about schizophrenia, and a practical and down-to-earth approach with patients and relatives. Previous experience working with people having chronic mental disorders is very important. Adherence to complex and sophisticated conceptualizations of mental disorders may interfere with learning behavioral family management techniques.

Behavioral family management can be offered to patients together with their relatives or can be offered separately. Both separate and conjoint sessions together can be offered as well. Some professionals feel that it is best to start the educational process shortly after the patient is admitted to a hospital in relapse, whereas others wait until the patient has stabilized on medication as an outpatient. Some educational programs are offered as "mini-marathons" lasting up to a full day, whereas others are spread out in 2-hour weekly programs. It does seem important to give relatives a chance to ventilate and abreact their strong feelings about the stress and strain of harboring a mentally ill person at home, and this may be best done without the patient present. Unless such abreaction is given vent, stored-up feelings can interfere with the later work aimed at more constructive goals and communication.

BASIC COMPONENTS OF BEHAVIORAL FAMILY MANAGEMENT

There are seven major components to behavioral family management:

- Engaging the patient and relatives in a collaborative, positive therapeutic relationship

- Conducting a behavioral or functional assessment of each individual and the family as a whole
- Providing education on the nature of mental disorders and their evidence-based treatments and rehabilitation that conveys realistic expectations to all family members regarding the psychosocial functioning of the person who is disabled
- Teaching family members to advocate for and meet their own needs by using services and resources available in the community as well as "getting a life" for themselves apart from the patient
- Providing training in communication skills, including expressing and acknowledging positive feelings, actively listening, making positive requests, expressing negative feelings directly without accusativeness, and taking a time-out from a tense situation
- Providing training in systematic and structured problem-solving
- Using special cognitive-behavioral techniques to help individual family members or the family as a group to overcome persisting symptoms, distress, dysphoria, disabilities, or motivational problems that do not respond readily to the first four strategies

The components can be viewed as *modular* since it is possible to customize the intervention to fit a variety of needs of patients and families, resources and constraints of a clinical site or mental health system, time for conducting the treatment, and competencies of practitioners. The modularity also offers flexibility in the delivery of the components to a particular family. For instance, it may be feasible to offer the educational component initially at the time of a patient's admission to the hospital and then, later, to engage the family in the remaining components when the patient has achieved stabilization of the illness. The components can be given in a variety of formats, including single families; multiple-family groups, seminars, or workshops; and patients together with or separate from their family members. Flexibility is desirable in considering how to use the components of behavioral family management, with the practical exigencies of families, practitioners, and clinical facilities determining how to deliver the treatment.

BEHAVIORAL ASSESSMENT OF THE FAMILY

The specific nature of the patient's and relatives' problems and goals should shape the scope and focus of behavioral family management. Therefore, it is essential to begin with a comprehensive and sensitive assessment of each person's needs in the family as well as the strengths and deficits of the family as a whole. The process of behavioral assessment and analysis is inextricably interwoven with the process of therapy and behavior change; accordingly, it continues throughout the duration of behavioral family management rather than being limited to the initial sessions. Analyzing and pinpointing problems, setting goals and priorities, and selecting interventions go hand in hand with monitoring of progress.

CLINICAL EXAMPLE

Lily was 32 years old, married with three young children, when she experienced her third relapse of mania followed by a deep depression. Each of her episodes was triggered by smoking marijuana. A functional analysis revealed that she felt that her children were "out of control" and that she did not know how to discipline them, deferring to her husband. Lily stated that she wanted more than anything to be a good parent. Her husband was a "take charge" person who tried to protect his wife from any stress. He didn't realize that marijuana was a stressor and would smoke it with her. Their marriage was on the verge of collapse as her husband and children felt helpless and abandoned when she became euphoric and grandiose and went on spending sprees.

As a result of the functional assessment, her psychiatrist referred her to a dual diagnosis treatment center for her marijuana abuse, arranged for a local agency to register her for a course in parent training with subsequent customized consultation, and engaged Lily and her husband in behavioral marital therapy to improve their communication and problem-solving capacity. At the same time that he prescribed mood-stabilizing and antidepressant medication, the psychiatrist engaged Lily in behavioral activation therapy to speed her recovery from depression.

Since the patient and relatives may come to a therapist for family intervention with little or no previous contact, a method for collecting and sorting information efficiently should be available. Each member of the family should be assessed for his/her behavioral assets and deficits, self-defined problems and goals, reinforcers, and motivation for change. These assessments can be carried out using a variety of questionnaires, interview formats, therapist observation, or self-monitoring by the individual. Meeting individually for at least one session with each member of the family, or for a portion of a session, helps the rapid assembly of these data and fortifies the development of the therapeutic alliance.

Meeting with the family as a whole permits assessment and analysis of family strengths and deficits, their problem-solving styles, and their ability to communicate. The power structure (e.g., who makes the decisions), status, and role of the family members can be assessed through questionnaires, role-plays, structured family interaction tasks, and naturalistic observation of the family process. For example, family questionnaires are available that inquire about the patterns of decision making and the degree of satisfaction that members of the family have about the existing mechanisms for allocating family resources (Stuart 1980).

CLINICAL EXAMPLE

Paul, a 29-year-old single, unemployed clerk, was discharged from his fourth hospitalization in a psychiatric unit of a general hospital after an exacerbation of his schizophrenic disorder. He had been ill for 6 years but functioned reasonably well living at home with his parents between relapses. Recently, however, his relapses had become more frequent despite good adherence to his antipsychotic maintenance medication.

Questionnaires and interviews with Paul and his parents revealed a clear pattern of decision making: decisions were made by default by his mother, who tended to ignore or emotionally withdraw from entreaties made by Paul and his father for family action or family activities. For example, it was decided that Paul would return to live at home with his parents after his most recent hospitalization when suggestions by Paul and his father that he obtain his own apartment went unresponded to by his mother, who also kept the checkbook and would have had to write out a check for the first month's rent. Further observation of the family together revealed that there was little mutual acknowledgment of feelings and opinions expressed by one or another of the family members. Each member of the family would reliably fail to receive feedback for ideas or emotional expression. To obtain a better grasp of how the family members perceived problems, the therapist asked each individual to describe something that had happened during the past week that was a source of tension or distress. The therapist then determined the extent to which each person shared the feelings and the way concern and coping were expressed by others.

As a result of this assessment, a goal was set to focus on the importance of a shared approach to decision making for matters that affected everyone in the family, such as where Paul might live. Moreover, prime among the communication skills in which the patient and family would have to receive training were active listening and making a positive request.

Besides the training in communication skills, the family assessment leads to the identification of problems that one or more of the family members are struggling with and that can become grist for the behavioral family management mill. These problems can be stressors within the family system, such as the negativism and social withdrawal of a young adult with schizophrenia with which the parents are trying to cope, as well as those emanating from outside the family, such as financial or housing problems.

Interview instruments or questionnaires are available to assess the quality of the emotional relationships among patient and relatives (Leff and Vaughn 1985; Mueser and Glynn 1999). Questions center around the patient's and relatives' perception of the development of the mental disorder; their understanding and views about the disorder; conflicts, quarrels, and irritability; the family time budget; management of household tasks and responsibilities; and subjective attitudes expressed by family members about one another. In evaluating the family interaction relationships, the therapist looks for signs of unrealistic expectation for improvement and functioning, criticism, intrusiveness, and emotional overinvolvement.

Are there deficits in communication between parents and their young adult schizophrenic son who secludes himself in his room? How well do the family members deal with a major problem, such as unexpected denial of Social Security benefits to the sick relative? Are the family members spending excessive time together, to the exclusion of their own, independent needs for recreation and socialization? Are relatives inadvertently reinforcing maladaptive or symptomatic behavior in their sick family member through overprotectiveness and oversolicitousness? A major aim of the family assessment and behavior analysis is to take the "temperature" of the family emotional climate and specify the individual and interpersonal problems, deficits, and assets that contribute to the "fever."

A highly productive way of gaining an assessment of the abilities of a family to engage in constructive communicating and problem solving is to identify a problem or issue that each member has endorsed as being current and marked by disagreement. The therapist then can ask the family members, who are being observed in a session, to spend 5 minutes attempting to solve the problem or reach a consensus. What unfold in front of the therapist's eyes are the capabilities and deficiencies of the communication and problem-solving style of each family member and of the family as a whole. More detailed descriptions of how to conduct behavioral assessment and analysis are available in Chapter 4 ("Functional Assessment") of this manual and in publications by Keefe and colleagues (1978), Arrington and colleagues (1988), Mueser and Glynn (1999), and Phillips (2005).

Whatever the problems are, the assumption of the therapist, shared with the family, is that the family is coping with the problems as best they can, given their present resources and capabilities. The aim of behavioral family management and the responsibility of the therapist are to enhance the family's capacities through goal setting and education about the nature of the disorder and how to obtain needed treatment, rehabilitation, and communication and problem-solving skills training.

LEARNING EXERCISE

Reinforcers are people, places, things, and activities that are enjoyed, preferred, selectively chosen, and interacted with frequently. Reinforcers serve to motivate behavior by strengthening the attitudes and actions of an individual that immediately precede them and elicit their occurrence. For example, going to a movie or a sporting event after a productive day at work tends to increase future productivity. The most common reinforcers are social in nature, such as praise, warmth, friendliness, and acknowledgment from friends, coworkers, teachers, supervisors, and relatives.

It's important, in family management of serious mental disorders, to identify reinforcers for each member of the family, especially for the patient with the disorder, since loss of intrinsic motivation and interests is often a core characteristic of the disorder. One way to identify reinforcers that can be used to selectively strengthen desired behavior and progress toward goals is to survey each member of the family for his/her current preferences for people, places, and objects. With one of your current patients, ask the following questions to elicit that person's idiosyncratic reinforcers.

* Among your personal contacts each week, who do you spend most of your time with? With whom would you like to spend more time?
* Where do you spend most of your time? In which room of your home? What activities do you prefer to engage in? What would you like to do more often?
* What would you like to have more of? What foods, drinks, possessions, hobbies, clothes? When you have money, what do you spend it on?

EDUCATING THE FAMILY ABOUT SCHIZOPHRENIA

The element common to all of the forms of family intervention with disabling mental disorders is education about the nature and treatment of the disorder. This education can be given in many different ways; for example, some therapists and clinics offer half-day or full-day "survival skills workshops" to relatives and patients with serious mental disabilities. The aims of the workshop are to give information; familiarize families with available treatment, rehabilitation, and social services; connect the patient and relatives to the clinicians and the agency for continuing care; and promote social support among the families. Other formats are equally effective in accomplishing these aims, such as meeting with relatives and the patient separately for education; providing the education in brief increments as part of an ongoing family therapy program; conveying education through self-help and advocacy organizations like NAMI; and providing educational seminars for multifamily groups.

Educational efforts are facilitated by high-quality media for translation of technical information to a layperson's level of comprehension. This is particularly important for families with limited education or in cases in which literacy is marginal. Videotape productions on schizophrenia have been produced, and diagrams, brochures, and informational handouts are useful supplements to verbally transmitted information. The content of the education focuses on what is currently known about the disorder in question and its causes, course, and treatment. In Tables 6.6 and 6.7 are exhibited informational topics and practical advice for patients and their relatives provided through educational videos, PowerPoint or overhead presentations, handouts, brochures, and booklets.

CLINICAL EXAMPLE (continued)

Paul and his parents came weekly for three sessions on education about schizophrenia. When the symptoms of the disorder were discussed, he spoke openly about the fear and dread he had of his "voices"; surprisingly, his mother confided that she had had a "nervous breakdown" many years before that had required a brief psychiatric hospitalization. The therapist encouraged Paul and his mother to "compare notes" and discover the similarities and differences in their symptoms. Paul's father, who had been aloof and distant from Paul's illness heretofore, took a more active interest as he learned about the biobehavioral roots of schizophrenia. In particular, he seemed to grasp the biological basis of schizophrenia from the diagrams of synapses and neurotransmitter receptors offered during the educational sessions.

During the educational sessions, the therapist turns the patient and the relatives into the real "experts," by soliciting their experiences and personalizing the learning experience. When the symptoms of the disorder are

---

● **TABLE 6.6**

Informational topics on schizophrenia and antipsychotic drugs provided to families and patients in educational sessions

SCHIZOPHRENIA

1. Schizophrenia is a serious, disabling mental disorder that affects 1% of the population throughout the world, with its most common onset in late adolescence and early adulthood. Both males and females are affected equally, although the age at onset is later, on average, for women—possibly because of the protective effects of female hormones.

2. The symptoms of schizophrenia include delusions (strange, bizarre, and false beliefs), hallucinations (usually voices that are experienced as alien people speaking to the patient or about him/her), abnormalities in thought and speech (incoherence or skipping from topic to topic), flat emotional expressiveness (blunted spontaneity in facial expression and tone of voice), emotional and social withdrawal, and apathy with loss of interests and motivation.

3. The exact causes are unknown, but genetic influences are present, the structures and functions of the brain are often abnormal, and the chemical messengers (neurotransmitters) that are responsible for voluntary and rational thinking and behavior may be imbalanced.

4. As with any medical disease, a variety of social and environmental events can worsen the symptoms of the disorder by overstimulating the brain. These include financial stressors, losses of important relationships, conflicts in relationships producing tension, and disappointments and frustrations at work or school.

5. Protective factors can combine to reduce the symptoms, relapses, and cognitive impairments of schizophrenia. Examples of protective factors are regular adherence to appropriate types and doses of medications, supportive family relationships, abstinence from alcohol and illicit drugs, regular visits to a psychiatrist, and participation in rehabilitation such as supported employment and social skills training.

6. Recovery from schizophrenia is possible but is more likely when the individual has had a) successes in social, academic, and occupational functioning prior to the onset of the illness, b) short periods of time when antipsychotic medication was not being used, c) a relapse prevention plan based on detection of early warning signs of relapse, and d) treatment and rehabilitation services that were comprehensive, continuous, coordinated, collaborative, consumer-oriented, consistent, connected to the individual's phase of disorder, and competently and compassionately delivered.

7. One of the most important factors in promoting recovery and wellness is a collaboration among the patient, family members, and mental health professionals. Better outcomes ensue when all "team members" work together to identify problems, break them down into small obstacles that can be overcome, and learn skills for illness management, communication, and problem solving.

(continued)

● TABLE 6.6 *(cont'd.)*

ANTIPSYCHOTIC MEDICATIONS

1. Regular, reliable, and daily use of antipsychotic medications is the mainstay of treatment of schizophrenia. It may take some time for the family and patient, working together with the psychiatrist, to find the best type, dose, and combination of medications. Collaboration and sharing information about the benefits and side effects of any medication among all stakeholders is the best route to successful use of medication.

2. It's not possible to predict in advance which medication is best for any one patient. The best predictor is the initial subjective response to the first few days of a new medicine. If the patient feels "bad" and distressed after the first week, that particular medication may not be worth continuing. It's almost always possible to find a type, dose, or combination of medications that the patient will find helpful. In choosing a medication, either first- or second-generation antipsychotics may be considered; having such a large number of medicines is an advantage, since each person may have a different response to the same medication.

3. Antipsychotic medications that are considered first-generation drugs have neuromuscular side effects that can be intrusive—especially the tormenting restlessness that is called *akathisia*. A delayed side effect that may appear many years after using these first-generation drugs is called *tardive dyskinesia*. Second-generation antipsychotics often have hazardous metabolic side effects, including weight gain, diabetes, and abnormalities of cholesterol and other blood lipids. Patients and families need to be knowledgeable about these side effects, how to recognize them, and what to do about them. An ounce of prevention is worth a pound of cure.

4. Side effects are at their peak when a patient starts a new medication, then they gradually subside. On the other hand, the therapeutic or beneficial effects of most psychotropic drugs—like those for schizophrenia—gradually accumulate and may not be fully evident until 1 or more months. Therefore, it bears to be patient in waiting for that date when the therapeutic effects surpass the side effects.

5. Most side effects are mild and not dangerous (e.g., dry mouth, some dizziness or sedation). Consulting one's doctor may lead to some practical suggestions, such as chewing sugar-free gum or carrying a water bottle if dry mouth is the problem.

6. Street drugs (e.g., amphetamines, narcotics, cocaine, marijuana) can only make an existing mental illness worse; in fact, using amphetamines or cocaine can produce an illness indistinguishable from schizophrenia.

7. Medications cannot teach patients how to live better; thus, medications must be combined in complementary ways with psychosocial treatments and rehabilitation. Too much medication can cause side effects like sedation that may interfere with rehabilitation. On the other hand, if a patient gets into a treatment program that is overstimulating with expectations for performance that are too high, stress will increase and the medication dose may also have to be increased to prevent a relapse.

> ● TABLE 6.7
>
> **Guidelines for coping with challenging, difficult, and unexpected situations involving a relative with schizophrenia or another disabling mental disorder**
>
> **Have realistic expectations for your mentally ill relative**
>
> 1. *Accept the illness while always looking for ways to find positive qualities of the patient.* Although hope for improvement is important, it must be realistic. The family must accept the illness and its disability, recognizing that treatment does not guarantee success. Treatment and rehabilitation can work, but going slowly is often faster than trying to get too much done too quickly. The patient is not the same as the illness—always find the positive things that the patient does and says.
>
> 2. *Set goals that can be readily achieved.* Be realistic about what your relative can accomplish. You can learn this gradually over time, but always start with minimal expectations, and let yourself be pleasantly surprised when a small activity is performed. Goals should be limited in scope, very concrete and easy to describe, and attainable.
>
> 3. *Reward small signs of progress.* If a task or goal is complicated and difficult to complete, break it down into smaller units. Use a personal yardstick by comparing this month's accomplishments to last month's. Don't compare current functioning with how the person functioned before the illness. Reward yourself and your relative with praise for success when the task is completed or for just "hanging in."
>
> **Learn to communicate effectively**
>
> 1. *Keep it cool.* Frustration and tension are normal, but tone these emotions down. Disagreements and conflicts are normal, but turn down the emotional temperature at such times. Give yourself time to cool down by separating what has made you angry from the person who did it. Take a time-out if things get hot.
>
> 2. *Give 'em space.* Privacy and time alone are valuable and important as a coping method for everyone in the family. It's OK to offer companionship and opportunities to participate in activities as a family, but it's also OK to refuse. A person with a serious mental disorder is easily overstimulated and stressed. Having time alone can be important in buffering stress.
>
> 3. *Keep it simple.* Say what you have to say clearly, calmly, positively, and briefly. Repeat communications if necessary because "information processing" is dysfunctional in schizophrenia.
>
> **Use problem solving as an everyday routine**
>
> 1. *Solve problems step by step.* Make changes gradually. Work on one thing at a time. Sit down together and do some "brainstorming" before rushing into a response or solution to a problem. Problems are normal; how you deal with them makes the difference.
>
> *(continued)*

● **TABLE 6.7** *(cont'd.)*

2. *Carry on business as usual.* Reestablish family routines as quickly as possible after a relapse or hospitalization. Stay in touch with your family members and friends and ask for their assistance—if only to lend you their ear for sympathetic listening. Keep your friendship circle intact; social support is important for everyone.

3. *Set limits.* Everyone needs to know what the rules are. A few reasonable rules about simple courtesy and responsibilities in sharing a household keep things calmer. No one should tolerate rude, destructive, threatening, or aggressive behavior. Everyone in the family must read from the same page on basic expectations for social interaction. A "family contract," written with the help of a mental health professional, can help to keep the peace.

described, each person in the family gives his/her own perspective on the specific symptoms of the patient in the family. Some patients are surprised that anyone would want to know about how they coped with the distressing and fearsome symptoms. Relatives show gratitude that a professional would spend time going over the basics of knowledge of the disorder or even explain the rudimentary facts of mental illness, its genetics, and how it is diagnosed. Many of these educational sessions have a cathartic effect, and families learning the material together often form spontaneous mutual help and support groups that long transcend the end of the family educational program.

TRAINING IN COMMUNICATION SKILLS

While psychoeducational approaches to family management can give information, promote cognitive mastery over the illness, demystify mental disorders, permit emotional abreaction, and facilitate social support, a more active effort at inculcating skills to patients and relatives is necessary for enduring effects on stress reduction, relapse prevention, social adjustment, lower family burden, and improved quality of life. Behavioral family management represents a skills development approach to patients and relatives alike.

Two of the skills required by patients and relatives who are coping with a chronic and severe mental disorder are effective means of communication and constructive problem-solving techniques. As was noted earlier in the section of this chapter on stress and relapse, the tensions and conflicts that embroil patients and relatives in high–expressed emotion households can have deleterious effects on both. Since communication and problem-solving skills are not taught in schools, it is only through incidental learning from influential models that anyone learns such skills for use in human relations. The aim of behavioral family management is to provide training in these interactional skills so that stress and relapse may be reduced while social adjustment and quality of life may be enhanced. The flow chart depicted in Figure 6.2 (discussed earlier in this chapter) highlights the mechanism involved in reducing relapse through training in these skills.

KEY COMMUNICATION SKILLS

In almost all areas of human relations, the interactions between individuals are mediated by generic skills for expressing emotions and obtaining instrumental and affiliative needs:

- Initiating positive statements and suggestions
- Acknowledging positive actions of others
- Making positive requests of others
- Actively listening and responding empathically
- Expressing negative feelings constructively
- Taking a time-out to cool down

If the discrete verbal and nonverbal behavioral components of these skills can be pinpointed, it would be far easier to teach the skills to patients and relatives. The assumption of behavioral family management is that by building behavioral competencies in communication through repeated practice, the subjective, internalized emotional congruence experienced by the individual will gradually develop. As an example of the specific verbal and nonverbal components inherent in communication skills, those relevant for "making a positive request" are listed in Table 6.8. Since a core deficit in many seriously mentally ill patients is lack of initiative and motivation, learning how to effectively request actions and responses can be helpful for relatives in overcoming obstacles induced by the patient's behavioral inertia and apathy.

When family members want to request a change for the better from some unpleasant, disagreeable, or disturbing behavior, it is important that they start by identifying the specific behavior that is objectionable. A family member must state exactly what he/she has seen or heard the patient doing or saying, while avoiding labeling or interpreting the patient's motives. Putting negative labels on the person instead of sticking with the annoying behavior per se can close the door on communicating and problem-solving. This is followed by describing the negative impact that the behavior has had on the family member. For example, a family member could say, "When you cursed me three times just now, it made me feel really bad and scared.

> **TABLE 6.8**
>
> **Verbal and nonverbal components of the communication skill "making a positive request."**
>
> - Look at the person.
> - Use a pleasant facial expression and tone of voice.
> - Say exactly what you would like him/her to do or say.
> - Tell how it would make you feel if he/she complied with your request.
> - In making positive requests, use phrases like
>   - » "I would like you to _____."
>   - » "I would really appreciate it if you would do _____."
>   - » "It's very important to me that you help me with the _____."
>   - » "It would relieve me of a burden if you would_____."

It's important to me that you don't curse." This is much more likely to bring about the desired change than if the family member said, "You have a dirty mouth. If you don't stop that, you'll have to live somewhere else."

CLINICAL EXAMPLE (continued)

After four sessions of education on schizophrenia, Paul and his parents were ready to begin training in communication skills. Training began with the skill "acknowledging positive actions in others," because it boosts family morale and builds good feelings for later training in managing anger, irritation, and frustration. Each person in the family group was given a chance to practice—under the direct supervision of the therapist—the correct use of verbal and nonverbal elements in this communication. For example, Paul was coached to make better eye contact and to say with more vocal emphasis, "Dad, when you let me use your car last night to drive to the movie, I really felt good. It gave me a boost with my friends to be able to offer them a ride instead of bumming a ride from them."

Paul's father chose to compliment his wife on her cooking and home redecorating but needed some modeling from the therapist in coming to the point quickly and in being specific about what he liked. Paul's mother had a knack for this particular skill and required very little instruction. During the next weeks, Paul and his parents practiced this communication skill daily through a homework assignment called "Catch a Person Pleasing You." The diary or log used to prompt and record the homework on this communication skill is shown in Figure 6.4, with the particular entries made during the course of 1 week by Paul's mother included. It should be noted that in practicing communication, family members are encouraged to use the skills with a variety of people, both inside and outside the family. This widespread use of the communication skill aids its durability and generality.

Communication Skills Training
"Giving Positive Feedback"

Date	Person who pleased you	What exactly did they do that pleased you?	What did you say to them?
MON	Paul	Washed the family car	Told him how nice the car looked
TUES	Husband	Complimented my hairdo	Gave him a kiss!
WED	Neighbor	Loaned me some butter	Thanked her
THUR	Paul	Went to the State Dept. of Rehabilitation	Told him how pleased I was that he was interested
FRI	Paul	Took his medication without a reminder	Said it relieved me of worry
SAT	Husband	Went grocery shopping for me	Let him know it gave me some free time
SUN	Sister	Phoned me long distance	Showed excitement in my voice

EXAMPLES:

Looking good	Working in yard	Going to work	Being considerate	Attending treatment
Being on time	Being pleasant	Offering to help	Going out	Making phone call
Helping at home	Having chat	Tidying up	Showing interest	
Cooking meals	Making a suggestion	Making bed	Taking medicine	

FIGURE 6.4 Diary form used in behavioral family management to encourage and reinforce all family members in practicing the communication skill "giving positive feedback." Each day, Paul's mother noted at least one pleasing event or comment initiated by another family member to her and what she said to acknowledge how that positive action made her feel.

FAMILY THERAPIST AS TEACHER AND TRAINER

Behavioral family management is a highly structured, goal-oriented, and competency-based treatment requiring an active, directive therapist. In many ways, the behavioral competencies of the therapist more resemble those of athletic or drama coaches than they do the skills of a traditional psychotherapist. Structuring the session is important if the goals of behavioral family management are to be met. The competent therapist as educator paces the session (much as an orchestra conductor paces a performance) and sets rules and guidelines that establish clear expectancies for the learning of desirable behavior and interactions of family members. Figures 6.5 and 6.6 show the behavioral family therapist actively conducting a session where the family members are using their communication skills for problem solving. The behavioral family therapist actively intervenes to prompt and shape adherence to the agenda set for a particular session. For example, if family members violate the rule "no blaming is allowed," the therapist must consistently interrupt and redirect any blaming statement to a constructive alternative.

Behavioral family management also places a heavy emphasis on instigating behavior change in the home environment. Success in generalizing skills learned in a session into the home requires open and trusting collaboration between therapist and family members, compliance with homework assignments, and positive changes in the family interactions made quickly and early in the series of sessions. Compliance with homework is abetted by the therapist's emphasizing the importance of the task, gaining commitment from the family members to do the assignment, anticipating potential excuses or obstacles in the completion of the assignment, and providing adequate prompts for doing the assignment in the home itself.

Failure to complete homework assignments is cause for problem solving (e.g., asking questions such as "What interfered with your practicing communication at home this week?"), not extensive rationalizations or excuses. In the first place, if the behavioral family therapist does not regularly and predictably inquire about the last homework assignments at the start of each new session, how can there be any expectation that homework will be done? If students in schools were not held accountable for their homework—let's say in getting feedback and marks for them after they are reviewed by the teacher—how could they be expected to complete their homework? The therapist carries the responsibility for motivating generalization of what was learned in treatment sessions into the family home and the family's everyday interactions. If necessary, family members should be required to complete their homework assignments during a therapy session.

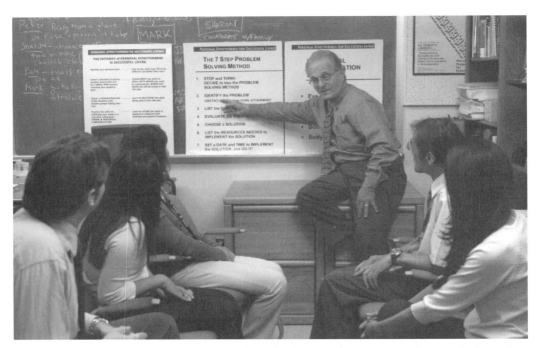

FIGURE 6.5 A behavioral family therapist teaches a family to use their communication skills in the service of problem solving.

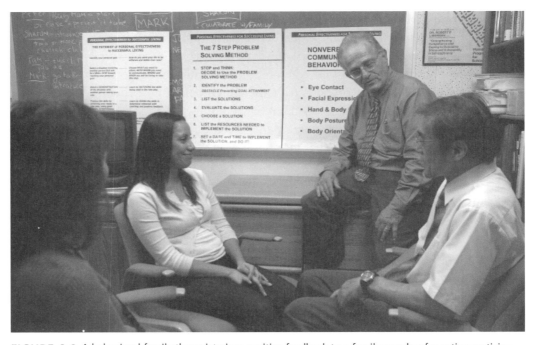

FIGURE 6.6 A behavioral family therapist gives positive feedback to a family member for active participation in the learning of problem-solving skills.

EXAMPLE

In using a problem-solving approach to improve homework completion, the following questions can be used to get patients and their family members to discover for themselves how they can facilitate their generalization of communication and problem-solving skills into everyday life.

THERAPIST: What interfered with your practicing communication at home this week?

FAMILY MEMBER: We just were too busy. So many things came up that we didn't expect.

THERAPIST: Can you think of ways to create a special time for your homework that would not be "invaded" by emergencies or other problems?

FAMILY MEMBER: That's a hard one. We just run out of time.

THERAPIST: Let me suggest some possibilities for completing your homework each week. I'll write them on the board, and we'll consider the feasibility of each one. I'd like you, Mrs. Smith, to be our scribe and take notes.

- Set aside time BEFORE eating each night
- Set an alarm clock for the same time each night and do the homework then
- Take a break from your evening dinner for the homework assignment
- Let me make a phone call to you each night to remind you to do the assignment
- You call me each morning and report to me on your previous day's homework

THERAPIST: OK, let's roll up our sleeves and do some problem solving.

A good behavioral family therapist is a good teacher. In explaining principles and guidelines to patients and relatives, therapists frequently overestimate their capacity for processing information. Even highly educated patients and relatives, because of the stress they are experiencing and other intrinsic learning disabilities, need information that is transmitted simply and clearly in their own language. Frequent repetition is required, along with inquiries that ascertain how well the therapist's communications are being decoded by family members. In addition, the therapist must make sure that patients and relatives are learning to communicate through guidance of principles rather than simply enacting specific verbiage in response to the expectations of the therapy program.

Keeping the patient and relatives on track during structured sessions can be facilitated by the therapist who evokes a positive climate at the start of

LEARNING EXERCISE

To expose yourself to the active and directive skills required in effective behavioral rehabilitation with persons having mental disabilities, try out the following steps in a therapy session with one of your current patients or families. Adapt the methods to your own comfortable style and to the nuances of the therapeutic relationship; however, be prepared to feel some discomfort and awkwardness in being a behavior therapist if your past clinical work has been primarily nondirective and psychodynamic.

- Start by giving the patient and/or family members a rationale for learning one of the communication skills, for example, "acknowledging positive actions by others." Explain how this communication skill will reduce stress and tension in relationships, reinforce the positive features of others, and make others feel good about themselves.

- Ask the patient and/or relatives to repeat, in their own words, the rationale you've just given and to embellish the rationale from their own experiences in giving or receiving positive acknowledgment from others.

- Demonstrate the skill by taking the role of the patient and/or one of the relatives who needs to learn the proper way of expressing this communication. For example, you might say (if taking the role of a relative of a person with schizophrenia), "It really made me relax and feel more optimistic when I noticed that you had taken your medication without any reminders last week."

- Instigate a behavioral rehearsal in which the patient or the family member emulates your demonstrated or modeled expression of positive acknowledgment. Encourage the person to incorporate the behaviors that were modeled into his or her own inimitable style.

- Prompt and coach the person who is going through the behavioral rehearsal. This will require you to get out of your seat and position yourself close to the person performing the behavioral rehearsal. Coaching may involve using hand signals or gestures, giving verbal cues (e.g., "Good, keep up the eye contact"), and kneeling or standing close to the person to provide emotional support.

- When the rehearsal is finished (and, incidentally, keep it brief—not longer than a few minutes at most), provide abundant positive feedback for the person's efforts in using the communication skill. The feedback you give should be specifically focused on the component behaviors that were well communicated. For example, you might say to your patient or family member, "You made good eye contact and spoke with a warm tone of voice when you complimented his attire."

- Adopt a "shaping" attitude, which means looking for and responding to small signs of improvement in the patient's or family member's ability to express feelings and needs. The awkward and halting efforts seen initially will give rise to greater fluency in patients and relatives as repeated rehearsal and positive feedback are provided in the course of skills training.

each session and who clears away distracting and intrusive preoccupations of the family members. For example, an effective behavior therapist starts each session by effusively greeting the patient and relatives, acknowledging positively their attendance, smiling, and putting them at ease with small talk. The therapist solicits information regarding any crisis facing the family since the last meeting and specifies how and when attention will be given to it. If the family group is expected to complete homework assignments, then they must be reinforced for doing so by having the homework focused on as soon as possible in the therapy session. Review of the quality and quantity of completed homework provides an opportunity to reinforce approximations to successful in vivo use of the communication skills being taught and to determine which family members will require attention to remediate deficiencies implicit in the evaluation of the homework. Just as homework begins each session, it ends the session as well.

LEARNING EXERCISE

You may do this exercise through self-observation or by observing one of your colleagues who is attempting to practice behavioral rehabilitation techniques. Check each of the competencies listed below if you observe it being done.

- Actively helps the patient and family in moving from global problems toward setting and eliciting specific goals.
- Assists the patient and family in building possible scenes for behavioral rehearsal in terms of "What emotion, problem, or communication?" "Who is the interpersonal target?" and "Where and when?"
- Orients and instructs patient and family to promote favorable expectations from behavioral family management before role-playing begins.
- Structures role-playing by setting the scene and assigning roles to client and family members.
- Engages the patient and family members in behavioral rehearsal—gets the client and family to role-play with each other.
- Models for the patient and family appropriate and alternative modes of communication and problem solving.
- Prompts, coaches, and cues the patient and family during the role-playing, being out of a seat and providing close support.
- Gives patient and family positive feedback for specific behaviors.
- Gives patient and family corrective feedback for specific deficits and suggests alternative behaviors.
- Ignores or suppresses inappropriate behavior.

- Gets physically within 1 foot of the patient and family during role-playing.
- Suggests an alternative behavior, communication skill, or strategy for a problem situation that can be used and practiced during the behavioral rehearsal or role-playing.

TRAINING IN PROBLEM SOLVING

Once the family unit has gained some experience in the various skills of communicating, using the verbal and nonverbal elements described thus far, the therapist can proceed to the teaching of systematic problem solving. The communication skills serve as building blocks for efforts at problem solving: Without the ability to listen to each other, acknowledge positive efforts, make positive requests of each other, and express unpleasant feelings noncritically, family members will not be able to engage in constructive problem-solving.

What are the problems that face patients and relatives who are dealing with a serious mental disorder? They include all the stressors and painful events of everyday life plus the special burdens added by a pervasive and unrelenting illness, marked by symptoms and disability. The following problems are particularly common in families harboring a chronically mentally ill relative. It should be noted that each problem affects all members of the family, albeit to different degrees and in different ways.

- Social withdrawal, irritability, suspiciousness, erratic eating and sleeping patterns, mood swings, and aggression
- Excessive supervision, nagging, and monitoring of the patient
- Poor grooming and self-care and lack of initiative or desire to participate in activities
- Frustration in obtaining needed help from professionals in a timely and sufficient manner
- Stigma of mental illness felt with friends, siblings, relatives, co-workers, and others in the local community
- Lack of appropriate housing and vocational alternatives for the person with the mental disorder
- Frustration and obstacles in obtaining disability benefits through the Social Security Administration and state vocational rehabilitation agencies

The key role of the problem-solving phase in the overall behavioral family management approach is depicted in Figure 6.7. While elements of the problem-solving sequence in Figure 6.7 are implicitly used by everyone, a

Step 1. **Stop and think! How do you solve problems?**

A problem is an obstacle that prevents you from reaching one of your personal or family goals. When faced by a situation where you don't know what to do, stop and think how to proceed using the problem-solving method.

Step 2. **What is the problem? Use good communication skills while you are problem-solving.**

Discuss with your family members what **obstacles are interfering** with your reaching some important **personal or family goal.** Break big problems down to smaller ones because then it is easier to reach your goal because the obstacles are smaller. Define the problem by writing down the goal and the obstacles after coming to an agreement with your family members.

_____

_____

Step 3. **List all possible ways that the obstacles can be removed and the goal reached.**

Using "brainstorming," list all possible alternatives that may solve the problem. Don't make any judgments about the feasibility of any of the alternatives yet—write down even "bad" or "silly" ideas. Get everyone in the family to contribute suggestions.

1. _____ 2. _____
3. _____ 4. _____
5. _____ 6. _____

Step 4. **Evaluate the alternatives.**

Discuss among the family the advantages and disadvantages of each of the alternative ways identified in Step 3 for solving the problem. Is the alternative feasible? Will it solve the problem? What combinations of alternatives might be most successful in reaching your goal?

	Advantages	**Disadvantages**
1.	_____	_____
2.	_____	_____
3.	_____	_____
4.	_____	_____
5.	_____	_____
6.	_____	_____

For each alternative, do the advantages outweigh the disadvantages?

Step 5. **Choose one or more of the alternatives that are most practical, feasible, and likely to succeed. Reach a consensus among the family members using good communication skills.**

Write down the chosen alternative way you've decided to solve the problem.

_____

_____

Step 6. **Plan how you and your family will implement the alternative(s) that you've chosen. Set a date and time to carry out the plan and DO IT!**

What resources (time, objects such as maps and pencil and paper, transportation, telephone, e-mail, money, other people to help) will you need to solve the problem? Consider how to cope with hitches in the plan. Practice what you will say, to whom, when, and where—use a role-play to practice. Write down the plan.

_____

_____

Step 7. **Review the progress you've made in carrying out the plan.**

Consider what you've been able to accomplish with each step of your problem-solving plan. Each member of the family should give praise and positive feedback for progress, even efforts. If the plan does not work, consider using other alternatives or else return to the beginning and identify a different problem and goal that might be easier to reach.

FIGURE 6.7 Problem-solving worksheet used by family members to reach their personal and family goals in behavioral family management and its derivative family treatments for the seriously mentally ill. The seven-step problem-solving process is guided by the therapist during weekly sessions and continued during family meetings at home between sessions.

highly structured and systematic teaching of the entire sequence is especially important with the seriously mentally ill, for two reasons. First, unless the training is thorough, with overlearning of the steps and sequence, the information-processing deficits of persons with schizophrenia and the stress experienced by their relatives will inevitably interfere with effective problem solving. Second, the problem-solving strategy taught in this phase of behavioral family management will serve as the principal vehicle for generalization and durability of clinical gains beyond the direct intervention period itself. Thus, careful and systematic training in problem-solving skills—built upon previously learned communication skills—becomes the single most important component in the behavioral family management approach to chronic mental disorders.

CLINICAL EXAMPLE (continued)

Paul and his parents presented the problem of Paul's lack of privacy as the problem they wished to work on. Paul described it first as coming from the smallness of their home and the presence of a nephew who lived with them and tended to tease and provoke Paul. In addition, Paul complained that his parents' dissension and arguments would invariably draw him into their conflict, heightening his stress and exacerbating his symptoms. Paul's father, conceding that Paul did lack privacy, felt that the nephew was a major source of the difficulty. Once all family members had a chance to reflect on the problem and to contribute to its clarity and specificity, the therapist asked Paul to serve as scribe and began to generate alternatives for solving the problem.

Paul's mother suggested soundproofing Paul's room; his father suggested that Paul could try jogging or puttering around with house chores to get his mind off the stress. Paul countered with an idea for renovating an old spare room in an unattached section of the home that would place him farther away from others in the family. He also thought that listening to music through headphones might help. Paul's father indicated that Paul could visit his aunt for periods of respite, as she lived nearby. Several other alternatives were presented before the family evaluated each alternative. A consensus was reached on the desirability of renovating the spare room, and the renovation was begun during the next month. Paul's father was a handyman with tools, and Paul launched the renovation by making a positive request for his father's assistance in the project.

LEARNING EXERCISE

Using a problem from one of your own clinical or personal domains, go through the problem-solving sequence. Choose a problem that has been relatively difficult to resolve in the past. See if you can make the problem-solving sequence work for you. When you generate alternatives, it is important to suspend judgment and evaluation of consequences, because this prematurely closes down the essential steps for learning the method. Simply brainstorm any and all options that come to mind. Later, when you move to the evaluation stage, you can consider the feasibility, practicability, and appropriateness of each alternative.

In the actual training of problem-solving skills, each session begins with the therapist soliciting the report of previous problem-solving efforts by the family unit. This comes from the homework assigned from the last session. If the problem previously pinpointed has not been adequately dealt with, the family is asked to consider continued work on that problem before proceeding to another one. In all cases, however, the family members are given the responsibility to designate problems and their priority for solution. Using a worksheet similar to the outline depicted in Figure 6.7, the family works through each of the problem-solving steps. One member of the family takes a turn at being the "scribe" for the family unit and fills in the spaces on the worksheet as the family generates alternatives, weighs pros and cons of each alternative, and works toward an implementation plan.

SPECIAL BEHAVIORAL TECHNIQUES

Professionals experienced in the use of behavior analysis and therapy are able to interpolate these methods into the behavioral family management approach. Specific problems faced by one or another family member may not be remediable through the modules listed earlier (i.e., behavioral assessment, education, communication skills, and problem solving); they may require more focused and definitive interventions drawn from the repertoire of a skilled behavior therapist. Examples of problems that have responded to behavioral techniques include phobias, psychogenic pain, enuresis, extreme social withdrawal, and aggression. Social skills training techniques, elaborated in Chapter 5 ("Social Skills Training"), are frequently employed by professionals in the course of behavioral family management to improve the social functioning and role skills of individual family members.

CLINICAL EXAMPLE (continued)

Paul was stabilized with fluphenazine and was attending behavioral family management with his mother and father when he complained about his difficulty in meeting peers at the local community college he had enrolled in. He was making good progress in learning communication skills in the family sessions, so the therapist decided to set aside some time at the end of one session to offer social skills training on meeting fellow students. Paul readily agreed to role-play approaching a female student after class. He received coaching and modeling from the therapist on how to initiate a greeting and an invitation to study together over coffee in the school cafeteria. After repeating the role-play twice, Paul felt ready to carry out an assignment to approach the young woman the next day in class. He was given a small assignment card by the therapist to remind him to make good eye contact, speak with a firm tone of voice, and use gestures.

LEARNING EXERCISE

Do you have a patient or client who might be suitable for behavioral family management? Even patients with disorders other than schizophrenia can benefit from this modality. Once you've selected a potential patient in your mind, consider the value of offering that patient social skills training in the context of the behavioral family management. One major advantage of linking social skills training with behavioral family management is the promotion of autonomy and individuation. It has been shown in families with a member who has schizophrenia that experience high levels of stress and strain, that less than 35 hours per week of face-to-face contact between the patient and his/her relatives can reduce the likelihood of relapse. So, social skills training can have a dual benefit: moving the young adult patient toward greater independence while at the same time reducing stress within the family environment.

For the patient you've chosen, what interpersonal scene would you formulate for use in social skills training? With whom would the patient interact? Over what social or instrumental need? What would the patient's short- and long-term goals be in that situation? What additional consultation and training would you require before initiating social skills training with that patient?

Adaptations of Family Management for the Mentally Disabled

In the past 25 years, a diversity of approaches have emerged for educating and empowering families of the seriously mentally ill. The origins of these interventions have likewise been diverse: community mental health programs, psychiatric hospitals, veterans hospitals, academic research centers, self-help organizations, and consumer advocates. The methods described for behavioral family management have been adapted for use in multiple-family groups, with teams for assertive community treatment, in consumer-run programs, and for a patient population with a variety of psychiatric disorders: bipolar disorder, depression, panic and agoraphobia, eating disorders, and obsessive-compulsive disorder. Many of these evolving family services have been documented as effective in empirical studies.

Varying in objectives, extensiveness, and breadth, these services draw their inspiration from the same five basic components of behavioral family management: assessment of family, education, training in communication skills, use of problem-solving steps, and special techniques or elements for achieving additional goals. The most successful programs have addressed 15 principles (Table 6.9), identified through a consensus of experts brought together by the World Fellowship for Schizophrenia and Allied Disorders (World Fellowship for Schizophrenia 1999).

MULTIPLE-FAMILY GROUPS

With interest and experience in multiple-family groups and a desire to adapt behavioral family management to that mode of treatment, William McFarlane, M.D., requested consultation and training from the therapists of behavioral family management at the UCLA Clinical Research Center for Schizophrenia and Psychiatric Rehabilitation. The earliest developmental work on behavioral family management actually was done in multifamily groups during the mid-1970s in London and Los Angeles (Liberman et al. 1980, 1984a, 1984b).

In McFarlane's now well-validated and widely used approach, several families with their mentally ill relatives meet together led by one or more professional clinicians. The frequency of the meetings varies, but the overall aim is to have the families serve as a supportive social network that organizes and coordinates most of the mental health services—except medication—needed by the patients. The multifamily group provides:

> ● **TABLE 6.9**
>
> **Guidelines for working with families that have a member with a disabling mental disorder to facilitate his/her recovery**
>
> Mental health professionals working with families that have a member with a disabling mental disorder can facilitate the recovery of the patient. This is expedited by strengthening families' capacities to cope with stress and collaborate with practitioners who are offering services to their relative. The 15 principles listed below serve as guidelines to practitioners.
>
> 1. Coordinate all elements of treatment and rehabilitation to ensure that everyone is working toward the same goals in a collaborative, supportive relationship.
> 2. Pay attention to both the social and the clinical needs of the patient.
> 3. Ensure optimum medication management.
> 4. Listen to families' concerns and involve them as equal partners in the planning and delivery of treatment.
> 5. Explore family members' expectations of the treatment program and expectations for the patient.
> 6. Assess the strengths and limitations of the family's ability to support the consumer.
> 7. Help resolve family conflict by responding sensitively to emotional distress.
> 8. Address feelings of loss.
> 9. Provide relevant information for the patient and his/her family at appropriate times.
> 10. Provide an explicit crisis plan and professional response.
> 11. Help improve communication among family members.
> 12. Provide training for the family through structured problem-solving techniques.
> 13. Encourage family members to expand their social support networks and to participate in family advocacy and self-help organizations (e.g., NAMI).
> 14. Be flexible in meeting the needs of the family and be sensitive to cultural and ethnic differences.
> 15. Provide the family with easy access to another professional in the event that the current treatment relationship with the family ceases.

- Engagement of families and patients in a group mediated by an alliance with experienced, knowledgeable, and empathic professionals.
- Education about schizophrenia, its presumed causes, and the protective and stress factors that determine the course of illness.
- Guidelines for coping with the illness as a family and advocating for needed services.
- Practice in solving problems that are connected with the illness.

- Pursuit of vocational and social rehabilitation for the patients through the efforts of the cohesive, supportive, and increasingly capable family members.
- A mini–social network in which families help one another in tangible ways to reach recovery-oriented goals.

Multifamily groups offer indefinite, long-term services—spirited by competent and compassionate clinicians—including the full range of psychosocial treatment and rehabilitation. High levels of cohesion are established through the development of long-term social networks of family members who share a common cause for promoting recovery in their loved ones. One of the most impressive results of the networking is the "job club" that family members form, tirelessly seeking employment for whoever needs it from among the mentally ill relatives of the group members. In fact, the employment outcomes are among the very best in vocational rehabilitation of the mentally ill.

The multifamily group treatment model has been disseminated widely throughout the United States and foreign countries, with evidence of cross-cultural efficacy. In one study of this modality when offered in a randomized, controlled trial to English- and Vietnamese-speaking families together with their schizophrenic relatives, individuals from both cultural groups that participated in the family treatment experienced substantially fewer relapses, lower symptoms, and better vocational outcomes (Bradley et al. 2006).

FAMILY-ASSISTED ASSERTIVE COMMUNITY TREATMENT

By connecting the therapeutic elements of the multifamily group to a coordinated team providing in vivo outreach services of assertive community treatment, there is an amplification of the effectiveness of the multifamily group alone (McFarlane et al. 1992). The assertive community treatment clinicians provide crisis intervention, job development and job finding, encouragement, and assistance for graded increases in responsibilities for community living by patients while collaborating at the same time with families. With use of a combination of these two evidence-based interventions, relapse rates are substantially lowered and vocational outcomes improved.

FAMILY-FOCUSED TREATMENT FOR BIPOLAR DISORDER

As a graduate student and postgraduate fellow at the UCLA Clinical Research Center for Schizophrenia and Psychiatric Rehabilitation, David

Miklowitz, Ph.D., adapted the techniques of behavioral family management for the special problems and needs of persons with bipolar disorder (Miklowitz and Goldstein 1997). His interest in designing a family treatment for bipolar disorder was sparked by his finding that families with few coping skills and high "expressed emotion" needed an educationally based treatment to reduce their stress. An effective family-focused intervention would empower them to manage the manifold problems and turmoil that accompanied episodes of mania and depression in their loved ones. This diagnosis-specific approach, termed *family-focused treatment,* has been shown in controlled studies to be an evidence-based practice for bipolar disorder. Family-focused treatment includes 21 sessions delivered over 9 months to patients and their family members together. Family-focused treatment has been shown to reduce relapse rates and rehospitalization, produce better medication adherence, and strengthen the capacity of the family to effectively manage daily life with their ill relative.

Given the lifelong susceptibility of persons with bipolar disorder to recurrences of manic and depressive episodes, family-focused treatment aims to assist patients and their relatives to:

- Understand the stress-related, biological nature of their disorder and gain conceptual mastery over the prospects of relapse by learning about protective factors.
- Develop a relapse prevention contract based on their becoming familiar with the warning signs or prodromal symptoms to relapse.
- Practice using their relapse prevention contract with a well-defined emergency activation strategy when warning signs emerge.
- Accept the need and understand the value for long-term, maintenance, prophylactic mood-stabilizing medication.
- Learn how to cope with stressors that unavoidably crop up in family life, including use of alcohol, marijuana, and other illicit drugs.
- Acquire communication skills that can then be used to solve problems, large and small.

Patients and relatives together are taught to keep a chart that tracks daily moods on a 6-point scale from -3 (severely depressed) to 0 (normal) to $+3$ (manic). On the same chart, the participants record use of medication, hours of sleep, stressors, and symptoms such as irritability, social withdrawal, or inflated self-esteem. Overcoming obstacles to maintaining a consistent sleep/wake cycle is one of the most important problems to solve because of the protective function of proper sleep in forestalling manic relapses.

INVOLVING FAMILIES IN SERVICES FOR THE SERIOUSLY MENTALLY ILL: A VIDEO-ASSISTED MODULE

Developed in collaboration with NAMI, this video-assisted program was designed for mental health professionals with little or no experience in collaborating with family members in the treatment of persons with schizophrenia and other disabling disorders (Liberman et al. 2000). A series of sessions commences with the engagement of family members in a partnership with clinicians to augment the impact of comprehensive services for the mentally disabled. The sessions include step-by-step procedures for teaching family members and their mentally ill relative essential communication skills, problem-solving skills, and how to use an integrated approach for persons with dual substance abuse and mental disorders. There are seven sessions, each comprising a set of competencies that the clinician is learning as he/she teaches a variety of skills to the family.

The program is flexible and can include the patient if it is deemed advisable. The decision to include the patient is primarily made on the basis of symptom and cognitive stability; in other words, if the patient is coherent, has sustained attention with little distractibility, and has no symptoms that would intrude on the learning process, then patient participation is desirable. The seven skill areas for the module "Involving Families in Services for the Seriously Mentally Ill" are listed in Table 6.10.

In session 6, families are taught how to cope with particular difficulties and challenges presented by patients with treatment-refractory disorders, dual diagnosis patients, aggressive patients, patients involved in the crimi-

---

● **TABLE 6.10**

Skill areas for the module Involving Families in Services for the Seriously Mentally Ill

1. Developing a collaboration with the family
2. Offering information on mental illness
3. Enhancing family communication and problem solving
4. Helping the family access and use the mental health service system
5. Helping the family meet its own needs
6. Helping the family cope with special characteristics of the patient
7. Managing confidentiality and cultural diversity

nal justice system, children, and individuals with a recent onset of mental illness. The competencies in session 6 mirror these challenges for the trainer. In session 5, practitioners acquire competencies for the following teaching skills:

- Connect families to community resources, including NAMI affiliates
- Relieve burden and grief that come from having a mentally ill relative
- Empower families to become involved in advocacy for their mentally ill relative's needs for treatment and rehabilitation as well as for obtaining a broader spectrum of mental health services for the community as a whole
- Encourage families to learn how to use stress management skills, maintain their social support network, and keep a life of their own apart from the mentally ill relative
- Use behavioral learning techniques to assist families to acquire and make use of educational materials wisely

The practitioner uses structured exercises for engaging the family and patient in the educational process. Interventions for reducing the family's emotional burden include ways to broaden their social support network. Training is accomplished by the mental health professional using a trainer's manual, with the family member and patient following a consumer's guide and a demonstration video that employs real family members and patients achieving the learning objectives set for each session. The following dialogue, used in session 5, aims to help a single mother to keep her own life goals alive to cope with the worries of what is happening to her son, who has schizophrenia and is living in a board-and-care home.

EXAMPLE

MS. SIMPSON: I just feel awful that Scott had to move out. You know, he got so paranoid that he threatened the neighbors, and my landlord said either Scott went or we both went. I certainly didn't have the money or energy to move. But I never wanted him in one of those places. And now I worry about him all the time.

CLINICIAN: You worry all the time?

MS. SIMPSON: Well, is he eating, losing weight, and getting along with his roommate? Is he smoking too much, drinking, or using marijuana? When we lived together I could watch him.

CLINICIAN: Sounds like it's a lot of stress for you. What happens when you worry too much?

MS. SIMPSON: I can't sleep. I just watch the clock in the middle of the night and worry.

CLINICIAN: Are you still going for a walk each evening?

MS. SIMPSON: No, I'm too busy. I don't get home from work until 8 P.M., and then it's dark and I try to reach Scott on the phone to see how he's doing.

CLINICIAN: Why do you get home so late?

MS. SIMPSON: Well, I'm preoccupied with Scott, amd it's so difficult for me to concentrate on my work and organize my time.

CLINICIAN: So it sounds like you need to figure out how to allocate your time a little better to make sure that you get your walk and connect with Scott enough to feel comfortable. Let's try to get Scott on the phone right now and see how he feels about your being so worried about him. Also, you need to contact your friends and relatives to get support from them now that they all know about Scott's illness.

FAMILY INTERVENTIONS IN EARLY PSYCHOSIS

Family services have been adapted to meet the particular needs of families with a young adult whose psychotic disorder is of recent onset or whose prodromal symptoms have prompted them to come for assistance. Considerable effort is expended to include families as collaborators in the treatment process, especially because of their high level of anxiety, concern, and confusion about the nature of their teenagers or young adults. For this reason, family members are invited to attend all meetings for treatment planning and medication management with their relative's psychiatrist. Staff members experienced in working with families are assigned to families as they enter the clinic program. Concern about the impact of psychosis on the family system is reflected by the overall goals to minimize the disruption to the life of the family, the adverse effects of demoralization and grief, and the high levels of burden. During six to eight sessions over the course of 6 months, family members, together with their ill relative, participate in education, although more frequent sessions are scheduled to help families to recognize and respond to early warning signs of relapse (for relapse prevention) and crises associated with the psychosis.

A flexible program of services is individualized to meet the special needs of each family and can include training in communication and problem-solving skills.

PSYCHOEDUCATIONAL APPROACHES

Less intensive than behavioral family management and its variants are a host of educational programs that have more modest aims. For these programs, primarily designed to offer time-limited lecture-discussion groups, mental health practitioners and advocates have crafted curricula that serve very much like the lesson plans used by schoolteachers. The best of these are refined during field trials and years of experience. Typically, they consist of a series of sessions with educational objectives for family members, with or without the presence of the patient, to learn about 1) the diagnosis, etiology, and influences bearing on mental disorders; 2) pharmacological and psychosocial treatments; 3) appropriate services available in the local community; 4) the importance of developing collaborative relationships with mental health professionals; and 5) ways of coping with the stress and challenges of living with a mental disorder. Research has shown that one of the main beneficial outcomes of psychoeducational programs that are offered by mental health clinics and other facilities is much more favorable attitudes by family members toward the clinicians serving their ill loved ones. These improved attitudes are translated into better communication, relationships, and detection of early warning signs of relapse.

Support and Family Education (S.A.F.E. Program)

A carefully structured workshop for delivering information and coping skills to family members and community caregivers of persons with severe mental disorders, the S.A.F.E. Program was developed and validated by Michelle Sherman, Ph.D., at the Oklahoma City Veterans Affairs (VA) Medical Center. She and her colleagues have held psychoeducational workshops for family members and other caregivers, consisting of 18 monthly sessions, led by professional clinicians, on a continuous, rotating basis for over 8 years with notable success. Unique among psychoeducators, Sherman included information on a variety of mental disorders, including posttraumatic stress disorder, consistent with the varied population of the VA Medical Center. A special feature of this program is the personalized attention that can be given to the participants, since the latter complete a questionnaire in advance of coming to the first session. The questionnaire elicits information from them regarding their experiences as caregivers during the previous month, their problems in coping with the mentally ill person, caregivers' level of distress, their understanding of mental illness, and their ability to take good care of themselves.

Each session begins with a review of the goals of the program and an empathic and mutually supportive discussion of the caregivers' problems and successes during the previous month. A 45-minute didactic workshop with active discussion is promoted by the clinician, who follows a detailed lesson plan. The workshop features role-plays of coping skills, discussion questions, video clips that highlight problems and solutions covered in the session, and handouts. The list of topics for each of the sessions is given in Table 6.11. One of the most important "draws" of the workshops is the opportunity they afford caregivers to throw questions about medication issues to a psychiatrist, who is always present. Given the slim opportunities for family members to meet with their relatives' psychiatrists, it is highly reinforcing for them to discuss their concerns and worries about medication with an expert. A representative of the local NAMI organization is also present to contribute to the discussion and to raise awareness of the mani-

● **TABLE 6.11**

Topics for each session of the S.A.F.E. workshops

1. What causes mental illness?
2. What can I do when my family member is depressed?
3. What can I do when my family member is angry or violent?
4. Communicating tips for family members.
5. Limit setting and boundaries with family members.
6. How can I take care of myself as caregiver?
7. Rights and responsibilities of patients, family members, and professionals.
8. What do we tell other people about mental illness?
9. Stress-busting tips for family members.
10. What do you do when your help is rejected?
11. Do's and don'ts in helping your family member.
12. Tips to help make the holiday season pleasant.
13. Posttraumatic stress disorder and its impact on the family.
14. Schizophrenia and its impact on the family.
15. Common family reactions to mental illness.
16. Problem-solving skills for families.
17. Creating a low-stress environment and minimizing crises.
18. Coping with the stigma surrounding mental illness.

fold resources offered by this self-help group as well as in the community as a whole. The sessions close with the distribution of small gifts to signify the leaders' appreciation for the participants' commitment to their ill relatives.

While the participation of patients together with their caregivers is often viewed as essential in family management services, when a workshop like S.A.F.E. has such a large amount of information and problem solving to accomplish in a limited time, it can be decided to hold separate psychoeducation groups for patients. It must be understood that the aims of the S.A.F.E. Program are to improve the coping skills of the family members, not to bring about clinical improvement in the patient. This is a key issue, because clinicians often neglect the protean needs of family members and other community caregivers. Biting off too much in the limited time frame that most mental health professionals have to educate caregivers is a recipe for failure.

EXAMPLE

One of the handouts offered by the S.A.F.E. program is used in the session "Stress-Busting Tips for Caregivers." It reveals the practical nature of psychoeducation that enables caregivers to use in their everyday life what they've learned from the workshop. The handout also exemplifies the use of humor in distancing caregivers' moods away from worry and gloom.

Everyday Survival and Stress-Busting Kit

Each item in your kit is to remind you:

Toothpick—to pick out the good qualities in others.

Rubber band—to be flexible; things might not always go the way you want.

Band-Aid—to heal hurt feelings, yours or someone else's.

Pencil—to list your blessings every day.

Eraser—that everyone makes mistakes, and it's okay!

Chewing gum—to stick with it and you can accomplish almost anything.

Candy kiss—that everyone needs a kiss or hug every day.

Tea bag—to relax daily and go over that list of your blessings.

Evaluation of the S.A.F.E. Program has been favorable, with significant increases in knowledge of mental illness and awareness of treatment and rehabilitation resources in the community and at the veterans hospital. Over time, attendance has increased from an average of 4 to more than 25 per session. As expected, a significant correlation was found between the number of sessions attended and the caregivers' ability to effectively manage the stressors and challenges of everyday life with their mentally ill relatives and community residents. The satisfaction of attendees with the program was astounding; the overall mean satisfaction rating was 18 out of a possible 20. The S.A.F.E. Program curriculum has been attractively packaged in the form of a manual for widespread dissemination and is available from a University of Oklahoma Web site (http://w3.ouhsc.edu/safeprogram).

> "To the world,
> you may just be
> somebody...
> but to somebody,
> you may be the
> world."
>
> APOCRYPHAL

EXAMPLE

Attendance at family education groups or workshops can be elicited in a variety of ways; for example, by phone or e-mail, personalized invitations when family members visit their relative who is hospitalized, at the time of admission to the hospital, or by letters. Here is an example of a letter that regularly resulted in high rates of attendance, most likely because it offered highly valued information or consultation opportunities about each family's concerns for their ill relative.

"It's time again for that once-in-a-month opportunity; the hospital's family education meeting. If you have a loved one in the hospital or if your family member is a former patient now living in the community, we look forward to seeing you. We have information to share with you regarding the progress of your hospitalized relative in his/her individualized treatment plan and on an educational topic related to serious mental disorders. This month, there will be opportunities for specialized consultations from Dr. K and Dr. L, who will answer questions that you have related to your relative with mental illness, whether hospitalized or now in the community."

Working With Families

Working With Families is another psychoeducational program that has been successfully disseminated to agencies throughout the United States, Japan, and other countries. It comprises three user-friendly manuals that enable practitioners to rapidly and competently teach family members and patients essential information about schizophrenia and its management: 1) *Schizophrenia: A Family Education Curriculum*; 2) *Schizophrenia: Family Education Methods*; and 3) *Family Skills for Relapse Prevention* (Amenson 1998). The manuals are designed to be used by mental health professionals, who can

> "In time of test,
> family is best."
>
> BURMESE SAYING

flexibly draw from the detailed lesson plans, handouts, and slide presentations in leading small or large groups of family members—with or without patients present. Created and produced by Christopher Amenson, Ph.D., and sponsored by the Pacific Clinics Institute of Pasadena, California, the credibility and effectiveness of the curricula are amplified by having consumers who have recovered from mental disorders and family members serve as co-leaders.

When used fully, the manuals provide the technical resources for a 12-hour course on schizophrenia, appropriate for family members, as well as paraprofessional caregivers who serve schizophrenia patients in a variety of community residences and mental health agencies. The topical content, amount, frequency, and duration of family education can be tailored to the special needs of the target population, psychiatric hospital, psychosocial rehabilitation center, mental health agency, or even private practice.

Demonstrating the potential for wide-scale adoption of this approach to family education, a three-phase training program was used to teach leadership skills to 39 social workers, psychologists, and nurses selected competitively from most mental health centers of the Los Angeles County Department of Mental Health (Amenson and Liberman 2001). In phase 1, participants received 20 hours of didactic training over a 7-week period. They were provided with an overview of research on family psychoeducation, methods for engaging and collaborating with families, skill-building exercises, and practice assignments to complete at their "home" clinics. Phase 2 consisted of six sessions, lasting a total of 18 hours, during which trainees became familiar with the manuals serving as technical support for their subsequent efforts in leading family groups at their own mental health centers. Surrogate classes were formed with five to six trainees, each of whom played the role of a family member while rotating responsibilities as "teacher" or group leader. Key skills that were learned included the ability to:

- Communicate interest in and empathy toward the audience.
- Demonstrate organization and knowledge of the material.
- Provide a conceptual map for understanding schizophrenia for the audience.
- Use stories, analogies, or personal experience to enhance learning.
- Use strong opening and closing statements.

In the final phase, each trainee took turns as a "practice teacher" for the others, who role-played an audience of family members. The practice teacher led one session from *A Family Education Curriculum,* using selected behavioral techniques drawn from the manual *Schizophrenia: Family Edu-*

cation Methods. After completing a competency test, the trainees started family education classes at their mental health centers. Supervision was provided by the master trainer, with positive reinforcement delivered for successes and problem solving for nettlesome difficulties encountered with their family groups. The trainees favorably evaluated the scope and methods used in their three- phase learning experience.

The training resulted in a doubling of the proportion of the trainees who actually led family education groups during the 9 months subsequent to their participation in the three-phase program compared with the 9 months before—from 44% to 87%. The number of family education groups given by the trainees almost quadrupled between the same 9 month periods, from 41 to 156. The success of this project for "training the trainers" can be attributed to the 1) persistent advocacy for family education services by NAMI–LA County; 2) support of top management of the county mental health department, which made family education a priority for all mental health centers; and 3) on-site consultation and feedback by the trainer at each mental health center that encouraged flexible adaptation of the curriculum and provided motivation to the neophyte leaders of the family courses.

Family-to-Family

After years of frustration with the failure of mental health service agencies to offer psychoeducation to families of the seriously mentally ill, NAMI took the bull by the horns and created its own, peer-led family education courses. Family-to-Family courses are organized and led by volunteers who are drawn from the membership of local NAMI affiliates in all 50 states. Lasting 12 weeks, the course is standardized with curriculum materials developed by the national headquarters of NAMI. Volunteers must first go through a demanding training process that enables them to acquire group leadership skills as well as knowledge related to major mental disorders and their treatments.

The main aim of the Family-to-Family program is to enable family members who attend the sessions to successfully transit through the stages of coping with the experience of having a relative disabled by a mental disorder. These stages include 1) comprehending and accepting the reality of the illness; 2) realizing that while cures are not available, effective treatment and rehabilitation are; 3) dealing with the anxiety, frustration, demoralization, and grief that constitute a common response to the disabling transformation of their loved ones; 4) accepting the illness, with realistic expectations for slow and gradual improvement with treatment; and 5) becoming advocates for the treatment needs of their loved ones. Priority is given to promoting the adaptation and well-being of family members, with the hope that salutary changes in the families will yield some indirect benefits to those with the mental illness. Evaluation of the Family-to-Family program has revealed increased knowledge about the causes and treatment of mental disorders, greater equanimity and confidence in coping with their relatives' illness, and improved savvy in dealing with local mental health services.

Empirical evaluations of the Family-to-Family course found that by 6–12 months after completing the program, the participants had become significantly more knowledgeable about mental illnesses and the treatments available for them, empowered to manage family problems, with greater vitality in their emotional life. They had fewer negative views of their relationships with their ill relatives (Dixon et al. 2001b; Pickett et al. 2006). They also experienced less unhappiness and worry. As would be expected from a course that provided brief, time-limited lectures and discussion of general knowledge for family members alone, one would not have expected improvements in the course of illness of their ill relatives. Measurable benefits for the designated patient requires a broader curriculum that includes intensive training of skills in communicating, solving problems, and negotiating and collaborating with the practitioners who are the representatives of the mental health service system. The families did not gain improvements in family burden, self-esteem, depression, physical illnesses, mastery in their dealings with their mentally ill relatives, or supports from their social network. Only more extensive training customized to the needs and goals of families, such as that provided by behavioral family management, could be expected to bring about a broader array of improvements in their lives and the lives of their loved ones who are ill.

In addition to the Family-to-Family educational seminar, most NAMI affiliates around the country offer regularly scheduled "care and share" support groups that enable family members to discuss the many obstacles they encounter in trying to motivate their mentally ill loved ones in treatment as well as in finding and motivating mental health professionals and programs to provide adequate services. In these peer support groups, many family members learn that "we are not alone." While the social support and networking functions of the "care and share" groups are valuable, a considerable number of family members have told me that they drop out of the groups because they themselves are up to their ears with their own problems and don't want to hear more about the plight of others. To balance this conundrum, most NAMI groups invite mental health professionals to give monthly or bimonthly lectures on promising developments in the field of psychiatry, followed by questions and answers that can lead family members out of the quagmire and onto higher, more solid ground.

EXAMPLE

After completing a Family-to-Family course, Ms. Wasow, a single mother with an adult son who has schizophrenia, got up her nerve to approach a new psychiatrist who had been assigned to treat her son. Because her son continued to have delusions and hallucinations despite optimal pharmacology, Ms. Wasow was going to ask the psychiatrist to consider using the newly developed, evidence-based treatment called *cognitive-behavioral therapy for psychosis*. As she walked through the door to the mental health clinic, she tensed up, a residuum of many unpleasant encounters with mental health professionals in that building who had not wanted to talk with her about her ideas for her son.

She was mightily surprised to be greeted by a young woman doctor with a warm smile, an extended hand, and the words, "Oh, thank you for taking the time to meet with me." The mother was so taken back that she immediately showed the doctor some photos of her son that were taken before his illness.

"She asked me excellent questions that might provide information to guide her initial approaches to my son. She made me feel like an expert about my son, which I am in some respects, and I think I gave her useful information. We parted with expressions of mutual thanks and appreciation."

On her part, the young psychiatrist waited for the mother to leave, then found tears moistening her eyes. "I looked at the worn photograph. A boy of about ten . . . smiling . . . happy . . . full of life and all its possibilities. His mother glowed with pride as she described her son and his many hobbies: making pottery, fishing, and playing the guitar. When I met with her son, a soft-spoken man with eyes downcast and a thick beard hiding and protecting him, I said, 'Hello, it's good to see you again.' He replied, 'Hello,' and agreed to have our session while walking outdoors. As we talked, there was not much difference in his demeanor, but despite the limited exchange of words, I was able to grasp the richness and wholeness of this man and his life. He is a man with diverse interests, fond memories, and potential for the future, and he has a family who loves him.

"As a physician in this day and age with our 15-minute medical checks, it is so easy to lose sight of the wholeness of the person, to only see our clients as snapshots during that one brief moment in their lives, to forget the context, the life story. How fortunate I was to be given the gift of a broader perspective through the eyes of his mother. Psychiatrists and family members should automatically contact one another as step one. When they meet, a very useful exchange can ensue, where the family member is invited to tell the story of the patient's whole life, to bring alive a person in the fullness of his interests, desires, strengths, hopes, and personal goals."

LEARNING EXERCISE

You can work synergistically with NAMI groups in your locale or state and thereby promote the coping efforts of relatives of your patients and their collaboration with you. But it is first necessary that you make contact with such groups firsthand, get acquainted with their leadership and membership, and explore ways for mutual assistance. One concrete way to develop a working alliance with these groups is to offer to give a talk or lead an informal coping and support group in a discussion of mental illness. The families are always hungry to hear from psychiatrists, as most family members are deprived of opportunities to talk to the psychiatrists of their loved ones. This exercise is a prompt for you to locate at least one NAMI group near your place of professional practice and expose yourself to its activities and members. To locate the nearest group, check your phone book under National Alliance on Mental Illness or phone the national headquarters of NAMI in Arlington, Virginia at 703-378-2353.

▶ Summary

Families of patients with chronic mental disorders are ill equipped to manage the primary caretaking responsibilities that have fallen to them because of deinstitutionalization. Practitioners in hospital and community-based facilities for the severely and chronically psychiatrically disabled are only beginning to educate families about the nature of illnesses such as schizophrenia, to train them in specific skills that are helpful in coping with the long-term management of the mentally ill, and to provide support for the families burdened by the stress and tension of chronic illness.

For those handicapped mentally ill persons who live with or near their families, the importance of the family can scarcely be overstated. Family members often represent the patient's primary source of companionship, involvement in activities, and assistance in coping with day-to-day problems.

The responsibilities for providing case management for their mentally ill relatives often create stress and conflict within the family unit. Relatives can become overinvolved with a mentally ill family member who appears to be helpless to fend for himself/herself. Without support and education from professionals, relatives can also lack the understanding of the nature of chronic schizophrenia that enables them to lower their performance expectations of the patient to a more realistic level.

Schizophrenia can be considered a stress-related illness, and tension in the home, when accompanied by frustration, disappointment, criticism, intrusiveness, and demoralization, can contribute to an emotional climate that fosters relapse. An increase or reappearance of psychotic symptoms in a person who is biologically vulnerable to schizophrenia can be an outcome of the precarious balance between the amount of life stressors and the problem-solving skills of the individual and his/her family system. Too much stress—such as that resulting from criticism or overinvolvement with a relative—or too few coping and problem-solving skills can lead to symptomatic exacerbations.

The goals of behavioral family management are to reduce tension and stress in the family system by transmitting to the patient and his/her relatives a clear understanding of schizophrenia or other major mental disorders in lay terms, to teach problem-solving and communication skills, and to increase the patient's adherence to antipsychotic medication and psychosocial rehabilitation programs. A further aim of behavioral family management is to enhance the social adjustment and quality of life of the patient and relatives through teaching them the functional skills for meeting their needs and obtaining required mental health and social services.

Behavioral family therapy is highly structured and systematically employs principles of learning and behavior change. However, it is conducted in a nurturing manner by therapists who aim to maintain a warm and encouraging learning environment for the patient and relatives. The therapist's firm and directive, yet gentle and supportive, style keeps the family on track through the various educational objectives inherent in the therapy. In the initial phase of behavioral family management, information is presented to families in a didactic format, with the use of visual aids and handouts on the nature, course, and treatment of schizophrenia. Family members are asked to share their perceptions and experiences, and the patient is encouraged to discuss symptoms as the "expert" in that area. Schizophrenia is presented by the therapist as a disorder marked by severe problems in living—working, self-care, socializing, thinking, and feeling. Education on the etiology and treatment of the disorder is tailored to the level of sophistication of each family. The educational process, offered in a supportive manner, helps families to lighten their burden of guilt, overresponsibility, confusion, and helplessness. Relatives become less judgmental, intrusive, and critical of the patient's behavior and learn to set more realistic goals for themselves and the mentally ill family member.

Since the stress of chronic mental disorders poses continuing challenges for problem solving over the long haul, patient and relatives alike are helped to learn how to communicate effectively with one another and the world around them. Effective coping, communicating, and problem solving together have the potential for reducing impairments and disabilities of major mental disorders, reducing the burden of illness on the family, and maximizing social and instrumental role functioning. Communication and problem-solving skills are taught systematically by providing a rationale for each targeted skill, step-by-step instruction in the use of the skill, demonstrations, and practice through behavioral rehearsal and homework assignments aimed at generalization and overlearning. Unqualified praise for each step taken toward acquiring and using the skills and knowledge imparted in behavioral family management reinforces the learning process.

Results from well-designed and controlled outcome studies suggest that behavioral family management and its analogues can reduce family stress, burden, and relapse. Marked improvements in social functioning can accrue to patients and relatives alike. Optimism can be gained from the impact of family-based approaches to psychiatric rehabilitation when therapies harness available principles of learning and methods for facilitating interpersonal relationship skills. Much progress can be expected by expanding family involvement in the community management of schizophrenia and other chronic mental disorders. It is obvious that family members having extended contact with a patient have the potential for magnifying the impact of mental health services. By teaching patients and relatives a conceptual and factual understanding of mental illness and how to better cope, communicate, and solve problems, mental health professionals can increase their efficacy in a manner that will prove cost-effective.

A broad-based consumer advocacy movement comprising family members and patients will no longer accept a passive role in treatment and rehabilitation of the mentally ill. Mental health professionals will have to obtain training and experience in working collaboratively with families if they want to avoid being marginalized by a powerful and parallel system of self-help in education, coping with the illness, personal and social supports, advocacy, and assertiveness. Families and patients are determined to take control of their illnesses and lives with or without the help of professionals. The use of family education in routine clinical practice is alarmingly limited, despite the fact that various forms of psychoeducation are evidence-based and packaged in forms that are user-friendly.

The consumer movement is person-centered and recovery-oriented. Members of this unstoppable movement will continue to insist that they be involved as active participants in diagnosis, treatment planning, use of pharmacological and psychosocial treatments, and the full range of rehabilitative services. When families become collaborators in treatment, their stress levels and burnout are reduced and their morale is lifted, and they become more effective "extenders" of professional services.

The best outcomes ensue from intensive and long-term treatment of the whole family when education about mental disorders and their treatments is combined with training of communication and problem-solving skills and expansion of the supportive social networks of families. The results are remarkable, with rates of relapse and rehospitalization lower by two- to five-fold when compared with medication, case management, and supportive therapy. Better adherence to treatment is noted, as well as improved family, social, and vocational functioning. Research has documented superior benefits for behaviorally oriented family therapy as compared with customary treatments in the following disorders: schizophrenia, bipolar disorder, major depression, alcoholism, agoraphobia, eating disorders, and obsessive-compulsive disorder.

Longer-term treatment is usually held weekly for 3 months, biweekly for 6 months, and then monthly for 2 years. Sometimes multiple-family groups continue on indefinitely to maintain and further the improvements that have been attained. There is every good reason to offer family support and training in coping skills on a continuing, indefinite basis, just as psychiatrists provide with medication. Recovery will become the rule rather than the exception as educational programs for families evolve with the guidance of empirical evaluation and are integrated with medication and illness management, social skills training, supported employment, and assertive community management.

▶ Key Points

- Family members are of enormous importance in promoting recovery by their mentally ill loved ones. When families are not equipped with coping skills by mental health practitioners, the stress, frustration, and emotional and financial burdens of caregiving are overwhelming. Because schizophrenia and other mental disorders are stress-related biomedical illnesses, a lack of coping skills has adverse consequences on the patient as well as the family.

- When the emotional temperature rises within families "living on the edge," mentally ill members also experience stress and show higher rates of relapse and poor functioning. When mental health professionals reach out to families and offer them support and coping skills in dealing with intransigent and mystifying symptoms and disability, mentally ill relatives experience significant reductions in relapse.

- It is essential for practitioners to be educated about the absolute necessity of reaching out and involving families in diagnosis, functional assessment, illness management, rehabilitation planning, and supporting the treatment and rehabilitation services being provided to their ill members.

- Family interventions have been well documented as effective and evidence-based when they provide education about mental illness and its treatments, communication skills, and use of their know-how and skills in solving the problems that inevitably surface in family interactions.

- Key communication skills for reducing stress in families include:
  » Active listening.
  » Giving positive feedback for adaptive behavior.
  » Making positive requests, not advice, instructions, or demands.
  » Expressing frustration, stress, sadness, and annoyance in constructive ways.
  » Taking time out from heated interactions.

- Effective family services help relatives and patients alike to use communication skills in everyday problem solving. The problem-solving steps that make up effective coping and stress management are:
  » Identifying a family problem as one or more obstacles interfering with achieving mutually agreed-upon goals.
  » Brainstorming alternative ways to remove those obstacles.
  » Weighing the pros and cons of each alternative, in terms of feasibility and utility for achieving the goal.
  » Selecting one or more alternative methods and planning their implementation.
  » Evaluating the benefits resulting from the problem-solving efforts.
  » Giving mutual positive feedback for success and recycling the procedure for the next problem that emerges within the family.

- Family advocacy groups have developed and disseminated specific self-help programs that have been shown to be helpful to families in coping with the burden of severe mental illness within their midst. These groups include:
  » Family to-Family educational seminars.
  » Peer-to-Peer educational seminars.

- » In Our Own Voice education for the public and for mental health professionals.
- » Care and Share groups in many locales around the United States.
- » Political advocacy for improved mental health services and research.

- Adaptations of behavioral family management have been broadly conceived and empirically evaluated, following the principle of "re-invention" of innovations to better fit the patient population, nature of the disorder, and constraints and resources in each locality.

- Effective analogues include multiple-family therapy, family-focused therapy for bipolar disorder, and brief educational programs that were designed for and found helpful in groups of family members who were baffled by harboring a mentally ill person in their home and were unable to obtain comprehensive psychoeducational assistance from their local mental health centers and privately practicing psychiatrists.

- The Family-to-Family education program has a standardized curriculum, and its trainers are volunteers from the local affiliates of NAMI. The program has been favorably evaluated and is offered widely in the United States.

- While psychoeducation can be helpful to all patients as well as relatives, the benefits do not extend much farther than improved collaboration with mental health professionals and some attenuation of the worry and stress of the family members.

- The recovery movement and the Internet will continue to encourage clinicians to adopt services for families and patients that will convey to them what is known by professionals. Informed families with coping skills can amplify the effectiveness of professionals' treatment of the mentally disabled, with the result that more patients will achieve recovery and participate more fully and normally in their family and community life.

▶ Selected Readings and Educational Videos

Backer T, Liberman RP: Living on the Edge [video with discussion guide]. Available from Available from Psychiatric Rehabilitation Consultants, PO Box 2867, Camarillo, CA 93011–2867 or www.psychrehab.com.

Backer T, Liberman RP: What Is Schizophrenia? [video with discussion guide]. Available from Available from Psychiatric Rehabilitation Consultants, PO Box 2867, Camarillo, CA 93011–2867 or www.psychrehab.com.

Bernheim K, Lehman A: Working With Families of the Mentally Ill. New York, WW Norton, 1985

Budd R, Hughes I: What do relatives of people with schizophrenia find helpful about family interventions? Schizophr Bull 23:341–347, 1997

Coursey R, Curtis L, Marsh D: Competencies for direct service staff members who work with adults with severe mental illness: specific knowledge, activities, skills, bibliography. Psychiatr Rehabil J 23:8–92, 2000

Cuijpers P: The effects of family interventions on relatives' burden: a meta-analysis. Journal of Mental Health 8:275–285, 1999

Dixon L, Lyles A, Scott J, et al: Services to families of adults with schizophrenia: from treatment recommendations to dissemination. Psychiatr Serv 50:233–238, 1999

Dixon L, McFarlane W, Lefley H, et al: Evidence-based practices for services to families of people with psychiatric disabilities. Psychiatr Serv 52:903–910, 2001

Falloon IRH: Family Management of Schizophrenia. Baltimore, MD, Johns Hopkins University Press, 1986

Falloon IRH, Liberman RP: Behavioral family interventions in the management of chronic schizophrenia, in Family Therapy in Schizophrenia. Edited by McFarlane WR. New York, Guilford, 1983, pp 117–140

Falloon IRH, Boyd J, McGill C: Family Care of Schizophrenia. New York, Guilford, 1984

Falloon IRH, Boyd JL, McGill CW, et al: Family management in the prevention of morbidity of schizophrenia. Arch Gen Psychiatry 42:887–896, 1985

Goldman HH: Mental illness and family burden: a public health perspective. Hosp Community Psychiatry 33:557–560, 1982

Goldstein MZ (ed): Family Involvement in the Treatment of Schizophrenia. Washington, DC, American Psychiatric Press, 1986

Intagliata J, Willer B, Egri G: Role of the family in case management of the mentally ill. Schizophr Bull 12:699–708, 1986

Lefley HP: Family Caregiving in Mental Illness. Thousand Oaks, CA, Sage Publications, 1996

Lefley H (ed): Family Coping With Mental Illness: The Cultural Context. San Francisco, CA, Jossey-Bass, 1998

Liberman RP, Glynn SM, Backer TE, et al: Involving Families in Services for the Seriously Mentally Ill: A Video-Assisted Treatment Module for Families, Patients and Practitioners. Available from Psychiatric Rehabilitation Consultants, www.psychrehab.com, PO Box 2867, Camarillo, CA 93011.

McFarlane WR: Multifamily Groups in the Treatment of Severe Psychiatric Disorders. New York, Guilford, 2002

Miklowitz DJ, Goldstein MJ: Bipolar Disorder: A Family-Focused Treatment Approach. New York, Guilford, 1997

Morey B, Mueser KT: The Family Intervention Guide to Mental Illness. Oakland, CA, New Harbinger Publications, 2007

Mueser KT, Gingerich S: The Complete Family Guide to Schizophrenia: Helping Your Loved One Get the Most Out of Life. New York, Guilford, 2006

Sartorius N, Leff J, Lopez-Ibor J, et al (eds): Families and Mental Disorders: From Burden to Empowerment. Chichester, UK, Wiley, 2005

Snyder KS, Liberman RP: Family assessment and intervention with schizophrenics at risk for relapse, in New Developments in Interventions With Families of Schizophrenics (New Directions for Mental Health Services, No 12). Edited by Goldstein MJ. San Francisco, CA, Jossey-Bass, 1981

Vaughn CE, Snyder KS, Freeman W, et al: Family factors in schizophrenic relapse. Arch Gen Psychiatry 41:1169–1177, 1984

▶ References

Amenson CS: Schizophrenia: A Family Education Curriculum, Family Education Methods and Family Skills for Relapse Prevention. Pasadena, CA, Pacific Clinics Institute, 1998

Amenson CS, Liberman RP: Dissemination of educational classes for families of adults with schizophrenia. Psychiatr Serv 52:589–592, 2001

Arrington A, Sullaway M, Christensen A: Behavioral family assessment, in Handbook of Behavioral Family Therapy. Edited by Falloon IRH. New York, Guilford, 1988, pp 78–106

Bradley GM, Couchman GM, Perlesz A, et al: Multiple-family group treatment for English- and Vietnamese-speaking families living with schizophrenia. Psychiatr Serv 57:521–530, 2006

Butzlaff R, Hooley J: Expressed emotion and psychiatric relapse. Arch Gen Psychiatry 55:547–552, 1998

Dixon L, McFarlane W, Lefley H, et al: Evidence-based practices for services to families of people with psychiatric disabilities. Psychiatr Serv 52:903–910, 2001a

Dixon L, Stewart B, Burland J, et al: Pilot study of the effectiveness of the Family-to-Family education program. Psychiatr Serv 52:965–967, 2001b

Fadden G, Bebbington P, Kuipers L: Caring and its burdens. Br J Psychiatry 151:660–667, 1987

Falloon IRH: Family Management of Schizophrenia. Baltimore, MD, Johns Hopkins University Press, 1986

Falloon IRH, Boyd JL, McGill CW, et al: Family management in the prevention of morbidity of schizophrenia. Arch Gen Psychiatry 42:887–896, 1985

Falloon IRH, Held T, Coverdale JH, et al: Family interventions for schizophrenia: a review of long-term benefits of international studies. Psychiatric Rehabilitation Skills 3:268–290, 1999

Hatfield AB: What families want of family therapists, in Family Therapy in Schizophrenia. Edited by McFarlane WR. New York, Guilford, 1983, pp 41–65

Hatfield A, Lefley H (eds): Families of the Mentally Ill. New York, Guilford, 1987

Hooley JM: Expressed emotion and psychiatric illness: from empirical data to clinical practice. Behav Thera 29:631–646, 1998

Imber-Mintz L, Liberman RP, Miklowitz DJ, et al: Expressed emotion: a clarion call for partnership among relatives, patients and professionals. Schizophr Bull 13:227–235, 1987

Jungbauer J, Angermeyer MC: Living with a schizophrenic patient: a comparative study of burden as it affects parents and spouses. Psychiatry 65:110–123, 2002

Keefe FJ, Kopel SA, Gordon SB: A Practical Guide to Behavioral Assessment. New York, Springer, 1978

Leff J, Vaughn CE: Expressed Emotion in Families. New York, Guilford, 1985

Lehman A, Kreyenbuhl R, Buchanan R, et al: The Schizophrenia Patient Outcomes Research Team (PORT): updated treatment recommendations 2003. Schizophr Bull 30:193–217, 2004

Liberman DB, Liberman RP: Involving families in rehabilitation through behavioral family management. Psychiatr Serv 54:633–635, 2003

Liberman RP: Behavioral approaches to family and couple therapy. Am J Orthopsychiatry 40:106–118, 1970

Liberman RP: Behavioral methods in group and family therapy. Semi Psychiatry 4:145–156, 1972

Liberman RP, DeRisi WJ, King LW: Behavioral interventions with families, in Current Psychiatric Therapies. Edited by Masserman J. New York, Grune & Stratton, 1973, pp 175–182

Liberman RP, Wallace CJ, Vaughn CE, et al: Social and family factors in the course of schizophrenia: toward an interpersonal problem-solving therapy for schizophrenics and their relatives, in Psychotherapy of Schizophrenia: Current Status and New Directions. Edited by Strauss J, Fleck S, Bowers M. New York, Plenum, 1980, pp 21–54

Liberman RP, Falloon IRH, Aitchison RA: Multiple family therapy for schizophrenia: a behavioral approach. Psychosocial Rehabilitation Journal 4:60–77, 1984a

Liberman RP, Lillie FJ, Falloon IRH, et al: Social skills training and behavioral family management for relapsing schizophrenia. Behav Modif 8:155–179, 1984b

McFarlane WR, Stastny P, Deakins S: Family-aided assertive community treatment, in Effective Psychiatric Rehabilitation. Edited by Liberman RP. San Francisco, CA, Jossey-Bass, 1992, pp 43–54

McFarlane W, Dixon L, Lukens E, et al: Family psychoeducation and schizophrenia: a review of the literature. J Marital Fam Ther 29:223–245, 2003

Miklowitz DJ, Goldstein MJ: Bipolar Disorder: A Family-Focused Treatment Approach. New York, Guilford, 1997

Mueser KT, Glynn SG: Behavioral Family Therapy for Psychiatric Disorders. Oakland, CA, New Harbinger Publications, 1999

Mueser KT, Glynn SM, Liberman RP: Behavioral family management for serious psychiatric illness, in Family Interventions in Mental Illness (New Directions for

Mental Health Services). Edited by Hatfield AB. San Francisco, CA, Jossey-Bass, 1994, pp 37–50

Perlick DA, Rosenheck RA, Clarkin JF, et al: Impact of family burden and affective response on clinical outcome among patients with bipolar disorder. Psychiatr Serv 55:1029–1035, 2004

Phillips A: Behavioral assessment, in Encyclopedia of Behavior Modification and Cognitive Behavior Therapy: Adult Clinical Applications, Vol 1. Edited by Hersen M. Thousand Oaks, CA, Sage Publications, 2005, pp 82–110

Pickett SA, Cook JA, Steigman P, et al: Psychological well-being and relationship outcomes in a randomized study of family-led education. Arch Gen Psychiatry 63:1043–1050, 2006

Pitschel-Walz G, Leucht S, Bauml J, et al: The effect of family interventions on relapse and rehospitalizations in schizophrenia: a meta-analysis. Schizophr Bull 27:73–92, 2001

Psychiatric Rehabilitation Consultants: Medication Management Module and Symptom Management Module. 2007. Available from Psychiatric Rehabilitation Consultants, PO Box 2867, Camarillo, CA 93011-2867 or www.psychrehab.com.

Sherman MD: The Support and Family Education (SAFE) Program: mental health facts for families. Psychiatr Serv 54:35–37, 2003

Stuart RB: Helping Couples Change: A Social Learning Approach to Marital Therapy. New York, Guilford, 1980

Tarrier N, Barrowclough C: Providing information to relatives about schizophrenia. Br J Psychiatry 149:458–463, 1986

Tessler RC, Gamache GM: Family Experiences With Mental Illness. Westport, CT, Auburn House (Greenwood Publishing Group), 2000

Vaughn CE, Snyder KS, Freeman W, et al: Family factors in schizophrenic relapse. Arch Gen Psychiatry 41:1169–1177, 1984

World Fellowship for Schizophrenia and Allied Disorders: Principles for working with families, in Families as Partners in Care Program. Toronto, World Fellowship for Schizophrenia and Allied Disorders, 1999. Available from www.world.schizophrenia.org.

CHAPTER 7

Vocational Rehabilitation

7

Vocational Rehabilitation

Each morning sees some task begun,
Each evening sees it close;
Something attempted, something done,
Has earned a night's repose.

LONGFELLOW, "THE VILLAGE BLACKSMITH"

WORK IS valued and needed by mentally disabled persons as much as by all other citizens. Having a job confers many of the same benefits to all workers. In particular, a mentally ill person who goes to work each day:

- Gains dignity, satisfaction, and personal validation for being productive.
- Has opportunities to socialize and interact with co-workers.
- May become friendly with co-workers and enjoy recreational and social activities with them outside of the workplace.
- Has opportunities to vicariously learn social and problem-solving skills by observing co-workers and supervisors during their interactions.
- Gets the benefits of planned and scheduled routines and tasks that displace symptoms of depression, anxiety, worry, and psychosis.
- Experiences increases in self-confidence, self-esteem, self-responsibility, empowerment, and hope for the future—if depression, anxiety, and psychosis lift after obtaining employment and sufficient tenure on the job provides an experience of success for the individual.
- Can experience improved cognitive capacities because of the job's requiring concentration, memory, problem solving, and decision making.
- Earns money that is a generalized reinforcer that can be exchanged for many of the essentials (e.g., food, housing) and discretionary pleasures of everyday life.
- Can protect against relapse, since employment often serves as a protection against stress and neurocognitive vulnerability.

- Acquires a personal status, role, and identity as a "worker" that have important exchange value when meeting people and feeling good about oneself.
- Participates in emotional, attitudinal, and behavioral experiences that are consistent with recovery, health, and normality.

While having a job confers dignity and self-respect to the individual, it also does much more. Work enables us to arise each day with purpose and function. The sunrise, alarm clock, and time card are signals to us that our labor is needed and valued—by ourselves and by those who gain from what we produce. Moreover, having the responsibility for punctuality and regularity of attendance at work adds motivation, structure, and routines to our lives that otherwise would be empty and drab.

Work, by itself, lends respectability to each person; in addition, it is important to recognize the value of all forms of work, not just the ideal jobs that are found in the wider society. It may be said that work is the only human activity that can be pursued for 8 hours or longer each day. We can't eat or drink 8 hours a day. We can't play games for 8 hours a day. We can't make love 8 hours a day. But we can work and benefit from our work for 8 or more hours a day. This capacity for work very likely has evolutional significance, being hardwired into our brains and bodies through our long-ago ancestors. Those among them who were successful in working at obtaining food, making tools, and building homes survived longer and passed their genes onto succeeding generations.

The importance of work for the mentally disabled has been recognized for 200 years since the advent of moral treatment. Psychiatrists of the nineteenth century believed that "prayer, good manners, and occupied hands and minds" were important for rehabilitation. Inactivity was considered a contributing factor to psychiatric illness. Nature abhors a vacuum, and when a person is doing nothing, symptoms tend to rush in to fill the person's life space. "Idleness is the devil's workshop" has a cogent meaning for persons with schizophrenia, mood disorders, and other disabling mental conditions.

Psychiatric hospitals offered patients a variety of paid occupations, viewing work as therapy. Unfortunately, the jobs made available to institutionalized mentally ill patients were primarily for the convenience of the hospital and its staff. Through their labor on farms, food service, furniture repair, laundering, and grounds maintenance, patients contributed to the financial support of mental care rather than to their own rehabilitation and normalization. However, even jobs artificially created by patronizing superintendents and staff of state psychiatric hospitals yielded some benefits to the institutionalized mentally ill. Not the least of these benefits were the behavioral activation, daily and weekly structure, modest salaries, and sense of accomplishment.

▶ Continuum of Vocational Rehabilitation

The dignity of work extends to the mentally disabled wherever they are employed. It is presumptuous for practitioners and researchers who promote evidence-based vocational programs such as supported employment to derogate the value of work by those who are employed in *sheltered workshops, segregated work enclaves, transitional jobs,* or *consumer-run enterprises.* We look through the lens of our own cultural and socioeconomic biases when we view competitive employment in the marketplace as the best vocational activity for *all* persons with mental disabilities. Having a continuum of vocational services makes the fit between person and job more likely. Individualization of vocational planning and placement is echoed by Henrik Ibsen's words: "Different people have different duties assigned to them by Nature; Nature has given one the power or the desire to do this, the other that." The wide variety of vocational programs available for persons with mental disabilities empowers patients to:

- Participate in consumer-initiated decision making in the choice of vocational activity.
- Move from one to another type of vocational rehabilitation depending upon their performance, psychiatric symptoms, life outside of work, and personal satisfaction. Of course, the availability of different forms of vocational rehabilitation in one's own community also determines choice and mobility in the genre of work experience.
- Choose work with guaranteed, secure, long-term tenure instead of supported employment in the competitive sector with its inevitable turnover.
- Have access to some type of vocational activity in communities where supported employment is not available.

The increasing availability of evidence-based supported employment is a boon to mentally disabled patients because it opens opportunities for real work with the status, salaries, and normative experiences that are consistent with recovery. Developmentally disabled persons—who often have severe brain impairments and low levels of functioning—have enjoyed employment opportunities in normal workplaces for more than two decades. It is past the time for similar opportunities to be made available to mentally disabled persons—especially since current concepts of severe mental illness point toward a neurodevelopmental etiology that has common roots with developmental disorders.

Even when supported employment is well provisioned with well-trained job coaches, employment specialists, and job developers, this modality has been able to recruit only one-half of the mentally disabled who are receiving services in various types of mental health facilities. Furthermore, only one-half of those entering such programs actually obtain employment. For those who are successful in beginning a job in the competitive work sector, there is a high rate of turnover, with less than one-half sustaining their employment beyond 6 months or so. Thus, supported employment is not for everybody. There is a spectrum of alternative forms of vocational rehabilitation, including transitional employment, work enclaves, consumer-run enterprises, and satisfying volunteer opportunities. These alternatives have documented effectiveness in helping mentally disabled persons secure various types of jobs that offer productivity, money, social contacts and cohesiveness, and pride and contentment. Moreover, there is less worry by the patient that earned income will jeopardize the protection of Social Security and Medicaid or Medicare benefits.

Therefore, just as in other realms of treatment, vocational services should be bent to fit the person, not vice versa. Vocational rehabilitation at its best customizes work experiences according to the interests, preferences, abilities, symptoms, deficits, and resilience of the mentally disabled, within the opportunities, resources, and availability of jobs in the local area. The spectrum of vocational rehabilitation for the mentally and developmentally disabled is shown in Table 7.1. "Evidence-based" is not solely a concept of statistically significant benefits derived from average results to large numbers of patients in research studies. Services should also be valued and utilized for the "evidence base" of the benefits they confer to a particular patient. We should not fit all of our patients into a procrustean bed.

▶ Work Assessment and Readiness

Assessment of vocational activity is interwoven with rehabilitation decision making. Thus, assessment methods can 1) inform us regarding predictors of successful employability and sustained employment, 2) enhance a person's readiness for work, and 3) provide feedback to the patient as well as the rehabilitation team on how well work is being performed.

> • TABLE 7.1
>
> **Spectrum of services for the mentally and developmentally disabled in the world of work**
>
> •
>
> - Training of work tasks and errorless learning
> - Prevocational training and work adjustment
> - Sheltered workshops
> - Transitional employment
> - Work enclaves and work crews
> - Consumer-run enterprises and prosumers
> - Supported employment
> - Training in workplace fundamentals
> - Job Club
> - Occupational training and independent employment
> - Job maintenance
> - Supported education

ASSESSING PREDICTORS OF VOCATIONAL SUCCESS

Prediction is useful primarily when making decisions about enrolling a person in a particular form of vocational rehabilitation. So, knowing the characteristics of the person and his/her social environment at the time of rehabilitation planning can be informative—especially in league with the patient's phase of illness and own preferences. If the person's attributes reflect an unfavorable prognosis for work and he/she has not reached a plateau in the stable phase of the disorder, the clinician may wish to 1) delay vocational placement until the patient stabilizes, 2) engage the individual in low-demand vocational activities, and/or 3) intervene with predictors that may be malleable.

It is unrealistic to expect characteristics of individuals and their social environments to predict long-term success at work, because so many things change with time. The person's phase of disorder may change prognostic factors such as negative symptoms, as well as his/her level of psychosocial functioning, social supports, and overstimulating or understimulating environments. The following personal and social characteristics may have significant positive effects on patients' success in getting and keeping jobs.

- Good cognitive functioning

- Realistic family support for working with a "cool" emotional climate in the home
- Prior work experience
- Good premorbid social and educational attainment and current social functioning
- Younger versus older adults
- Fewer and less intense mood, anxiety, conceptual disorganization, and negative symptoms
- Abstinence from illicit drugs and alcohol
- Expressed desire to work and willingness to expend effort to find work
- Few or no disincentives from Social Security or other disability entitlements

One important factor that influences the success or failure of attempts by severely mentally ill individuals to find and keep a job is the availability of staff members who have training and supervision in an active approach to job development, placement, and supports. These qualities of staff members are found in supported employment programs where the job coaches and employment specialists spend the vast majority of their time in the field with patients, employers, and work supervisors. These designated employment specialists also maintain ongoing collaborative contacts, problem solving, and communication with the patient's psychiatrist and other members of the treatment team. Mentally ill individuals who are successful in obtaining and maintaining jobs with the assistance of supported employment emphasize the personal qualities of their relationship with employment specialists (Becker et al. 2007). They attribute some of their success to emotional support; that is, having someone who encourages them to work, discusses stresses of working, and helps them get accustomed to the job. Helpful, practical elements in the supports provided by employment specialists include counseling on how to keep disability benefits while working part-time, finding jobs, practicing job interviews, and being accompanied to job interviews.

It is especially critical to match the patient's attributes with the type of job. Person–job fit has been shown to be a significant predictor of employment success in all occupations for persons without mental disorders—it is no different for the mentally ill. Thus, an individual with schizophrenia who is easily overstimulated will work better in a quiet location without the interference of noise, conversation, or other socially stimulating aspects of a job setting.

ENHANCING WORK READINESS

In addition to the predictors of work capacity, it is possible to enhance readiness to work through motivational interviewing. Table 7.2 lists questions that can be used to probe for personal readiness for employment so as to identify disabled persons who are more likely to engage in an arduous job search. In screening and preparing patients for participation in supported employment or alternative rehabilitation programs, vocational counselors meet with mentally ill patients who are receiving disability income and explain the benefits and costs of employment. These include incentives to work offered by the Social Security Administration, trial work periods, medical insurance, housing assistance, and continued support available from job coaches and the person's psychiatric treatment team. Benefits counseling helps to increase the earnings of individuals in supported employment. Another means of preparing patients for supported employment is a 2-day orientation group in which participants learn about the specific aims and procedures of supported employment. They can ask questions and have ambiguities, work incentives, and work disincentives clarified and work anxieties desensitized.

ASSESSING WORK PERFORMANCE

Psychiatrists and other allied mental health professionals can inquire periodically of their employed patients regarding their work experience. This line of inquiry may enable emerging problems to be pinpointed with appropriate interventions. Questions such as "How are you doing at work?" "Has your job changed in any way?" "Are you able to get your job done?" and "Do you worry about keeping your job?" are asked. Work performance of

● **TABLE 7.2**

Personal Readiness for Work Questionnaire

- What do you look forward to when you think about going to work?
- How will your daily life be changed when you get a job?
- Who wants you to go to work?
- Picture yourself doing the kind of work you might get. What are your thoughts and feelings?
- What does having a job mean to you?

mentally disabled persons can be reliably and readily assessed in vocational rehabilitation programs by simply measuring productivity and quality of a person's output. This measure predicts who gets and keeps a job. The Work Behavior Inventory provides six scales of work performance: social skills, cooperativeness, work habits, work quality, personal presentation, and over-all work performance. It can be used to give positive or corrective feedback to participants depending upon their performance.

▶ Training of Work Tasks and Errorless Learning

Learning tasks required by a job and performing those tasks at an acceptable level are basic to all occupations and requirements for continued employ-ment. Because persons with psychiatric and developmental disabilities have cognitive impediments to concentration, learning, memory, and judgment, it is essential that *special educational techniques* be used in teaching them to meet the criteria for their job description. Thus, whether the tasks are in prevocational, sheltered, transitional, or supported work, the use of behav-ior analysis will streamline and improve the learning and retention of work tasks. The basic principles and methods of behavior therapy were described in Chapter 2 ("Principles and Practice of Psychiatric Rehabilitation"). Here, we describe *task analysis,* which is the first step in teaching job skills. Task analysis organizes any work task into teachable steps and strategies for job coaches, employment specialists, supervisors, or employers.

The tasks are broken down into small, functional component steps—an essential starting point for persons with cognitive deficits. The steps may be presented to an apprentice employee one at a time or several at a time. Most tasks involve multiple pieces of learning—groups of steps that are connected to one another in some way. Separating dishes and utensils and operating a dishwasher in a cafeteria are an example. If the steps are sequential, the training may use *chaining*—presenting the steps in a predetermined order. *Backward chaining* can be done by presenting the last step in a group of steps until the learner performs it, then the next-to-the-last step or groups of steps, and so on, until the task has been learned. *Forward chaining* begins with the presentation of the first step in the chain until the learner has learned it, then the next step or group of steps in the chain, and so on, until the task has been learned. Positive or corrective feedback is given by the trainer at each step in the learning process. Each step is performed repeat-edly until there are no errors.

The learning of work tasks is made as efficient as possible to compensate for the learning and memory deficits of persons with severe mental and developmental disorders. The training procedure is organized to reduce the number of errors made by the worker while learning each element of a job task, as each error becomes a counterproductive learning experience. The trainer models or demonstrates each step in the task, and then the learner performs each step. Cumulative training of all of the steps in the complete task proceeds in a forward-chaining sequence. Performance of each component step is overlearned to achieve a high level of performance proficiency and resistance to forgetting. This form of precision teaching is far more effective and produces more reliable and durable performance than typical, trial-and-error learning.

▶ Prevocational Training and Work Adjustment

Prevocational training, also known as *work adjustment,* aims to expose and teach individuals to adjust to basic expectations for participation in simulated work settings. Levels of participation are gradually increased, as is the complexity of the tasks. If participants show progress in their interaction with co-workers and supervisors, as well as in the quality and rate of completion of assigned tasks, the amount of supervision can be gradually faded back to levels more akin to those provided in normal jobs.

Teaching of vocational and social skills, as well as personal hygiene and grooming, is done incrementally in classes and during task activities. The aim of these programs is to involve individuals who have been unemployed for many years in vocational counseling or work activities that teach skills such as regular attendance, punctuality, appropriate personal appearance, building stamina in the workplace, and harmonious interactions with co-workers and supervisors.

Time spent in a prevocational work adjustment program may be counterproductive, however. Patients who spend weeks or months in preparatory vocational sessions are significantly less likely to subsequently obtain competitive employment than those who are placed on a real job without preparation. Thus, in a controlled study, patients who were randomly assigned to participate in preparatory counseling of the "Choose-Get-Keep" vocational rehabilitation program popularized by the Boston University Center for Psychiatric Rehabilitation had lower employment rates than patients who were assigned to supported employment (Bond et al. 2001b).

Work adjustment is a dignified alternative for individuals who demur from opportunities to be involved in more competitive work situations. This approach may also be helpful to mentally disabled individuals who have failed in their efforts at transitional or supported employment, feel demoralized, and are adamant about not wanting to reconnect with employment specialists, counselors, or job coaches. While 60% of the seriously mentally ill verbally express interest in working, less than half actually take advantage of work programs when offered. In some ways, these individuals make a decision to "retire" from the workplace at least for the time being. For such individuals, work adjustment may provide an accommodating environment, a routine to structure their days, cohesion and fellowship with others, and a satisfying and productive work milieu.

While work adjustment is beneficial for people with a variety of diagnoses, in recent years veterans and others with posttraumatic stress disorder have appeared to be particularly drawn to work adjustment programs.

● **EXAMPLE OF BEST PRACTICE**

A particularly fine work adjustment program, utilizing farming and livestock management, achieved good results with schizophrenia patients in Japan (Fuller et al. 2000). A similar approach, with horticulture as its modality, is operated at the Veterans Affairs (VA) Greater Los Angeles Healthcare Facility. On the grounds of the hospital, space is allocated for the growing of flowers, vegetables, and fruit trees. A greenhouse serves the purpose of introducing patients to simple but gratifying tasks of preparing soil, planting seeds, and cultivating, transplanting, fertilizing, and watering plants. On a weekly basis, patients, accompanied by staff members or volunteers, go to street fairs and markets to sell flowers and vegetables grown in the program.

On the basis of patients' level of cognitive and task functioning, as well as personal inclinations, assignments are made to activities in the Horticulture Program that vary in requirements for complexity, social skills, and independence from supervision. Because inpatient stays at the VA hospital are so short, the program primarily caters to outpatients, many of whom are followed for years in the various psychiatric clinics. This program has been particularly useful for veterans with posttraumatic stress disorder, who find serenity in the quiet, natural environment and satisfaction in seeing the work of their hands grow and bear fruit, vegetables, and flowers.

Their symptoms are antithetical to successful adaptation in competitive or even transitional employment: interpersonal hypersensitivity, suspiciousness, distrust, anger, emotional flashbacks, impulsivity, and drug and alcohol abuse. For individuals who are unemployable because of severe symptom and functional impairments or because they are not interested in normal work settings, this type of low-key work is better than no work at all. Where work adjustment programs are available, seriously impaired persons may gradually overcome job-related social anxieties, withdrawal, and hostility, eventually gaining an appetite for a job in the wider community. Prevocational programs continue to be used by occupational therapists working with psychiatric inpatients. Structured and unstructured art, ceramics, crafts, and other activities are used to gauge and strengthen prevocational skills such as initiative versus passivity, working independently versus need for supervision, and sustained attention versus distractibility. The information is shared with the attending psychiatrist, who can use it in making decisions regarding medication, privileges, and discharge readiness.

▶ Sheltered Workshops

As we enter the twentieth-first century, sheltered workshops have become anachronistic for the mentally ill in the United States. They are still used, however, in areas where the local economy does not offer sufficient jobs for the nondisabled citizenry, much less for those with serious disabilities. Charitable agencies that run shops with secondhand merchandise often employ mentally and developmentally disabled persons to sort, repair, and sell furniture and clothing. The medical centers sponsored by the Department of Veterans Affairs continue to offer a work program to physically and mentally disabled veterans called *Compensatory Work Therapy*. Similar to many other sheltered workshops, rehabilitation staff obtain contracts from local businesses for piecework such as fabricating, packaging, assembly, connecting electronic parts, computer repair, and sorting and labeling.

The work is carried out in facilities segregated from normal employment. While these jobs are often boring and repetitive, they enable individuals to structure their days, experience a sense of accomplishment, and earn money that supplements veterans pensions and Social Security benefits. In fact, studies carried out with veterans who have had schizophrenia for many years have shown that various types of sheltered work are associated with improvements in symptoms and social functioning as well as increased likelihood of gaining subsequent competitive employment.

❱ Transitional Employment

In transitional employment, an individual participates in occupations that have direct relevance to specific jobs in the community. The occupational activities are usually located in mental health sites, such as psychosocial clubhouses or rehabilitation agencies. For example, at an integrated service agency in Long Beach, California—*The Village*—members of the organization have jobs on site in food service, word processing, and accounting (Chandler et al. 1997). Retail sales at a secondhand clothing shop offer transitional work opportunities to members of the Step Up on Second Street rehabilitation agency in Santa Monica, California. In Hokkaido, Japan, a rehabilitation program offers training to its participants in gathering and processing seaweed, which is an important local industry in which mentally disabled "graduates" of the training program can apply for jobs.

● EXAMPLE OF BEST PRACTICE

The Eden Express Restaurant in Hayward, California, is owned and operated by a nonprofit agency for training disabled patients in the full range of jobs available in food services—hosting and reserving tables, waiting on and busing tables, dishwashing, and preparing and cooking food (Backer et al. 1986). In the context of staffing a restaurant, the clients also learn regular attendance, punctuality, good grooming and personal appearance, communication skills with customers, problem solving with co-workers and supervisors, and ability to take constructive criticism. All of these skills are learned in the context of a business that must be profitable to remain open. Thus, the Eden Express has a dual function: to offer vocational rehabilitation to clients and to serve the community as a viable enterprise.

The various job tasks at the Eden Express are organized into a hierarchy of difficulty based on degree of complexity and amount of stress. Trainees master less demanding jobs first—like dishwashing—before moving to jobs, such as waiting tables or cashiering, that are more challenging. The supervisors at the restaurant are experienced restauranteurs who also have contacts with other restaurants in the community where jobs can be sought for graduating trainees. Toward the end of their training, participants learn to prepare résumés and job applications to ready them for their job search. Because food service jobs are often part-time, it is possible for trainees to earn salaries that supplement but do not jeopardize their Social Security benefits. Sixty percent of participants who completed their training in the Eden Express obtained jobs in the competitive work sector of their community. Two-thirds of these individuals were still working at their jobs 6 months afterward (Backer et al. 1986).

▶ Work Enclaves and Work Crews

Work enclaves and crews are a special version of transitional employment. Individuals learn a wide variety of skills for a natural workplace while they are laboring for pay at a real job site within the competitive sector of the community. These settings may include factories, clothing stores, department stores, farms and landscaping, street cleaning, and janitorial crews. The distinction between work enclaves and more naturalistic jobs comes from the segregated nature of the work enclaves. Those going through this type of vocational rehabilitation are closely supervised by mental health staff while working together as crews or in enclaves and separated from other workers who are not in the rehabilitation program. In addition, their salaries are lower because the cost of their rehabilitation supervisors must be subtracted from the overall income received by the enclave. Working for months or years in a transitional employment job has the drawback of reducing the likelihood of getting a job in the "real world of work." This may result from the comfort, supports, and cohesiveness that derive from working in the same organization that also provides recreational, social, and food services.

▶ Consumer-Run Enterprises and Prosumers

At the Portals Rehabilitation Agency in Los Angeles, members of the club run a bakery called the Corporate Cookie, which sells its products to thousands of executives and staff working in the high-rise office buildings in the area. A network of self-help, peer-support clubs in the greater Los Angeles area hire recovered patients to serve as club coordinators and officers of the organization. The director of Project Return: The Next Step is a recovered patient who joined one of the clubs as a member when he was still in the process of being stabilized from his schizophrenia. In Sacramento County, California, consumers run their own psychosocial clinics under county contracts. They provide a variety of services to mentally ill patients, including a full spectrum of skills training modules from the UCLA Social and Independent Living Skills Program. Other consumer-run businesses have included janitorial and gardening services (Fairweather et al. 1969), catering services, florist shops, and restaurants.

The term *prosumers* refers to persons who are employed by the local mental health authority as "professional caregivers" while at the same time being "consumers" of mental health services themselves. These individuals have made good recoveries from their mental illness and are hired to work as case managers, consumer advocates, and liaisons. Sacramento County in California employs more than 300 prosumers, the most in any county of the nation. Scholarships are given to patients in this county who wish to participate in a 2-year certificate program on psychosocial rehabilitation that is sponsored by a local community college.

The most successful consumer-run enterprise is the Fairweather Lodge, named after its founder, social psychologist George Fairweather (Fairweather et al. 1969). After working for a year in an enclave doing landscape maintenance with staff supervision, a group of mentally ill Californians moved into their own lodgings and converted their services into a bona fide, self-employed business providing landscape and cleaning services. This type of program was designed in the 1950s and 1960s by Fairweather and his colleagues, based on principles of social cohesion and social support. It was shown in systematic research to be quite effective in reducing rehospitalizations and improving the social adjustment of patients. Eventually, the Fairweather Lodge became an exemplar of consumer-run enterprises for vocational and social rehabilitation and was disseminated successfully to agencies throughout the United States.

EXAMPLE

A psychologist who was a customer of the Fairweather Lodge, a consumer-run housecleaning and janitorial service, described the quality of the work done in her home. "The gentleman who came to my home looked a bit strange and talked to himself the entire time he worked, doing my floors, bathroom, dusting, and washing my windows. He may have been mentally ill, but my kitchen, refrigerator, stove, and oven have never been cleaner than after he was finished."

There are three morals to this story:

- People with serious mental illness can meet high standards in their work and should not be stigmatized.
- Not all self-talk is tantamount to hallucinations—talking to yourself is often a means of concentrating on the task at hand, facilitating your attentiveness for task completion.
- Work can displace symptoms of mental disorder when the task is within the grasp of the individual and overlearned, as it focuses attention on actions outside of the person.

▶ Supported Employment

Supported employment is a mode of vocational rehabilitation that enables any disabled individual, no matter what the disability might be, to obtain a real job with dignity in the community. The supportive services for finding and keeping a job are wrapped around the disabled individual to compensate for the cognitive deficits, symptoms, social anxiety and awkwardness, strange behavior, and stigma that otherwise would reduce the person's job prospects to nil. These support services include work-related assistance and problem-solving provided by employment specialists and job coaches, as well as psychiatric and mental health services provided by personal support specialists (i.e., case managers), psychiatrists, and other members of multidisciplinary teams. The distinctive characteristic of supported employment is its emphasis on "place then train" rather than "train then place."

Fewer than 20% of the seriously mentally ill become employed when they have to find work on their own or through the assistance of conventional rehabilitation counseling. Thus, the employment rate of 40%–55% obtained by supported employment is quite impressive. When a new rehabilitation service can more than double the rate at which disabled persons can obtain jobs, statistics are not needed to qualify the service as "evidence-based." The most organized, widely used, and empirically validated form of supported employment is termed *individual placement and support* (IPS) (Becker and Drake 2003). Designed by Robert Drake and Deborah Becker at the Dartmouth Psychiatric Research Center, this program has become the quality standard for vocational rehabilitation throughout the United States. The ethos of normalization and community integration spawned supported employment as a keystone of habilitation of the developmentally disabled in the 1980s. It succeeded admirably in enabling mentally retarded individuals to live as participating citizens in their communities. There is every reason to hope that supported employment will benefit the mentally disabled in a like manner.

ASSUMPTIONS AND BASIC PRINCIPLES OF SUPPORTED EMPLOYMENT

Vocational rehabilitation should be considered an intrinsic component of mental health treatment, rather than a separate service. That is, the mental health agency must be responsible for coordinating and integrating employment services in a way that meets the needs of each individual patient. The most important point of departure for involving a disabled individual in supported employment is a clearly stated, well-considered desire of that individual to work at a job in the normal marketplace. Regardless of the obstacles that might have interfered with the individual's working in the past, the rehabilitation experts believe that their services can compensate for the individual's problems *if the individual truly wants to work.* While not all mentally disabled persons want to work, surveys have found that well over half do express a desire for some type of employment.

Verbal expressions of interest in working are just the starting point. During patients' orientation to supported employment, expectations for a working life are clarified through educational group and individual sessions. Examples of the specific concerns discussed in building realistic expectations for working are shown in Figure 7.1. Ultimately, "the motivational

GIVES and GETS Worksheet

Costs of Working	Benefits of Working
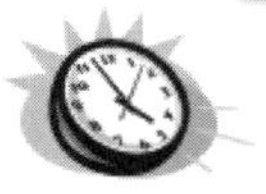 • Less free time • A change in my daily routine	• A productive way to fill my day • A structured and more rewarding use of my time
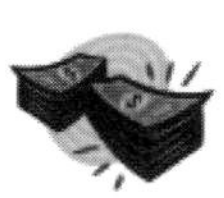 • Loss of Social Security • Cost of meals, clothes, transportation, etc.	• A way to get more money • Better meals, clothes, transportation, etc.
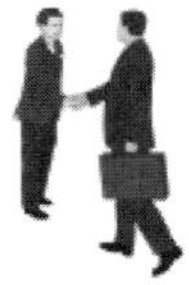 • Willingness to compromise with others • Willingness to follow the formal and informal "rules" of my workplace	• Positive, helpful, and rewarding social contacts • New friends
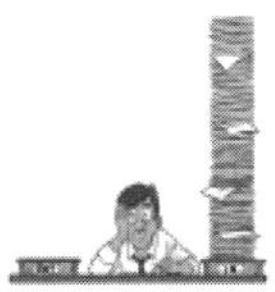 • Be productive and energetic, even when I don't feel like it • Follow routines for dress, hygiene, and use of tools	• Learn new skills that may help to advance my career • Pride in my appearance and ability to use tools and follow routines
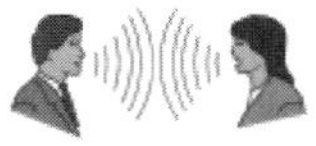 • I have to be flexible, enthusiastic, and willing to listen and to learn	• A satisfying feeling about myself and the knowledge I can do it!
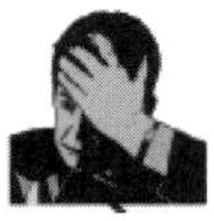 • Other costs and benefits	_____ _____ _____

FIGURE 7.1
Worksheet with systematic problem-solving exercises to help build realistic expectations and motivation for employment. Building realistic expectations and motivation for employment is fostered by systematic problem-solving exercises that focus on the specific benefits and costs of being employed. This worksheet is used with individuals or in a group and helps patients understand that the benefits may outweigh the disadvantages of a job.

rubber hits the road" when an employment specialist assists a disabled person who is expending the considerable effort required in searching for and obtaining a job. The procedural guidelines that undergird successful supported employment programs are listed in Table 7.3.

To effectively deliver supported employment, the employment specialist serves as a go-between for the employer, patient, mental health practitioners, and family. These liaison functions are depicted in Figure 7.2, underlining the importance of coordination of the various services and stakeholders. All involved must "read from the same page" if the patient is to succeed in getting and keeping a job. Given the various impairments that can intrude on a mentally disabled person's ability to sustain employment—cognitive deficits, upsurge in symptoms, stress, and stigma—it has

● TABLE 7.3

Policies and procedures for supported employment programs with high fidelity

- Type of job selected by and for the individual with a disability should be to the liking of the individual and fit that person's interests, preferences, skills, cognitive deficits, bizarre behaviors, and personal style.
- Employment specialists provide job finding, job development, and job placement services, and they, in league with job coaches, also may assist in task analysis and on-the-job training. How much of these services are done by rehabilitation workers and how much by the patients?
- There must be a close working relationship, marked by frequent and open communication, between the employment specialist and the other members of a mental health team (i.e., psychiatrist, social worker, nurse, and case manager).
- Advocacy, liaison, and collaboration between the employment specialist and the employer or supervisor are essential to the longitudinal process of follow-along supports to the patient.
- Patients are assisted in taking advantage of job accommodations.
- Employment specialist or job coach must be prepared to step in and perform the work of one of his/her patients if the latter is unable to come to the job or meet the expectations of the job and supervisor.
- Supports provided in this type of vocational rehabilitation must be available to the disabled worker indefinitely, because the disorders that have produced the disability are lifelong, with ups and downs, relapses and remissions, and periods of crisis and stability.
- Assistance with and instruction for transportation to and from the job are provided by the employment specialist.
- Family is involved as part of the rehabilitation effort to provide much-needed positive reinforcement and motivation for progress toward getting and then keeping a job.

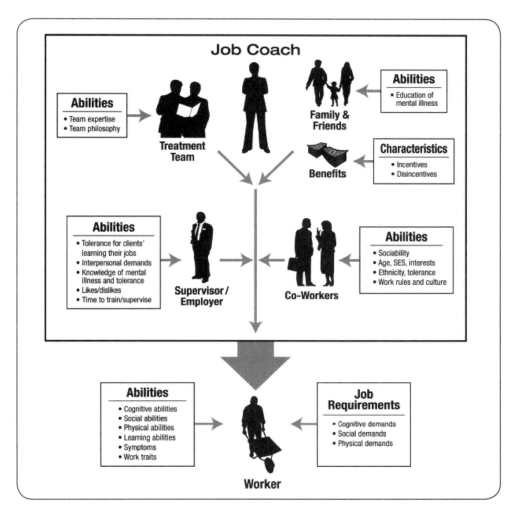

FIGURE 7.2 Program design of supported employment with employment specialist and job coach serving up to 18 patients each in job development, placement, and maintenance, with close liaison and communication with each patient's mental health multidisciplinary team. In this figure, the worker with a mental disorder has an array of abilities and impairments that must match with the requirements of the job. The individuals framed above the worker are those who are enlisted by supported employment to assist the mentally ill worker in obtaining and maintaining a job with success and satisfaction. The Job Coach, alternatively termed the employment specialist, is the central spoke in supported employment. The responsibilities of the job coach or employment specialist are to 1) serve as liaison with the patient's treatment team to ensure that the worker's needs for mental health treatment expertise are met along with the team's endorsement of work as an important goal to encourage; 2) educate the patient's family and friends so they will encourage and reinforce the patient's efforts in the world of work; 3) ensure that incentives exceed disincentives to motivate the patient to seek and sustain employment; 4) collaborate with the patient's employer to make accommodations for the special needs of the worker, to understand the nature of mental illness, and to provide time, opportunities, and support for the worker to learn the tasks of the job; and 5) engage in problem-solving with the patient worker to learn skills required to meet the social expectations of co-workers, work rules, and norms.

been a byword of the supported employment approach that employment specialists must be prepared to assist individuals who lose or leave a job to transition to another one. Transitions can take time, require changes in medication and other therapeutic interventions, and depend on sensitive, empathic, and motivating supports from the employment specialist. The keys to successful vocational outcomes in this modality are the professional and personal attributes of the employment specialist, including weekly or more frequent contacts between the specialist and the other members of the patient's multidisciplinary treatment team (Becker et al. 2007).

CLINICAL EXAMPLE

Bill was a 55-year-old man with schizophrenia who spent 25 years continuously in a state hospital located in a northern climate where the winters were fierce and the snow piled high. To enable patients and staff to move comfortably from one building to another, underground passageways were built and used frequently. After discharge and return to the city of his birth, Bill was arrested repeatedly for climbing into the city's sewers and walking underground from one part of the city to another. His mental health team discussed Bill's problem with their employment specialist. They brainstormed ideas that might lead to a paid job for Bill. Finally, the employment specialist said, "I know! What if Bill could get a job with the sanitation district that is responsible for the sewers?" When this option was explored with the human resources department of the sanitation district, Bill was hired to change the lightbulbs in the sewers. It was a win–win situation for Bill; he was able to continue his walking underground and simultaneously get paid for it.

Working alongside nondisabled co-workers in companies, offices, hospitals, and municipal agencies, patients participating in supported employment can identify with the role of nondisabled worker. Supported employment encourages community integration and destigmatization. Its benefits are equally applicable to individuals with mental illness, substance abuse, mental retardation, physical disabilities, or combinations of these.

RESEARCH ON SUPPORTED EMPLOYMENT

Just as supported employment has proven to be highly effective for a broad range of persons with mental retardation—even those with limited verbal skills such as adults with autism or Down's syndrome—it has also been validated as an effective, evidence-based program for mentally disabled adults. When the IPS model of supported employment is implemented in ordinary community support programs, mental health centers, and day treatment programs, higher rates of employment ensue for patients with a broad array of diagnoses. As expected, persons with cognitive impairments and schizophrenia have less success in IPS than do persons with less debilitating illnesses (McGurk and Mueser 2004, 2006).

Randomized, controlled trials of supported employment with a variety of traditional vocational services revealed significant advantages in getting and keeping jobs for patients assigned to supported employment (Bond et al. 2001a). In six studies, a *cumulative* mean of 55% of supported employment patients achieved competitive jobs at some time over 12–18 months, compared with 34% of those who participated in traditional vocational programs. In a 2-year, national, multi-site randomized trial of supported employment for 1,273 individuals with severe mental illness, the differences between supported employment and a variety of traditional types of vocational rehabilitation were statistically significant, favoring the supported employment condition (Cook et al. 2005). One might question whether the impact of supported employment was sufficiently great to make a difference from a clinical, vocational, or cost-effectiveness point of view. For example, in any one month, the percentage of patients gainfully employed in the supported employment condition varied from 20% to 25% versus 10% to 15% for the traditional programs, and average earnings were approximately 25% greater in the supported employment group.

Supported employment has been compared with alternative modes of vocational rehabilitation. Comparisons in randomized, controlled studies have been conducted with the "Choose-Get-Keep" job approach of the Boston University Center for Psychiatric Rehabilitation, services offered by psychosocial rehabilitation clubs, work enclaves, and standard vocational counseling with referrals to various rehabilitation programs in the community. In all of these comparisons, supported employment has shown superior outcomes in terms of number of persons who have been able to get employment, rapidity of getting a first job, number of hours or months working, tenure on the job, and income from work.

FIDELITY OF SUPPORTED EMPLOYMENT AS A FACTOR IN VOCATIONAL OUTCOMES

It doesn't take rocket science to know that the quality of any service, product, or program determines its value, impact, efficacy, and utility. In Chapter 5

("Social Skills Training") we learned that when social skills training hews to the principles and practices of motivational enhancement, social learning, behavior therapy, and generalization, patients more readily and thoroughly learn skills from the training and are able to use the skills in their everyday life. Similarly, when employment specialists follow the "gold standards" for implementing supported employment, their efforts are much more likely to yield jobs for their patients. There are three essential standards for ensuring the quality of supported employment. Employment specialists 1) spend the vast majority of their time in the community interacting with patients, employers, supervisors, and job sites; 2) do not have caseloads in excess of 18 patients; and 3) are fully integrated into their patients' mental health treatment teams. Training practitioners from mental health treatment teams to conduct supported employment on a part-time basis while they retain their clinical responsibilities in a mental health center will not lower the unemployment rate.

REALISTIC LIMITATIONS OF SUPPORTED EMPLOYMENT

To place the results of supported employment in perspective, it should be noted that in any one month, only 20%–35% are gainfully employed, reflecting the high turnover rate in terms of employed individuals losing their jobs. In fact, approximately 50% of patients who obtain jobs through supported employment programs are not working at those jobs 6 months after being hired. Twenty weeks, or approximately 5 months, is the average tenure in a job for those in supported employment, and it takes a long time for a person to obtain a job—approximately 6 months. While supported employment has been found to be more effective on most vocational measures than comparison approaches, it should be understood that the differences are not that great in absolute terms. For example, average earnings tend to be around $120 per month for individuals in supported employment versus $100 per month for those in psychosocial rehabilitation and standard local and state vocational rehabilitation services (Cook et al. 2005). Most studies of persons with schizophrenia and other disabling disorders find 5%–15% working at any one time; thus, supported employment has a statistically significant effect on employment but leaves much more to be accomplished with newer and stronger programs in the future.

If we are to avoid unrealistically rosy perceptions of supported employment, it's important to realize that the jobs in supported employment are almost all part-time, averaging less than 10 hours per week. This is not to diminish the personal, social, and financial value of supported employment, since it is meaningful to any person with a severe mental disorder to be able to obtain a job, irrespective of the number of hours and earnings. Being employed expands the role and personal and social identity of the person to that of a worker. It must be remembered that almost all individuals who enroll in supported employment are receiving Social Security benefits that would be jeopardized if they worked and earned beyond a modest income.

Most treatments for the mentally disabled have high specificity; that is, they are effective for delimited types of outcomes. Pharmacotherapy is effective for mood and psychotic symptoms, social skills training is effective for improving social competence and social functioning, and supported employment is effective for getting people jobs. This is especially true for persons with schizophrenia. Supported employment should not be expected to have rippling effects on other therapeutic outcomes—and it does not. Social adjustment, satisfaction with social relationships, symptom severity, quality of life, cognitive functioning, and self-esteem do not significantly improve during the 1- to 2-year duration of research studies of supported employment (Bond et al. 2001b; Mueser et al. 2004).

▶ Training in Workplace Fundamentals as a Supplement for Supported Employment

Regardless of the type of work restoration, mentally disabled persons need to learn how to deal with a range of challenges that confront any employee: knowing expectations for performance, anticipating and coping with stressors on the job, managing symptoms and medication while working, interacting with supervisors, and socializing with co-workers. Because of the wide range of work situations that may be encountered, patients benefit from adopting a flexible approach to problem solving when faced by novel dilemmas. The *Workplace Fundamentals Module,* one of the video-assisted training curricula from the UCLA Social and Independent Living Skills Program, offers repeated practice in problem solving for most situations encountered by individuals as they enter or reenter the world of work. The skill areas, containing the educational objectives for the curriculum, are shown in Figure 7.3.

The skills taught in the module make it particularly relevant for people who are engaged in a job search or those who have just been hired. If a person is ambivalent about obtaining a job, participation in the first skill area may serve as a preview of the requirements, expectations, and rewards that might be encountered in a workplace. The initial skill area brings the trainer or counselor together with participants for reviewing what mentally ill per-

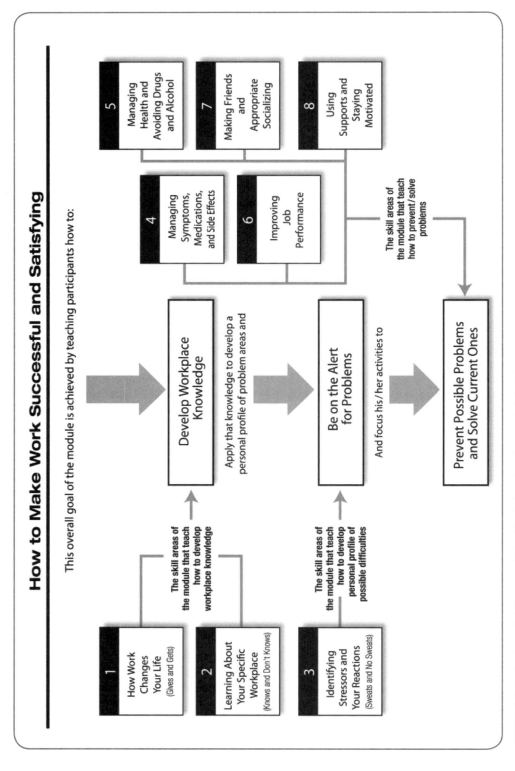

FIGURE 7.3 Goals and skill areas of the Workplace Fundamentals Module.

sons must "Give" to a working life as balanced by what they can expect to "Get" from work. "My Gives" are what the participant who works will have to do (get up early, go to work when I don't feel like it), and "My Gets" are the benefits that one receives from work (money, satisfaction from being productive). A video is shown of employed persons who discuss their own, individualized pros and cons of working. The video is followed by active questions and answers, previously shown in Figure 7.1, that individualize the work readiness, motivation, and expectations of the participants. A large body of research shows that setting positive, yet realistic, expectations can have a salutary effect on participation in treatment and rehabilitation. Also, a positive learning experience with the module can desensitize individuals who have apprehensions or concerns about the consequences of working.

In one situation from the module, an employee does not know how to do a particular task. She approaches her supervisor and asks him to demonstrate it for her, but he curtly refuses, saying he is too busy. The trainer asks the group members, "What would you do?" The participants in the module group then brainstorm various alternatives, consider their feasibility, weigh their pros and cons, and then decide on one or two options that may be effective in solving the problem. Each participant in the module receives a JOB (Job Organizing Book) printed as a large day planner. It is filled with blank worksheets that participants complete during their in vivo and homework assignments.

The module supplements supported employment but does not replace it. The leaders or trainers for the module do not help mentally disabled persons identify job leads, find jobs, prepare résumés, or participate in a job interview. Rather, the Workplace Fundamentals Module aims to equip participants with the capacity for solving the problems that inevitably crop up once on the job. In short, supported employment is the vehicle for assisting clients to obtain jobs, while the module aims to enable individuals to maintain their jobs and find satisfaction in their jobs by teaching skills that are instrumental to success and satisfaction on the job. By equipping persons with severe mental illness with the skills they will need to succeed on the job, this module fulfills three of the major stepping-stones to recovery: self-responsibility, empowerment, and personal growth.

One of the prime aims of the Workplace Fundamentals Module is to enhance the job tenure of participants in supported employment. In two studies, this seems to have been accomplished. One study was conducted in Santa Barbara, California, where patients were randomly assigned to the module plus supported employment or supported employment alone. Job tenure was more than 60% greater in the combined program, and the patients also reported significantly greater job satisfaction in this program

CLINICAL EXAMPLE

Jim, a 29-year-old man with schizophrenia, completed the Workplace Fundamentals Module, during which he was challenged repeatedly to engage in a structured problem-solving sequence. He became familiar with the identification of a problem as an obstacle that stood in the way of his goal and began to generate alternative ways to remove that obstacle or to set a new goal. Because of his pre-illness experience as a truck driver and desire to return to this line of work, his employment specialist coached him through the job search process. After 5 months of repeated disappointing job interviews, Jim obtained a job as a cross-country, big-rig truck driver.

Unfortunately, because of cognitive deficits, Jim encountered considerable difficulties finding his way to his destinations for unloading his truck and then getting back to the highway whence he came. No longer involved in supported employment and on his own, Jim used the problem-solving skills that he had learned in the module to meet his company's expectations for time limits on his scheduled routes. He developed a plan with his father to create "accommodations" for his cognitive difficulties. His father, adept at using the Internet and an online map site, communicated with him via cell phone for explicit directions to and from his delivery destinations. Subsequently, Jim compensated for his memory and visuospatial deficits by obtaining a GPS navigational device for his truck.

compared with supported employment alone. Knowledge and skills related to those taught in the module increased from 38% to 72% in the combined group after training versus from 40% to 51% in the supported employment–alone cohort. The skills did not significantly erode over an 18-month follow-up period (Wallace and Tauber 2004).

In a similarly designed study in Manchester, New Hampshire, average job tenure for patients in the combined program was 43 days longer, and the odds of their working were 42% higher, than those for patients in supported employment alone. The results from New Hampshire are even more impressive given the fact that they were obtained despite low attendance by patients in the module group (Mueser et al. 2005). A final study of combined supported employment and the module was carried out with young persons who had had onset of their schizophrenia within the previous 2 years. Of patients who participated in the module together with supported employment, 93% were able to successfully return to work or school within 1 year— more than twice as many as in a randomly assigned cohort of patients who received traditional vocational rehabilitation (Nuechterlein et al. 2005).

LEARNING EXERCISE

Consider for a moment when you began your current job or the one before it. What stressors did you encounter as you began to work that you were able to overcome because you either had the skills to remove certain interpersonal obstacles or were able to learn the requisite skills from co-workers, supervisors, or others? What coping and other personal skills did you use that enabled you to become successful in your work? What problems or stressors continue to "bug" you?

▶ Job Club

Some mentally disabled individuals, especially those who are not receiving disability pensions and who have been employed in the past, choose to obtain jobs on their own. The *Job Club* places the responsibility of finding a job on the patient, with the assistance of rehabilitation staff who are knowledgeable about employment opportunities in the locale and the vocational problems encountered by disabled persons. Emphasis in the Job Club is placed on skill building and goal setting and on providing a designated office or space where participants can use resources related to job finding and telephones for making job contacts, arranging job interviews, and making follow-up calls.

A basic tenet of the Job Club is that finding a job is a full-time job and patients are expected to participate in the club on a full-time, daily basis. In addition, by learning job-seeking skills and taking responsibility for the job search, patients learn independent employment-seeking skills that may be needed in finding subsequent jobs in the years to come. During the first week of participation in the club, patients learn basic job-seeking skills such as how to locate sources of job leads, look for a job, fill out job applications and résumés, use the telephone effectively, maintain grooming and dress appropriately, and participate in employment interviews.

Participants learn to not disclose their psychiatric problems on job applications or interviews, because that information is confidential and laws prohibit employers from inquiring about health matters unless the problem is directly related to the requirements of the job. However, the participants are briefed about their rights as disabled persons to request reasonable accommodations on the work site *after* they start a job. Reasonable accommodations might be requesting sick leave to see their psychiatrist during work hours or having a location at the job where the level of noise and conversation is limited. In the second week, patients begin a full-time job search and remain in the program until they find a job or leave the program unemployed.

Motivation to persist in the job search comes from abundant reinforcement from vocational counselors as well as from cohesion and a "buddy system" whereby two patients go out together to seek job leads and interviews. In some locales, state rehabilitation departments provide small amounts of money to participants contingent upon their meeting daily goals of phone calls for job leads and weekly employment interviews. Daily goal-setting exercises are also motivating because participants share their experiences and learn to break down large and seemingly unattainable tasks into more attainable objectives. A sample daily goal-setting and job-seeking log is shown in Figure 7.4.

CLINICAL EXAMPLE

Tony joined the Job Club after stabilizing from his recent relapse of schizophrenia. His work history was spotty, with transient jobs that he held intermittently over a 10-year period. As part of his delusional system, he was convinced that he contracted schizophrenia at the time when he had volunteered to give a pint of blood at a Red Cross drive. He felt the doctor had purposely taken out two pints of blood instead. His motive for joining the Job Club was to be able to save enough money to hire a lawyer to sue the doctor and get his pint of blood back.

Although he entered the Job Club with reservations about the counselors and his primary treatment team, he demonstrated a good attention span and quality of participation during the first week's training of basic job-finding competencies. In particular, he acquired excellent verbal and nonverbal communication skills for job interviewing after watching other participants go through their role-plays and receiving video feedback on his role-plays. He attended the Job Club every day and quickly picked up its routine of daily goal setting. He began searching for a job as a bookkeeper's assistant or bank teller because he had worked in jobs like that in past years. He was able to remain discreet about his symptoms, which were subsiding even as he participated in the club.

The first 2 months of job seeking were rough, and Tony became dejected after a number of job interviews failed to yield a job. With the daily positive reinforcement he received from the Job Club counselors, Tony persisted and subsequently found a position as a bank teller, remaining on the job for a full year. This vignette highlights the predictive value of a patient's past job history, social skills, and responsiveness to positive reinforcement.

Job Club Daily Log Form

Name: Chris Boyte Date: 8 / 9 / 06

Activities I will try to accomplish today:
- ✓ (1) Telephone Canvass Burbank
- ___ (2) Mail Application to ABC, Inc.
- ✓ (3) Review Want Ads
- ✓ (4) Call Rehabilitation Department

Time	Job Lead Source	Activity: In Person or Phone Contact, Résumé, Interview	Company Location: Name and Address, Phone Number	Name of Person Contacted	Type of Job	Results of Contact	Follow-up
9:00 A.M.	Yellow Pages	Telephone Contact	Help Temporary Services 11100 Wilshire Blvd. Tel. (213) 788-8883	Mr. Jones, Owner	Mechanic	Come In and Fill In Application	Yes
	Job Club Group Meeting	Telephone Contact	Help Temporary Services 11100 Wilshire Blvd. Tel. (213) 788-8883	Susan Employment Rep.	Photocopy Operator	No Job, Call Back Tomorrow	Yes
	N/A	In Person	Job Club Office	Don, Job Club Counselor	N/A	Help with Job Application	N/A
10:00 A.M.	N/A	By Self	Job Club Office	N/A	N/A	Continued Filling Out Application	N/A
	Previous Contact	Yellow Pages	Burbank Motors 876 Victory Blvd. Tel. (818) 237-4900	Alvin Rosen, Service Manager	Mechanic	Come In For Interview	Yes
	Previous Contact	Yellow Pages	Burbank Motors 876 Victory Blvd. Tel. (818) 237-4900	Alvin Rosen, Service Manager	Mechanic	To Call Back Tomorrow For Results	Yes

FIGURE 7.4 Daily log for setting goals in Job Club.

In several studies of the Job Club for individuals with mental disorders, the employment rate has varied from 29% to 90%, with the differences a function of the quality of the implementation of the program and the nature of the patient population (Tsang and Pearson 2001). At a VA hospital in Los Angeles, an evaluation of the Job Club revealed that 65% of patients obtained employment, 25% dropped out before getting a job, and 10% were deemed not ready for a job search (Jacobs et al. 1984). Participants included individuals with schizophrenia, recurrent major depressions, persistent dysthymia with major depressions periodically superimposed, bipolar disorder, dual diagnosis of substance abuse and a mental disorder, or a disabling personality disorder. This grouping of varied diagnoses is similar to that found in the mixed population who enroll in supported employment. It should be noted, however, that among the participants with schizophrenia, only 20% were successful in obtaining employment.

In a Job Club for Chinese patients with severe mental disorders in Hong Kong, intensive, social skills training was added. The skills training program covered many of the topics included in the Workplace Fundamentals Module. The skills taught were relevant to the interpersonal challenges experienced by disabled persons on the job. Follow-along services, inspired by supported employment, were also added to the Job Club format. Of those who received skills training and follow-along services, 47% were employed 3 months after the completion of the program. Receiving only skills training without follow-along services resulted in employment for 23% of the patients. Only 4% of the control group were employed at the 3-month follow-up (Tsang 2001). The Job Club is less effective with seriously disabled persons who have substantial negative symptoms, cognitive impairments, and limited work histories. For them, supported employment is the rehabilitation of choice, as it burdens them with far fewer task requirements and demands for planning and initiative. Once it becomes clear that each vocational rehabilitation program has specific efficacy for different subgroups of patients, rehabilitation practitioners will be able to match characteristics of the patient to the vocational program that best fits that patient's strengths, interests, and deficits.

▶ Occupational Training and Independent Employment

One of the key principles of psychiatric rehabilitation is individualization of goals and services for mentally disabled persons. This principle is no better illustrated than in the vocational sphere, where the great variation of patients' attributes requires use of the full continuum of the modes of rehabilitation. Some individuals can obtain training in specific occupations for which they have interest and ability, seek jobs on their own, and work successfully without services from vocational rehabilitation. Of course, they will require pharmacotherapy and a variable amount of skills training and supports from their psychiatrist and mental health team as they meet the challenges of a community-based training program, job search, and employment.

CLINICAL EXAMPLE

Eric, a 25-year-old man who was living at home with his parents, gradually recovered from 4 years of untreated schizophrenia during which he functioned at a severely regressed level. During his 3 years in a community-based rehabilitation program, he decided to take a 1-year course in welding because he had always had outstanding mechanical skills, crafting surf boards, restoring antique automobiles, and repairing yachts prior to his illness. Eric obtained his welding certificate and obtained a job in a small welding shop. Unfortunately, with the drying up of the aerospace and shipbuilding industries, there were no apprenticeship opportunities in the area; proprietors of welding businesses expected new workers to be capable journeymen. Eric experienced stress on this job, as the owner's expectations exceeded Eric's competencies. Eric's warning signs of relapse flared up, and using his emergency plan, he consulted with his psychiatrist. After careful consideration of the situation, they jointly decided that Eric should seek employment in a less stressful occupation. He quickly undertook a job search with the encouragement of his parents and psychiatrist and was hired as a picture framer in an art store. He handled this job exceedingly well, in part because he was able to work independently with a low level of social stimulation. Eric completed a work incentive program sponsored by the Social Security Administration, gave up his disability benefits, moved into his own apartment, and, at last contact, was still working at the same firm 8 years after obtaining the job.

▌ Job Maintenance

Because supported employment and transitional employment offer indefinite, ongoing supports, job maintenance is basic to those programs. Employment specialists, job coaches, personal support specialists, and vocational counselors need to be alert to some of the stressors and problems that often arise during a long-term effort at job maintenance. Some of these are not directly produced at the work site but affect the individual's performance on the job: stopping medication and having a relapse; change in medication, with new side effects that impair concentration or memory; alcohol or drug abuse; loss or change of a residence; change in psychiatrist or personal support specialist; and stress in the home with family, roommates, or landlord. Ultimately, effective follow-along services depend upon the resources available through the mental health and rehabilitation agencies in one's locale.

No matter how frequent or capable the follow-along services for job maintenance, some patients will lose their jobs or relapse. Neither the patients nor the professionals helping them should view these untoward events as "failures." Instead, the setbacks underscore the need to reintegrate the patient back into the appropriate level of services within mental health and vocational rehabilitation. Flexible levels of intervention by the psychiatric and vocational systems of service are essential to meet the changing needs of patients over the long haul.

The forms of intervention may vary, depending on the mental health resources available locally. While commitments for continuity of services are integral for supported employment and assertive community treatment, many persons with mental disabilities may benefit from less intensive intervention. Limited but strategically effective assistance may come from a patient's confidence in a 1) caring and competent psychiatrist who goes beyond medication management to encourage and provide supportive therapy for a return to a less stressful, part-time job; 2) psychologist who uses social skills training to assist the patient to improve communication with a supervisor or co-worker on the job; or 3) personal support specialist who persuades an employer to give the patient another chance after recovery from a relapse. This dynamic and fluid approach is no different for any of the areas of treatment and rehabilitation that serve mentally disabled individuals who may take occasional detours on the road to recovery. When all is said and done, success in a working life is largely a matter of practitioners and their patients hanging on after others have let go.

CLINICAL EXAMPLE (continued)

Tony had to leave his job at the bank after 1 year because of a sudden symptom exacerbation related to the death of his father and discontinuation of his medication. His psychiatrist scheduled extra sessions with intensive pharmacotherapy that restabilized Tony within 3 weeks. Referred back to the Job Club, Tony and the vocational counselors contacted his bank supervisor and worked out an Employee Assistance Program (EAP) that enabled Tony to resume work. The plan required Tony to meet biweekly with his psychiatrist and take injectable, long-acting antipsychotic medication. Tony, his psychiatrist, and the EAP counselor maintained communication with progress reports on a monthly basis.

▶ Improving Work Outcomes With Cognitive Rehabilitation

Because cognitive impairments of the mentally ill can interfere with their motivation for work as well as for learning and sustaining work performance (McGurk et al. 2003), computer-aided methods of cognitive training have been developed to remediate these impairments. Cognitive remediation has been used primarily with schizophrenia patients to elevate their ability for learning and mastering job requirements. One approach, termed *neurocognitive enhancement,* comprises computer-based training tasks with graduated levels of difficulty that require sustained attention, memory, category formation, planning, and strategies for problem solving. When participants achieve and sustain 90% correct responses on a particular cognitive task, they graduate to a more difficult level.

Neurocognitive enhancement improves working memory to a level consistent with that of normally functioning individuals, as well as thinking and flexible adaptation on the job. The computer-based training, however, is only one component of this vocational rehabilitation modality. Persons with schizophrenia who enroll in this program are simultaneously assisted by a vocational specialist who coordinates a comprehensive rehabilitation program that includes personalized goal setting, a weekly group meeting in which positive feedback is given for improvements in cognitive functioning and work performance, and support in getting and keeping a job. When computer-aided neurocognitive enhancement was added to supported employment, significantly greater benefits accrued to schizophrenia patients in the quality of their work performance, hours worked, and income earned in contrast with other patients who were randomly assigned to supported employment alone (Bell et al. 2007).

Similar benefits on vocational rehabilitation have been achieved by somewhat different software used for 24 hours of computer-based cognitive exercises. In this program, entitled Thinking Skills for Work, schizophrenia patients practice a broad range of cognitive functions, including attention and concentration, psychomotor speed, learning and memory, and executive functions. The computer exercises are designed to be enjoyable and motivating. Graded levels of difficulty are introduced as the individual reaches a preset threshold of successful learning for each task. Individuals who were randomly assigned to participate in Thinking Skills for Work plus supported employment achieved significantly better neurocognition, better retention in the program, greater employment rates, longer hours worked, and higher wages than their counterparts who participated in supported employment alone (McGurk et al. 2007).

With these promising results from computer-aided cognitive remediation, future prospects for employment are likely to be brighter for patients with schizophrenia and other disorders in which cognitive deficits limit successful outcomes of work rehabilitation. We may look forward to the day when persons with schizophrenia who wish to work can attain normal rates of employment with further research and development of cognitive remediation, linked with in vivo training of cognitive and social skills in the workplace plus supported employment.

▶ Supported Education

To help students with psychiatric disabilities achieve their educational goals, supported education provides assistance for students who are participating in mainstream schools and colleges, fully integrated with nondisabled students. This rehabilitation modality has the same general aims as supported employment but a different focus for its interventions. Counselors or rehabilitation specialists work with a small number of students, offering the following personalized on-site services:

- Assistance with developing educational goals and plans, college applications, financial aid, registration, orientation to campus settings, and benefits for disabled students
- Educational coaching and assistance for taking notes in class, participating in class, requests for time with teacher, developing good study habits, and obtaining extra time to complete tests and exams
- Availability of mentors and tutors; computers with adequate instruction and troubleshooting supports
- Liaison with college administrators, teachers, counselors, and campus mental health offices, as well as with the student's psychiatrist and mental health team

The education specialist or coach helps the student negotiate solutions to problems that inevitably arise, such as having to take incompletes for classes and temporary leaves when relapses occur. Another key area is assisting the student in socializing with other students. Educational support groups are offered, often with volunteers from the nondisabled student body to serve as models and "buddies" to help the disabled students to gain entry to college activities and experience comfort and satisfaction in locales where students "hang out." Supports and interventions are emphasized for keeping students in school and on their trajectory for longer-term, career goals.

Supported education has been favorably evaluated for both physically and mentally disabled students. In a controlled study, students with mental illness enrolled in a college-level supported education program were nearly twice as likely as those in the control group to be still in school or employed. The students who participated in supported employment also had a three-fold increase in their academic productivity as measured by completed courses.

▶ Work Incentives

The Social Security Administration has awakened to the fact that more than one-third of its disabled beneficiaries have mental or developmental disabilities, yet fewer than 5% ever leave the disability rolls. As a result, the agency has introduced incentives for disabled persons to return to work. The principal incentives are:

- *Earned income exclusion for persons receiving Supplemental Security Income (SSI).* Beneficiaries of SSI can earn up to $65 per month without losing any SSI payments. Beyond $65 per month, SSI payments are reduced on the basis of $1 for every $2 earned up to $600 per month. Thus, beneficiaries can accumulate more funds by working, earning income, and still retaining a substituted amount of their SSI payments.

- *Program for Achieving Self-Support (PASS) for individuals receiving SSI.* A PASS allows a disabled beneficiary to set aside income earned on a job for up to 2 years if an application form is filled out that describes how the income will be used to prepare the individual for self-support without SSI. A specific and clearly described plan for self-support and occupational development is required. Most mentally disabled persons will need assistance in completing the application and preparing the accompanying letter. The purpose is to encourage mentally disabled persons to become self-supporting workers with the assistance of vocational rehabilitation and then voluntarily give up their SSI. The earned income must be put in a designated bank account and can be used for purchasing a car, clothes, books, tools, and uniforms, or for paying tuition for occupational training programs, college, security deposit and first month's rent on an apartment, and any other expenses that can be set aside for the person's goal of supporting himself/herself without SSI. If the individual subsequently becomes disabled and stops working, SSI can be reinstated without filing a full-scale application to Social Security.

• *Trial work periods for individuals receiving Social Security Disability Income (SSDI).* The trial work period lets people test their ability to work for at least 9 months without affecting their disability benefits. They continue to get full benefits during the trial work period, no matter how much they earn. The trial work period can be broken down into periods less than 9 months as long as not more than 9 months are used over an interval of 60 months. If a person obtains long-term employment beyond the 9 months and goes off SSDI but subsequently becomes mentally disabled again, benefits can be resumed without filing another full-scale application for disability benefits.

• *Retention of Medicaid medical insurance after giving up disability benefits.* If a person takes a job that pays an amount beyond the threshold for any particular state's limit before stopping of SSI cash benefits, the individual is still considered disabled and can continue to receive Medicaid benefits as long as the health insurance is essential for maintaining health and well-being required for sustaining work. Thus, continued payments for psychiatric, rehabilitative, and medical evaluations and treatments will be made by Medicaid.

▶ Accommodations for Mentally Disabled Workers

The Americans with Disabilities Act of 1991 requires employers to make "reasonable accommodations" for workers with disabilities. Unlike the costly architectural changes and equipment purchases associated with accommodations for physically and visually disabled workers, most accommodations for workers with psychiatric disabilities are inexpensive or free. Such accommodations include flexible work schedules, time off for treatment appointments, and job restructuring to reduce stress. Accommodations that are helpful for the mentally disabled may require staff training, such as teaching a supervisor to provide positive and corrective feedback rather than criticism of performance to bolster the positive abilities and confidence of the worker with a psychiatric disorder. Another example would be erecting room dividers to give a private, quiet, and nondistracting work setting for a worker who has problems with concentration and sustained performance in a socially stimulating environment.

▌ Incentives for Rehabilitation Agencies to Improve Job Placement and Retention

Some state mental health agencies have introduced finanacial incentives for providers of vocational rehabilitation services based on the number of mentally disabled persons who are placed in jobs, retain their jobs, and have satisfaction with their services. One such program resulted in significant increases in job placements and retentions, closer liaison and collaboration between mental health and rehabilitation practitioners, and increased use of evidence-based rehabilitation such as supported employment.

▌ Summary

The role of worker is one of the most important ways to normalize the lives of persons with mental disabilities. Having the appropriate type of vocational rehabilitation that fits each person's preferences, needs, strengths, and phase of illness is the key to reestablishing a working life. A continuum of vocational rehabilitation opportunities provides opportunities to work for almost all persons with severe mental illness. This permits the essential individualization that enables "each bird to sing with its own throat." Supported employment is currently the "gold standard" for vocational rehabilitation because it helps individuals to obtain "real jobs" in the competitive marketplace without stigma and with ongoing and indefinite supports from an employment specialist.

Aided by equal opportunity legislation and work incentives available through Social Security, more mentally ill persons will find the door open to employment. The advent of evidence-based vocational rehabilitation services also expands possibilities for all those who want to work to have a reasonable chance to do so in regular jobs in the community. In the future, research and political advocacy will bring new advances and greater personnel resources in vocational rehabilitation, further enlarging openings in the workforce for the mentally ill and accelerating their progress toward recovery.

▶ Key Points

- Vocational rehabilitation has an extremely important part to play in promoting recovery of the seriously mentally ill. Having a job confers many benefits on all people, not just those with disability. Employment at some meaningful job—regardless of its status, hours required, or remuneration—provides a "worker" identity to the individual, which, in turn, enables a mentally ill person to join the ranks of nondisabled citizens in society. In addition, a job provides money to improve one's quality of life, opportunities to socialize and make friends, self-esteem, and self-efficacy. Working also introduces planned and scheduled routines, expectations, and activities into one's life that supplant the "social vacuum" associated with intrusive symptoms, indolence, apathy, depression, and demoralization.

- As in other rehabilitation modalities, vocational rehabilitation takes many different forms to fit the individual needs of the broad spectrum of persons with mental disorders. Persons with remitting disorders who have had good premorbid social competence are able to obtain jobs independently and work full-time. Supported employment, an evidence-based service, attracts the participation of a substantial minority of the seriously mentally ill, and half of those who enroll are able to obtain employment.

- Other vocational opportunities include firms run by the mentally ill themselves, jobs as consumer aides in mental health programs, and transitional employment in which mentally ill workers participate in bona fide job tasks, but in segregated locations with ongoing supervision by mental health staff.

- Predictors of successful work performance include good cognitive functioning, prior work experience, good premorbid social competence, family support, abstinence from illicit drugs and alcohol, and fewer disincentives from disability pensions.

- The nature of the vocational program also influences the likelihood that an individual will get and keep a job. In particular, great assistance comes from ongoing liaison by an employment specialist with the patient, the job supervisor or employer, and the mental health team responsible for psychiatric care. This permits the employment specialist or job coach to "teach the ropes" to the patient at the job site and provide problem-solving and clinical intervention when crises occur or symptoms flare up.

- New, novel interventions to improve vocational functioning—for example, cognitive training and errorless learning—are appearing that compensate for the cognitive impairments of seriously mentally ill persons that often compromise their success in a job.

▶ Selected Readings

Bell M, Bryson G, Greig T, et al: Neurocognitive enhancement therapy with work therapy. Arch Gen Psychiatry 58:763–768, 2001

Bond GR, Becker DR, Drake RE, et al: Implementing supported employment as an evidence-based practice. Psychiatr Serv 52:313–322, 2001

Cook JA, Razzano L: Vocational rehabilitation for persons with schizophrenia: recent research and implications for practice. Schizophr Bull 26:87–103, 2000

Drake RE, Becker DR: The Individual Placement and Support model of supported employment. Psychiatr Serv 47:473–475, 1996

Gold MW: Try Another Way Training Manual. Champaign, IL, Research Press, 1980

Jacobs HE, Kardashian S, Kreinbring RH, et al: A skills-oriented model for facilitating employment among psychiatrically disabled persons. Rehabil Couns Bull 28:87–96, 1984

Kern RS, Liberman RP, Kopelowicz A, et al: Applications of errorless learning for improving work performance in persons with schizophrenia. Am J Psychiatry 159:1921–1926, 2002

Mowbry CT, Brown KS, Furlong-Norman K, et al (eds): Supported Education and Psychiatric Rehabilitation: Models and Methods. Linthicum, MD, International Association of Psychosocial Rehabilitation Services, 2002

Oka M, Otsuka K, Ykoyama N, et al: An evaluation of a hybrid occupational therapy and supported employment program in Japan for persons with schizophrenia. Am J Occup Ther 58:466–475, 2004

Reger F, Wong-McDonald A, Liberman RP: Psychiatric rehabilitation in a community mental health center. Psychiatr Serv 54:1457–1495, 2003

Tsang HWH: Social skills training to help mentally ill persons find a keep a job. Psychiatr Serv 52:891–894, 2001

Wallace CJ, Tauber R: Supplementing supported employment with workplace skills training. Psychiatr Serv 55:513–515, 2004

Wallace CJ, Tauber R, Liberman RP: UCLA Workplace Fundamentals Module. Camarillo, CA, Psychiatric Rehabilitation Consultants, 1998 [Available from www.psychrehab.com]

▶ References

Backer TE, Liberman RP, King LW, et al: The Chronic Mental Patient Is Treatable and Rehabilitatable (video). Available from Psychiatric Rehabilitation Consultants, PO Box 2867, Camarillo, CA 93010; www.psychrehab.com, 1986.

Becker DR, Drake RE: A Working Life for People With Severe Mental Illness. New York, Oxford University Press, 2003

Becker D, Whitley R, Bailey EL, et al: Long-term employment trajectories among participants with severe mental illness in supported employment. Psychiatr Serv 58:922–928, 2007

Bell MD, Choi J, Lysaker P: Psychological interventions to improve work outcomes for people with psychiatric disabilities. Journal of the Norwegian Psychological Association 44:2–14, 2007

Bond GR, Becker DR, Drake RE, et al: Implementing supported employment as an evidence-based practice. Psychiatr Serv 52:313–322, 2001a

Bond GR, Resnick SG, Drake RE, et al: Does competitive employment improve non-vocational outcomes for people with severe mental illness? J Consult Clin Psychol 69:489–501, 2001b

Chandler D, Meisel J, Hu TW, et al: A capitated model for a cross-section of severely mentally ill clients: employment outcomes. Community Ment Health J 33:501–516, 1997

Cook JA, Leff S, Blyler CR, et al: Results of a multi-site, randomized trial of supported employment interventions for individuals with severe mental illness. Arch Gen Psychiatry 62:505–512, 2005

Fairweather GW, Sander DH, Maynard H et al: Community Life for the Mentally Ill: An Alternative to Institutional Care. Chicago, IL, Aldine, 1969

Fuller TR, Oka M, Otsuka K, et al: A hybrid supported employment program for persons with schizophrenia in Japan. Psychiatr Serv 51:864–866, 2000

Jacobs HE, Kardashian S, Kreinbring RH, et al: A skills-oriented model for facilitating employment among psychiatrically disabled persons. Rehabil Couns Bull 28:87–96, 1984

McGurk SR, Mueser KT: Cognitive functioning, symptoms and work in supported employment: a review and heuristic model. Schizophr Res 70:147–174, 2004

McGurk SR, Mueser KT: Strategies for coping with cognitive impairments of clients in supported employment. Psychiatr Serv 57:1421–1429, 2006

McGurk SR, Mueser KT, Harvey PD, et al: Cognitive and symptom predictors of work outcomes for clients with schizophrenia in supported employment. Psychiatr Serv 54:1129–1135, 2003

McGurk SR, Mueser KT, Feldman K, et al: Cognitive training for supported employment: 2–3 year outcomes of a randomized, controlled trial. Am J Psychiatry 164:437–441, 2007

Mueser KT, Clark RE, Haines M, et al: The Hartford Study of Supported Employment for Persons With Severe Mental Illness. J Consult Clin Psychol 72:479–490, 2004

Mueser KT, Aalto S, Becker DR, et al: The effectiveness of skills training for improving outcomes in supported employment. Psychiatr Serv 56:1254–1260, 2005

Nuechterlein KH, Subotnik KL, Ventura J, et al: Advances in improving and predicting work outcome in recent-onset schizophrenia. Schizophr Bull 31:530, 2005

Tsang HWH: Social skills training to help mentally ill persons find and keep a job. Psychiatr Serv 52:891–894, 2001

Tsang HWH, Pearson V: A work-related social skills training program for people with schizophrenia in Hong Kong. Schizophr Bull 27:139–148, 2001

Wallace CJ, Tauber R: Supplementing supported employment with workplace skills training. Psychiatr Serv 55:513–515, 2004

CHAPTER 8

Vehicles for Delivering Rehabilitation Services

Vehicles for Delivering Rehabilitation Services

No man is so tall that he never needs help to stretch
And none so small that he never needs help to stoop

OLD DANISH PROVERB

MOST INDIVIDUALS with disabling forms of mental and developmental disorders are in need of a comprehensive range of mental health and human services that fit their needs and meet their personal goals for optimal community functioning with a good quality of life. During earlier eras when the mentally disabled were treated in long-term psychiatric hospitals, comprehensive services were available under the aegis of the hospital. Each treatment ward, unit, or program provided the services of psychiatry, pharmacology, medicine and surgery, dentistry, nursing, social work, recreation, physical and occupational therapy, work rehabilitation, education, and, of course, daily life supports such as housing, laundry, grooming and personal hygiene, clothing, beds, and meals.

In the community, however, comprehensive services are not available under one roof. There is a profusion of agencies, personnel, and practitioners located in different places and operated by different administrations, sources of funding, policies, and procedures that are often poorly coordinated. Mentally disabled persons living in the community have their functioning undermined by fragmented services.

To remedy disjointed services, community-based mental health programs have attempted to organize themselves into *systems of service delivery*. Optimal treatment and rehabilitation of individuals with multiple needs and deficits requires a system, agency, or organization to ensure the accessibility, reliability, and availability of a comprehensive assortment of needed community-based services. Service delivery systems are vehicles for conducting assessments, providing and coordinating the needed services, offering crisis intervention and supports, and monitoring patients to ensure that desired outcomes ensue.

Interventions and services are provided by different practitioners and agencies; for example, one agency or practitioner might offer psychiatric medication, another, family education, and a third, supported employment. While not ideal, services offered by unconnected facilities and practitioners at different locales are a sociopolitical necessity. Traditional bureaucratic boundaries, mandated areas of responsibility, funding streams, and limited resources sometimes require "quilting" together the various service providers.

We know that comprehensive, continuous, and coordinated care is essential for rehabilitating the seriously and persistently mentally ill. Disjointed and episodic treatment that is available only at times of florid exacerbation or relapse is incompatible with rehabilitation and recovery. Because persons impaired by serious mental illness or developmental disability require long-term treatment that exerts a gradual and cumulative benefit over time, only services that are provided on a continuous basis will truly rehabilitate. Interruptions and discontinuites of care are among the most significant obstacles to establishing a favorable trajectory of progress and recovery.

Case management is the major vehicle for piecing together comprehensive and continuous services for individuals with mental disabilities. Varied organizational schemes have been designed to ensure the delivery and effectiveness of comprehensive, continuous, and coordinated services for community-based care of the severely mentally ill. Intensive and assertive case management, wraparound services, and integrated mental health care are described in this chapter. They differ in their format but share the same principles as listed in Table 8.1.

The clinical and organizational demands placed on all systems of service delivery can be visualized by the comprehensive, three-dimensional cube shown in Figure 8.1. One dimension of the cube is the type or phase of mental illness, as described in Chapter 3 ("Illness Management"). The second dimension consists of the modalities for comprehensive assessment, treatment, and rehabilitation that are functionally linked to the phase of a person's disorder: syndromal and functional assessment, pharmacotherapy, supportive therapy, cognitive therapy, social skills training, family education and supports, and vocational services. Programs and services for the community support and survival of patients are depicted in the third dimension. These include housing, social service entitlements, assertive community treatment, psychosocial clubs, day treatment centers, and residential treatment and rehabilitation.

● **TABLE 8.1**

Attributes of community care teams that provide personal support services (case management)

- Ensure accessibility to the full range of needed treatment and rehabilitation services delivered by a designated team or by a mental health center with a personal support specialist (case manager), ensuring that assessment, coordination, monitoring, and follow-up are provided. Provide round-the-clock emergency and crisis intervention, especially for nights and weekends.

- Consult with and coordinate services with agencies and practitioners external to the team or mental health center, such as housing agencies, the Social Security Administration, employers, schools, residential care operators, and state vocational rehabilitation departments.

- Give priority to persons with serious and disabling mental disorders of all ages and cultural backgrounds.

- Ensure that the focus of personal support services is on improvement in the realms of symptoms, work, education, peer relationships, family relations, community reintegration, personal hygiene, spiritual life, and recreation.

- Conjointly with patients and their families, set goals for community reintegration and recovery of patients in normal environments at work, schools, and homes and in social relationships.

- Ensure availability of personnel to meet the cultural and linguistic needs of patients and their families.

- Maximize the recovery model of treatment by building empowerment and self-responsibility, natural supports, and self-help through encouraging active participation by consumers in:
  - » Identifying their own relevant personal goals.
  - » Contributing to their own treatment plans.
  - » Collaborating with their treatment professionals in evaluating progress.
  - » Involving families and friends for generalization of improvement into the community.

- Offer flexible levels of intervention, from crisis services to long-term maintenance and reinforcement of stability and recovery.

- Acquire competencies for providing high-quality delivery of evidence-based services.

- Establish a fixed point of responsibility for personal support specialists working on treatment teams.

- During regularly scheduled team reviews of progress and problems of patients, give priority to promoting improved functional independence and symptom stability, as well as crisis intervention.

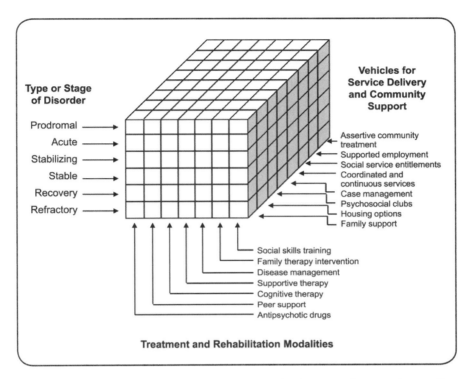

FIGURE 8.1 Three dimensions of coordinated services for delivery to the seriously mentally ill are depicted that ensure comprehensive, collaborative, competent, and continuous treatment. This comprehensive cube of evidence-based treatment practices, vehicles for service delivery, and community resources is matched to the type of stage of each patient's mental illness.

▶ Case Management: Personal Support Services

Traditionally, case management has been guided by a set of principles and procedures to ensure that patients are provided with assessment and treatment services to foster their integration into the community. However, the term *case management* carries a patronizing, paternalistic, and stigmatizing connotation. Patients and families do not want to be considered "cases" to be "managed." They prefer to be consumers of services that they have chosen in partnership with their clinicians. They look for specialized and technical assistance from mental health clinicians and agencies to achieve their own personal goals. A more apt term that is consistent with the dignity and empowerment of individuals with severe mental disorders is *personal support services.* The clinicians who provide such services can be identified as *personal support specialists.* In this manual, we prefer to use this latter term.

PRINCIPLES AND FUNCTIONS OF PERSONAL SUPPORT SERVICES

The principles undergirding personal support services are listed in Table 8.1. Adherence to the principles requires that personal support services be:

- Accessible.
- Continuous.
- Comprehensive.
- Coordinated.
- Flexible.
- Collaborative.
- Consumer-centered.
- Available through advocacy.
- Customized.
- Accountable.

Accessibility requires that patients neither experience undue delays before being evaluated and treated nor encounter insurmountable barriers to obtaining services. Examples of barriers are inadequate public transportation, lack of funds or other qualifications, homelessness, and communication problems resulting from cultural or language differences.

EXAMPLE

Because of the multicultural population of New York, Chicago, and cities of California, the public mental health systems in those places are required to include individuals who are fluent in languages such as Spanish, Russian, Chinese, Korean, Farsi, and Arabic. At one mental health center in California, the addition of two bilingual Latino personal support specialists led to a significant 150% increase in accessibility to services for Latino patients within 1 year.

One of the most important functions of personal support services is *crisis intervention,* an activity that is consistent with the principles of *accessibility* and *flexibility.* Most crises occur in the evenings or on weekends; therefore, if personal support services are to be available to patients who don't have their crises during office hours, modes of responsiveness need to be orchestrated on a 24/7 basis.

Some mental health systems of care use telephone services, others have evening and weekend phone numbers that go to clinicians manning a central "crisis and information" clearinghouse, and still others have calls routed to mobile emergency teams. To do justice to the principles of *continuity* and *collaboration,* agencies or clinics can equip members of treatment teams with beepers or cell phones and have the staff take turns for being "on call."

Comprehensiveness refers to the availability of the full range of services that are needed to maintain mentally disabled persons in the community and enhance their quality of life. Few mental health facilities that use personal support services are able to provide, under the same roof, all of the services needed by mentally disabled persons for stabilization of their illnesses and adjustment to the community. A variety of mechanisms are used to make comprehensive services available to individuals in their catchment area; for example, mental health programs often contract with other agencies that offer treatment and rehabilitation not within the ken of the responsible mental health authority. An alternative mechanism is the reliance on managed care "carve out" services provided by mental health insurers. A third mechanism, assertive community treatment, makes all services available under the aegis of a single mental health team. Assertive community treatment is currently considered "best practice" as a vehicle for delivering mental health services.

Customized services put into practice the aphorism "One suit does not fit all." Optimal case management or personal support services are *person-centered* and are responsive to the uniqueness of each patient. Doing justice to meeting the special needs of patients is challenging. Personal support specialists are almost always swamped by the diversity of patients, each of whom has his/her own interests, values, dreams for a better life, strengths, constellation of symptoms, and cognitive and functional deficits. To meet the challenge of individualization of treatment, clinicians should provide patients with services and supports that vary over time in their type and intensity and that are *flexibly linked* to the phase and severity of illness.

Services should not only fit patients' needs but also be orchestrated by the patients and their families. Patients are empowered by joining with their personal support specialists in making informed decisions regarding their rehabilitation. For patients to become informed participants in their treatment, practitioners must actualize a *consumer-centered* approach. Surveys of patients have documented that many of them are dissatisfied with the explanations of services that are given to them. They complain that information is not made available to them regarding how and why particular treatments exert their effects and what side effects they have.

The conundrum of educating patients is compounded by the passivity of most patients. In customary 15-minute clinical interviews, the typical number of questions asked by patients is zero. Therefore, personal support specialists, as well as other clinicians, must be competent as teachers. Teaching becomes treatment, as patients need to comprehend the nature of their disorders and services required for community integration and recovery. The educational role holds personal support specialists *accountable* for knowledgeable patients. Treatment outcomes are improved when patients receive encouragement to participate actively as members of their treatment team: learning about their illnesses, asking questions, receiving answers, and contributing ideas and preferences for the selection and implementation of their treatment plans. *Customized, consumer-centered, collaborative, and flexible services* will help patients to attain their personal goals and function as independently as possible.

CLINICAL EXAMPLE

James's schizoaffective disorder had stabilized, and he expressed a readiness to embark on rehabilitation. He and his parents had been encouraged from the beginning of his treatment to be active members of his treatment team. His psychiatrist, who was serving as his personal support specialist, discussed three alternative rehabilitation programs for James's consideration: a transitional living center, where he would receive vocational and independent living services; a psychosocial clubhouse; or a program involving participation in a series of social skills modules for acquiring abilities of friendship and dating, work, and recreation.

James declined these suggestions, instead choosing to work part-time in his father's business. He felt that the other options would stigmatize him. He wanted to remain on his previously chosen occupational trajectory, even if this meant creating accommodations for his current low capacities for performance and endurance. His father agreed with James. Although his psychiatrist was concerned about parental emotional over-involvement and unrealistically high expectations for James's functioning, he assented to James's wishes. Rehabilitation services then were deployed to provide consultation and supports to James and his father in the family workplace.

Advocacy comes into play for personal support specialists in a variety of situations, such as when a patient:

- Is rebuffed or unable to obtain some needed service, benefit, or civil rights.
- Encounters problems in reconciling with family or coping with a legal entanglement.
- Has needs that are not met by currently available services or existing policy or procedures.

Patients recognize, respect, and appreciate practitioners who go the extra mile as advocates. Advocacy strengthens the therapeutic alliance, improves adherence to treatment, increases motivation for change, and serves as a model that patients can emulate. Far from encouraging dependency, advocacy promotes the learning of self-assertiveness that is the raw material for progress down the road to recovery. The greatest benefits from successful advocacy come from matching services with patients and ensuring that the services are actually delivered.

EXAMPLE

Advocacy requires personal support specialists to depart from their routines, take time away from customary appointments, visit unfamiliar agencies and territory, and be assertive in novel situations.

- Visiting the local Social Security Administration office to appeal a rejection of a patient's benefit application or error in benefit payments
- Making a phone call and home visit to a patient's wife who has been alienated and estranged from her husband because of his use of cocaine and repeated relapses of schizophrenia—informing her of her husband's sustained sobriety, participation in rehabilitation, and desire to have a reconciliation
- Making a presentation at a school board meeting to support a family's request for financial support to enable their teenage son to attend an exemplary out-of-state residential treatment center

The diverse functions of personal support services place enormous demands on the treatment team and its individual practitioners. As graphically depicted in Figure 8.2, clinicians providing personal support services are in the midst of a five-ring "circus" of services that must be juggled, balanced, and delivered to patients, each of whom has different assets, deficits, symptoms, and personal goals. Most personal support specialists them-

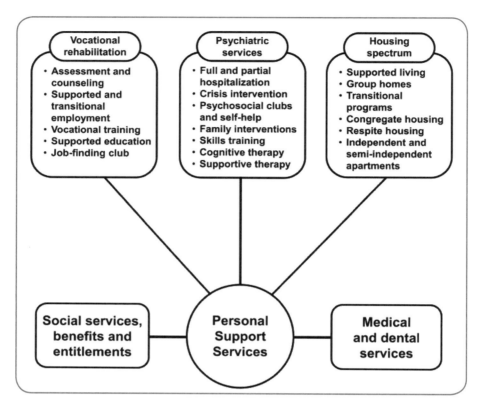

FIGURE 8.2 Spectrum of personal support services needed by severely mentally ill persons living in the community.

selves provide crisis intervention, supportive therapy, family contacts, and monitoring of the patient's clinical and community functioning. They have a major role in obtaining and renewing Social Security benefits, budgeting and managing money, securing appropriate housing, and ensuring access to psychiatric, medical, and dental consultation, psychosocial rehabilitation, and vocational rehabilitation.

PERSONAL SUPPORT SPECIALISTS

Personal support specialists are the most critical element in the effectiveness of a system of care. They serve as the human link between patients and the services that are available to promote recovery. The competencies required of personal support specialists are displayed in Figure 8.3. Having the competencies to perform the manifold responsibilities of this role is more important than the discipline or professional training of individuals. Armed with these competencies, any mental health professional—social worker, nurse, psychologist, occupational or recreational therapist, or psy-

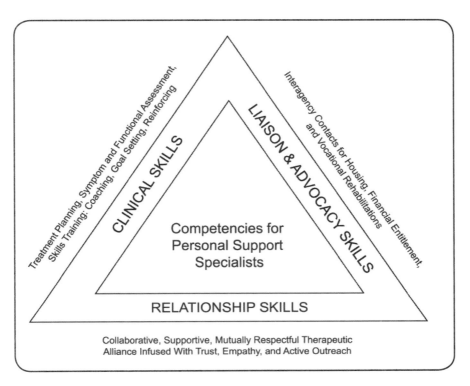

FIGURE 8.3 Competencies for personal support specialists (case managers).

chiatrist—can subserve the role of personal support specialist. However, in most venues, especially outside of major cities, paraprofessionals carry out personal support services because the agency cannot recruit and retain sufficient numbers of postgraduate-level professional clinicians. Fortunately, paraprofessionals can learn many of the requisite clinical skills and provide excellent service to patients. This is particularly true when the staff member has extensive experience working with the severely mentally ill, has competency-based training and supervision, and has the personal attributes that convey a collaborative and friendly style: warmth, genuineness, spontaneity, conscientiousness, empathy, and social skills.

Interpersonal skills are critical for mediating the functions and effectiveness of personal support specialists. As shown in Figure 8.3, *relationship skills* (for forming therapeutic alliances with patients and families), *clinical skills,* and *liaison and advocacy skills* combine to form a triad of competencies that distinguish excellence in case management or personal support services. Liaison and advocacy skills determine the ability of the personal support specialist to open doors to community resources, agencies, and other supports for meeting patients' needs. The effectiveness of a personal support specialist also depends upon the person's familiarity and personal contacts with the various service providers, both within and outside the agency. Who and what you know about community services can make the difference between patients receiving their needed rehabilitation services or not. As in any field of endeavor, the ability to communicate in a persuasive manner is decisive in securing the services that will keep patients on the road to recovery.

The complexity of coordinating services falls on or falls off the shoulders of personal support specialists, depending upon the scope and depth of their competencies. As can be seen in Figure 8.1 earlier in this chapter, patients receiving treatment in the community obtain the services they require for proceeding on the road to recovery only if personal support specialists and the multidisciplinary team can organize and deliver two dimensions of treatments and resources—treatment and rehabilitation modalities and resources for community support—in tandem with the patient's stage or type of illness so that treatments and resources are matched to a patient's needs as they change over time.

These challenging clinical demands are presented here not in a cavalier manner, but rather as a clear, clarion call to mental health stakeholders and policy makers who are attempting to reform their systems of services. In particular, the three dimensions of recovery-oriented services should be understood by managers, administrators, and politicians who hold the mental health purse strings and are responsible for putting their money where their rhetoric is. Their competencies in planning, organizing, decision making, and resource management are as difficult to acquire as those of personal support specialists. The clinical and organizational requirements for recovery in the community are sobering for those intoxicated by the purple prose of the "recovery movement."

HOUSING AS RESPONSIBILITY OF PERSONAL SUPPORT SPECIALISTS

While not an area of professional interest for mental health professionals, housing is of great importance to patients and their families. While its role in personal support services is clear from Figures 8.1 and 8.2, housing is at the very foundation of psychiatric rehabilitation and recovery from mental disability. Consider for a moment how you, the reader, would be able to function at college or in a job if you did not have a suitable place to live. Home is our point of departure for all the activities of our lives. It is no different for the severely mentally ill.

Too many severely mentally ill and dually diagnosed individuals are homeless or in jails and prisons. But a home is not simply having a "roof, a bed, and three square meals a day." Sadly, most mentally disabled persons in the United States reside in substandard board-and-care homes, nursing homes, or large, locked, and poorly staffed community facilities. Obtaining proper housing for their patients is a priority for personal support specialists. Housing with a pleasant environment, privacy, and appropriate supervision and activities is a prerequisite for living in the community with dignity and self-respect.

To be effective advocates for their patients' housing needs, personal support specialists must be knowledgeable of the spectrum of housing available in their communities. Know-how also extends to personal contacts and working relationships with the proprietors, managers, and staff of the various types of homes. For successful placements, the type of housing should be congruent with the phase of a person's mental disorder. In other words, the level of care and supervision available in a residence need to be compatible with the needs of the individual.

Personal support specialists offer continuity of care across the phases of a person's illness; thus, during an exacerbation of psychotic symptoms, a patient may benefit from a week or more of support, supervision, and security in a homelike crisis facility where a nurse is available and a consulting psychiatrist is "on call." As the psychosis stabilizes, the personal support

EXAMPLE

There are no stronger advocates for appropriate housing for the seriously mentally ill than their family members. In Los Angeles County, family members in various locales have banded together, raised funds, and purchased or constructed homes and apartments. Support for nonprofit housing has been provided by federal subsidies for apartment rentals, urban redevelopment, charitable organizations, the National Alliance on Mental Illness, the Mental Health Association, and the Los Angeles County Department of Mental Health. The spectrum of facilities now available includes crisis homes, transitional living, supported housing, and independent living. A longer-term, rehabilitation complex, *Homes for Life,* is noteworthy because it is a charitable, family-supported, nonprofit agency that has renovated and constructed two dozen homes and apartment buildings. *Homes for Life* offers varying levels of supervision and support services consistent with the needs of the mentally ill residents. The unique aspect of this program is its provision of a comfortable and familiar home for the lifetime of its resident.

specialist may be able to obtain housing for the patient in a board-and-care, foster, or group home where medication can be administered under supervision, meals are provided, and self-care skills can be encouraged.

Once in the stable phase, the patient will need the advocacy and liaison skills of a personal support specialist to move into a transitional or supported living home. Intermittent supervision and assistance are available in these residences, as the patient is expected to be able to function more independently. When the patient reaches the recovery phase and is fortunate enough to be receiving personal support services from a specialist with good advocacy skills, semi-independent or independent living apartments should be available. Patients' motivation to progress successfully through the continuum of housing is strengthened if they know housing with greater amounts of independence and personal choice will be available in the future.

MODELS OF PERSONAL SUPPORT SERVICES

Case management and *personal support services* are generic terms that encapsulate many different models and approaches to treatment planning, implementation, continuity, and consistency. However, "God is in the details," an aphorism that distinguishes different models of personal support services. Various models of personal support services (case management) can be categorized by their:

- Intensity, accessibility, and frequency of contact.
- Patient/staff ratio.
- Spectrum of services—relational support as well as specific treatments for vocational, dual diagnosis, and social skills training.
- Mobile outreach of services in the community and home.
- Use of individual personal support specialists who are assigned to specific patients versus having the entire team be responsible for all patients.
- Competencies and disciplines of the personal support specialists.
- Degree to which the host mental health program or team can offer the full range of needed services versus "brokering" services by making referrals to outside agencies.

In the least intensive model, personal support specialists may be assigned to serve 50–100 or more patients and serve as "brokers" for their patients, referring them to services without being able to follow up on the compliance or results with the referrals. Personal support is a very limited affair if the support specialist has more than 50 individuals to serve; this model is low on accountability, coordination, collaboration, accessibility, and effectiveness. Table 8.2 describes the types of personal support and treatment services that are available at the different levels of intensity of responsibility.

The best practice for personal support services is *assertive community treatment* (ACT), which has a patient/staff ratio of not more than 10:1, with the personal support functions shared by all members of its multidisciplinary team of 6–14 members. More than two decades of research and evaluation have shown benefits for patients served by ACT in reduced hospitalization, improved housing, greater patient satisfaction, and better quality of life (Stein and Santos 1998). Because ACT is by consensus of experts

● **TABLE 8.2**
Various levels of intensity and comprehensiveness of personal support services (case management)

MINIMAL, "BROKER" MODEL	COORDINATION MODEL	INTENSIVE ACT MODEL
Minimal liaison with service providers	Minimal liaison with families and service providers	Active liaison with families and service providers
Referrals for crisis services and hospitalization	Minimal advocacy for needed services	Advocacy and participation in developing needed supports and services
		Weekly or more frequent monitoring of patients
		Provision of most treatments using personalized services
	Intermittent supportive therapy	Frequent supportive therapy
	Coordination of crisis services with other service providers	Crisis intervention as needed, with emphasis on prevention of crises
Delimited following of patient through system of care	Modest following of patient through system of care	Following patient through system of care with personalized continuity of treatment
		Single point of accountability (with team)

Note. ACT= assertive community treatment.

the most thoroughly validated model of personal support services, it will be described in some detail in the next section.

▶ Assertive Community Treatment

Instead of trying to link services from a variety of disparate and disjointed providers, the ACT team is the primary provider of services. While there are variants of ACT depending upon its rural or urban locale, funding constraints, and ability to recruit and retain competent staff, the team consists of 10–14 staff who serve as a fixed point of responsibility for persons with disabling forms of mental illness (Stein and Santos 1998). Some teams serve specialized populations such as persons with schizophrenia, adolescents in transition to adulthood, young adults in the earlier and more acute phases of their disorders, homeless individuals, individuals who are high utilizers of mental health and social services, or persons with dual mental and addictive disorders.

The defining characteristic of ACT is its assertive outreach. ACT team members spend very little time in offices aside from team conferences, which take place daily to review the current status of the team's caseload and to share information so that each staff member is sufficiently knowledgeable to work with each of the team's clientele. Assertive outreach means providing services in the community locations where the patients live, learn, work, and spend their leisure time. This is a revolutionary movement in the delivery of services, since conventional services have been hospital- or clinic-based. Working alone in the community with clients is also challenging to staff members who may have concerns about their security and efficacy in unfamiliar locales. Thus, selection of staff for personal attributes that are compatible with risk-taking and relationship-building is of critical importance in mounting effective ACT. Training, using an apprenticeship or mentoring model, also helps to bring new staff up to snuff.

> "A desk is a dangerous place from which to watch the world."
>
> JOHN LE CARRÉ

CLINICAL SERVICES PROVIDED BY ACT

The team provides psychiatric assessment; medication; monitoring; supportive relationships; assistance with daily living tasks, including food, housing, and finances; liaison with families; and crisis intervention on a 24/7 basis. The spectrum of services offered by an ACT team is shown in Table 8.2. ACT teams assist patients in meeting all or most of their needs for community functioning from the day that they enter the program into the indefinite future, as long as they require intensive services.

A critically important feature of ACT is its delivering comprehensive services in a coordinated fashion by all members of a single team. When the team cannot provide a particular service, such as housing, then a team member advocates with the appropriate agency and collaborates with the patient to secure it. In addition, continuity of services is ensured by virtue of the availability of ACT staff 24 hours per day, 7 days per week. If a patient requires hospitalization for an acute episode, the team follows him/her, maintaining contact throughout the hospitalization period. As the single locus of responsibility for delivering services, each ACT team is where the "buck stops" and accountability begins and ends.

ACT can be viewed as serving its patients in a continuous manner across space and time, as well as responding to their needs for services in psychiatric, medical, and functional domains of community life. Because the effectiveness of ACT depends upon the fidelity with which its key principles are implemented, criteria for quality assurance of this modality have been developed for agencies that wish to adopt ACT and use it competently. Criteria used to determine the quality of ACT include "Team members spend 80% of their time working in the community with patients," "Team members provide four or more contacts and direct services averaging 2 hours per week per patient," and "There is a half-time psychiatrist for every 50 patients; the psychiatrist participates in team meetings and provides continuing education to the team members."

ACT offers many advantages for the treatment of mental disabilities, especially when individuals have marginal adjustment to the community, are at risk for relapse or rehospitalization, refuse to attend a mental health center or clinic, or are homeless and abusing illicit drugs or alcohol. The great advantage of ACT as a treatment approach for individuals with persistent or frequently relapsing mental disorders comes from the comprehensive, continuous, collaborative, coordinated, and consumer-oriented services ACT aims to provide. An ACT team assumes accountability for effective and timely provisions of personal support services. ACT aims to provide:

- Commitment and sensitivity in helping mentally ill persons to formulate and progress toward realistic personal goals.
- Interactions with patients in natural and more relaxed sites in the community that build trust and strengthen the therapeutic relationships.
- Reductions in dropouts and missed appointments because clinicians go to the patients rather than vice versa.

- Daily reviews of each patient by the ACT team to ensure that patients won't fall through the cracks.
- Continuity of team members with their cadre of patients, which promotes trusting, supportive, and empowering qualities inherent in human relationships.

All of these qualities of ACT are important for sustaining the arduous efforts of staff and patients alike in managing serious and persisting mental disorders. What better way to infuse hope into a therapeutic relationship than by the diligence and skill of an ACT team that knows that the road to recovery is paved with perseverance. The organizational design of ACT is shown in Figure 8.4.

Do all seriously and persistently mentally ill persons need to be served by expensive, resource-rich ACT teams? From the perspective of flexible individualization of services, one of the basic principles of rehabilitation (see Chapter 2, "Principles and Practice of Psychiatric Rehabilitation"), we

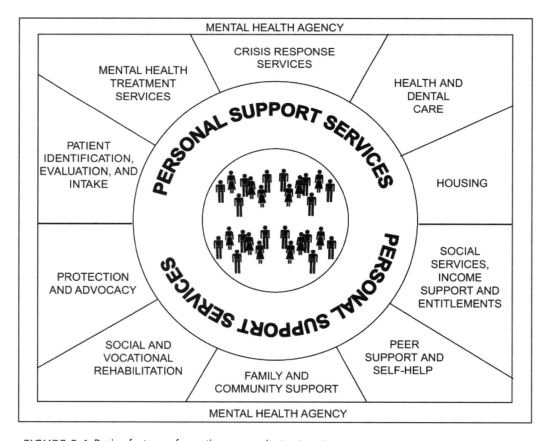

FIGURE 8.4 Design features of assertive community treatment.

would expect a more flexible approach depending upon each patient's needs. Unstable patients at high risk for relapse, neglect, homelessness, rehospitalization, or criminalization and incarceration would obviously benefit from the intensive outreach services of ACT. However, there is increasing evidence that only a minority of mentally disabled persons require ACT services (Salyers et al. 1998; van Veldhuizen 2007).

Once stabilized and moving on the road to recovery, patients should be given every opportunity to experience self-reliance, adherence to treatment, illness self-management, and shared decision making. Phase-linked treatment permits stable patients to shift from intensive monitoring and intervention to rehabilitation services that are delivered with a recovery orientation. This flexible approach gradually shifts the focus of treatment from keeping persons afloat in the community to involving them in vocational, educational, social, and recreational services consistent with each patient's personally relevant goals. Given the meager evidence that ACT reliably improves the social and vocational functioning of its clientele, rehabilitative services would appear to better meet the needs of many patients moving along the road to recovery (Mueser et al. 1998). However, the organization and delivery of rehabilitative services that are comprehensive, coordinated, continuous, consumer-oriented, and evidence-based may need to borrow and adapt many of the features that underlie the orchestration of ACT.

EFFECTIVENESS OF ACT

The evidence for the effectiveness of ACT has come primarily from the program repeatedly demonstrating its ability to reduce the hospitalizations of its patients, thereby extending patients' tenure in the community (Stein and Santos 1998). Patients receiving ACT services also report better subjective quality of life than individuals receiving conventional case management. The effectiveness of ACT depends in large measure on the quality of its services. Programs can assure quality and optimal clinical results by periodic checking of the degree to which ACT team members adhere to the fidelity of the ACT model (Bond and Salyers 2004). Using a fidelity scale is a boon for maintaining high-grade ACT services. For two decades, evaluations of patients and their family members who participated in ACT have indicated that more frequent contacts do not, by themselves, produce consistent therapeutic changes in stress and burnout of the family or in symptoms, work, or social competence of the patients (Mueser and Bond 2000; Test 1992). In recent years, however, new components—employment specialists, family education, and dual diagnosis services—have been added to the ACT team and promise to increase the breadth of ACT's impact.

● EXAMPLE OF BEST PRACTICE

Consistent with the emerging concept of recovery, a National Consensus Statement on Mental Health was crafted by clinicians, patients, families of the mentally ill, members of advocacy organizations, researchers, and state and federal officials: "Mental health recovery is a journey of trans-formation enabling a person with a mental disorder to live a meaningful life in a community of his or her choice while striving to achieve his or her full potential." What better way to achieve a meaningful life than to become empowered to become one's own personal support specialist? Resilience, personal strengths, enfranchisement, hope, and self-responsi-bility are not automatic accompaniments of living and coping with severe mental illness; rather, they are hard-earned through setting one's personal goals, learning skills and abilities necessary to attain one's goals, and striv-ing with stepwise success to achieve them. By using social skills training, clinicians on ACT teams can promote independent functioning of their patients while also increasing the efficiency of their services.

To accelerate the recovery process, the UCLA Psychiatric Rehabilitation Program uses training in personal effectiveness to equip patients to be their own personal support specialists. Actualizing the concept of helping people to help themselves, patients learn how to get their own needs met that are directly related to their personally relevant goals. This approach also fills the lacunae in most service systems due to insufficient personal support specialists. Most often delivered in groups—but also effective in family and individual contexts—this training encourages participants to identify specific interpersonal interactions occurring in the next week that, if accomplished, would bring the individuals closer to their longer-term personal goals. Examples of personal goals that have been achieved by patients in this program are:

- Returning to college and completing a bachelor's degree.
- Providing support, transportation, and physical assistance to one's mother with terminal cancer.
- Passing a Red Cross life-saving exam and working as a swim instructor at a YMCA.
- Getting a job at a country club parking cars.
- Applying for and obtaining subsidized housing.
- Obtaining a part-time job as a horticulturist.
- Moving into an apartment after 10 years of homelessness.
- Selling one's art at a weekly public gallery.

The procedure of training starts with a series of incremental and short-term goals leading, in this example, to a patient's overall goal of "making more friends." Weekly short-term goals were:

- "Attend a Bible class where there would be others who share my interest in religion."
- "Sign up for instruction in an activity at the local recreation center."
- "Join a local Sierra Club and go on its weekly hikes with other members."
- "Call a friend from high school with whom I've stayed in contact and invite him to join me for coffee or a movie."
- "Ask my personal support specialist if she knows anyone on her caseload whom I might enjoy getting to know."

The acronym SMART (**S**pecific, **M**eaningful, **A**ttainable, **R**ealistic, and **T**ransfer into one's real life) can be used to recall the attributes of setting goals that can be set week by week. In assisting the patient to choose interactions that are attainable short-term goals, the ACT staff can ask, "What might you be able to do this week that will be a step toward your overall goal?"; "With whom do you need to interact to achieve the goal?"; and "When and where will this interaction take place?" The active and directive teaching techniques used to teach patients how to implement and attain their weekly goals are the same as those used in social skills training as described in Chapter 5 ("Social Skills Training").

In using personal effectiveness for 35 years to empower more than 850 patients to responsibly make choices for more meaningful lives, we have noted the successful completion of an average of 67% of weekly behavioral assignments and 58% of long-term personal goals (Liberman and Kopelowicz 2002). Figure 8.5 shows the percentage of personal goals that were attained by patients from two psychosocial rehabilitation programs, one employing training in personal effectiveness and the other using more conventional supports. Even 24 months after the end of the patients' participation in the groups, personal effectiveness enabled them to achieve more of their personal goals, whereas there was an erosion of personal goals attained in the standard psychosocial rehabilitation program (Austin et al. 1976). As patients learn to chart their own journey toward recovery, they continue to depend upon the guidance and support of the clinician who is their personal support specialist; however, when patients are empowered by social skills training, their relationship is more like that of a student to a life coach than a patient to a therapist.

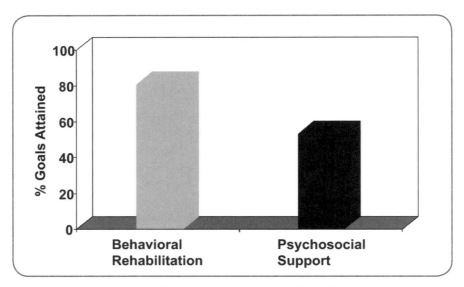

FIGURE 8.5 Goal attainment by patients in two psychosocial rehabilitation programs. *Source.* Data from Austin et al. 1976.

With regard to the relative efficacy of ACT, equally effective personal support services are achieved by other models of service that offer the full range of treatments without the specific configuration of ACT. Alternative modes of service that have achieved excellent outcomes are *intensive personal support services (case management), integrated mental health care,* and *wraparound services.* As repeatedly emphasized in earlier chapters, treatment services for the seriously mentally ill must be linked to the phase or severity of an individual's illness—symptoms, cognitive status, and psychosocial functioning; therefore, the intensity and type of case management or personal support services should vary as the individual's needs change. Intensive case management or ACT may be desirable when a person is having severe symptoms, unwilling to visit a mental health center for services, homeless, or functioning poorly in the community. However, it is entirely appropriate to make a joint decision with the patient to shift to a less costly and intensive level of support services when the individual has reached a stable phase of his/her disorder, is voluntarily adhering to medication regimens and psychosocial treatments, has insight and awareness of the need for continuing treatment, and has access to rehabilitation services.

▶ Integrated Mental Health Care

Vehicles for psychiatric treatment and rehabilitation are being redesigned to deliver services through the framework of primary care. These developments are the result of new mechanisms of financing mental health services as well as creation of closer links of organized psychiatry to the medical field as a whole. With the unsustainable, spiraling costs of health care, it is virtually certain that psychiatric services will be refocused to become more efficient and accessible through consolidation and coordination with the general health care system (Weist et al. 2001).

Specialized mental health services will continue to be needed for the seriously mentally ill, but these can be delivered within the context of primary care, multispecialty clinics, and group practices (Degruy 2006). Only a minority of psychiatrically disabled persons currently receive specialized mental health services, in part because of the inaccessibility of these services in the community, the scarcity of trained and experienced practitioners working in the public sector, and the underdiagnosis of psychiatric disorders by primary care physicians. As hospital care for all medical and psychiatric disorders continues to decline, replaced by ambulatory services, psychiatrists and allied mental health professionals will be increasingly called upon to serve in *consultant* roles in close contact and collaboration with primary care physicians and their practices. This role as consultant is not altogether different from the long-standing consultation-liaison role of psychiatrists with hospital-based physicians and medical, pediatric, and surgical teams (Regier et al. 1993).

In most developed countries of Europe, Canada, and Australia, there are many fewer psychiatrists per capita than in the United States. Accessibility of psychiatric services, including early identification and intervention for recent-onset mental disorders, is realized by close collaboration with primary care physicians and practices. Given the fact that family physicians are often the portal of entry of the mentally ill to initial contact with the health care system and provide more drug treatment to mentally ill persons than mental health specialists, a closer integration with mental health professionals is a rational direction for the future of psychiatry. Integration will also have the salutary effect of reducing stigma of mental illness, thereby reducing the time between onset of illness and initial treatment.

Surveys in European countries have documented that over 75% of family physicians are satisfied with their collaboration with psychiatric specialists, and over 90% would like even closer working relationships with mental health professionals and mobile outreach teams, as well as more education on psychiatric diagnosis and treatment (Strathdee and Williams 1984). Twenty-five percent of patients with chronic schizophrenia have their illnesses treated by primary care doctors in western European countries, Canada, and Australia (Falloon and Fadden 1993). The critical question is not whether integration with primary care medicine will rapidly increase, but rather what will be the nature and form of the integration.

MODELS FOR DELIVERY OF INTEGRATED MENTAL HEALTH CARE

Integration of mental health specialists—nurses, psychologists, and psychiatrists—into the regular, clinical staff of primary care practices has been increasing, with laudable results. Patient satisfaction is high and stigma is low. Significant numbers of patients are properly diagnosed, educated about their mental illness, and effectively treated.

Interdisciplinary treatment of the mentally ill in primary care settings is aimed at expanding high-quality, coordinated mental health and medical services to the large majority of currently unserved or ill-served mentally ill persons. This approach to integrative treatment is termed *collaborative care*. Successful models of collaborative care are characterized by having mental health professionals work in close proximity to primary care physicians and clinics to accomplish:

- Systematic care management by a nurse, social worker psychologist, or psychiatrist to assure reliable detection and diagnosis, development and coordination of a treatment plan, patient education, monitoring and close follow-up for adherence to the treatment plan, and modifications of treatment as needed.
- Consultation between a mental health care manager and the primary care physician and his/her adjunctive medical staff to assure consistency and coordination of mental health and medical services.

Collaborative care has been found to accelerate therapeutic benefits among sicker patients, extend services to ethnic minority groups, permit early intervention to forestall relapse, and improve quality of care (Halpern et al. 2004). Primary care physicians and nurses have appreciated easier access to mental health specialists, expert consultation on diagnosis and treatment options, and the continuity of caring for their patients (Felker et al. 2004).

A variety of mechanisms have been crafted to ensure the success of integrated treatment (Katon et al. 1996). For example, when psychiatric nurse practitioners use quantitative scales to measure the severity of symptoms of mood and psychotic disorders, passing on these data to the primary care physician leads to more informed decisions regarding pharmacotherapy (Katon et al. 2002). Tool kits for clinician and patient education make it possible for primary care nurses and physicians to improve compliance with evidence-based

> "As documented in the President's New Freedom Commission on Mental Health, "the mental health and medical systems are separated in many ways that inhibit effective care. Treatable mental or medical illnesses are often not detected or diagnosed properly and effective services are not provided."
>
> UNUTZER ET AL. (2006, P. 37)

treatments (Wells et al. 2000). To be sure, challenges to the collaborative care model require frequent and mutually respectful communications between the mental health and primary care teams as well as efforts to set positive yet realistic expectations for treatment outcomes with patients.

INTEGRATED MENTAL HEALTH CARE FOR AN ENTIRE COMMUNITY

England has adopted an integrated care model for mentally ill persons based on involving mental health specialists within the existing framework of primary health care. In one English county, the supports available to patients by the family, other caregivers, and general practitioners and their allied health personnel were preserved and extended by four multidisciplinary mental health teams that were integrated within the four primary care centers in the county. Crisis intervention and long-term rehabilitation were provided in the natural habitat, making full use of community resources in gaining access to employment, education, social, and recreational facilities that are provided to all of its citizens (Falloon and Fadden 1993). The design of this form of integrated mental health care is graphically shown in Figure 8.6.

The major difference between this integrated approach and ACT is the key importance of ongoing and accessible consultative services for primary care physicians from a multidisciplinary mental health team. The team is available to evaluate and offer needed specialty treatment to patients referred by the primary care physician, but the physician maintains longitudinal responsibility for the medical and psychiatric needs of his/her patients. In addition, the mental health team provides education and support for patients, family members, informal caregivers, family practitioners, nurses, and agencies in the community. Within the constraints of their abilities and disciplines, each professional person is trained to participate as a full member of the team through use of medication management, stress management, skills development, detection of early signs of relapse, supportive services, and advocacy.

The core members of the multidisciplinary treatment teams are trained in the competent delivery of diagnostic and assessment services and evidence-based treatments for the seriously mentally ill—including persons disabled by mood and anxiety disorders. All members of the team are cross-trained in these modalities to ensure consistency and continuity. For community nurses and family practitioners, the emphasis is on recognition of early stages of mental disorders and targeted pharmacotherapy. The flexible deployment of staff permitted by this model makes it possible to offer intensive rehabilitation wherever and whenever needed.

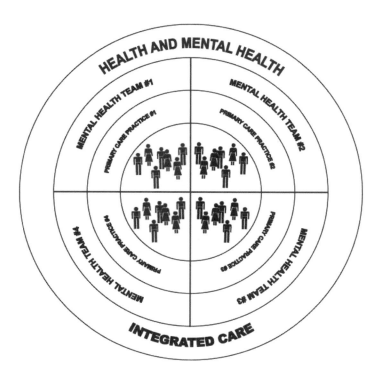

FIGURE 8.6 Design features of integrated mental health services. The distinctive mechanism is a mental health consultation and treatment team that works with primary care physicians or other frontline providers of services to make certain that the needs of the individual are met. Challenging patients beyond the expertise of the primary care physician or clinic are taken as patients by the team for direct services—at least until their disorder has stabilized. The team emphasizes training of the primary care providers so the latter can perform more and more of the services with less and less supervision, consultation, and intervention by the personal support, mental health consultation, and treatment team. The team offers indefinite, round-the-clock services to primary care providers, since new patients continuously arise who need consultation, and "veteran" patients may have relapses or complications that necessitate consultation or direct treatment by the team.

The role of family members, friends, clergy, and other informal supporters in the community is essential to the success of integrated care. Educating them to be members of the care team enables them to provide optimal support for those with mental illnesses. Patients are also accorded team membership through training in the nature and treatment of mental disorders, coping with emergent or persistent symptoms, and relapse prevention. The mission of the integrated team is to ensure that every person, no matter how severe his/her disabilities, can lead a full and satisfying life in the community.

Evaluation of integrated mental health care revealed a marked reduction of hospitalization, with an average of one bed used per 100,000 population. The number of relapses per year was a low 18% for schizophrenia and 15% for mood disorders. What may be the most impressive outcome of integrated care was a mean of 0.75 new cases of schizophrenia per 100,000 population identified in the county over a 4-year period—a 10-fold reduction from expected cases based on epidemiological surveys. An explanation of this striking example of mental health prevention may come from the program's emphasis on early case finding. With integration of the mental health specialists in family practice teams, a yearly average of 11.25 cases of individuals with prodromal symptoms of psychosis per 100,000 population were identified and effectively treated. The cost-effectiveness of this unique vehicle for delivering mental health care has been documented in an economic analysis (Falloon and Fadden 1993).

● **EXAMPLE OF BEST PRACTICE**

The Village Integrated Service Agency in Long Beach, California, blends multidisciplinary case management teams with community-based services and a clubhouse with a psychosocial recovery philosophy. Each team of seven staff members, called *personal service coordinators*, serves 92 members. Psychiatrists on the team work in close collaboration with local primary care physicians and hospitals to secure regular medical evaluations and treatments as needed. Coordinators spend approximately 60% of their time outside the clubhouse, where they accompany members to workouts at a gym, movies at the mall, dancing at a nightclub, and help them find apartments, buy and cook food, and apply for jobs. As in other rehabilitation programs, strengths are emphasized in the workplace, during community outings, and at Village meetings. Rather than a focus on formal training to build skills, the therapeutic emphasis is on "learning by doing." The Village has been empirically documented as more effective than standard mental health services, which lacked integrated services to meet the comprehensive, continuous, coordinated, and consumer-oriented needs of patients (Chandler et al. 1998).

▶ Wraparound Personal Support Services

For youths with major mental disorders, persons with head injuries, and individuals with developmental disabilities, specialized personal support services are necessary for mainstream life in the community. Their needs call for more continuous rehabilitation—more correctly, habilitation—at home, in school, or at work and in social and recreational activities. Best practices for these populations are called *wraparound* services or systems of care (Koegel et al. 1996).

A system of care for children and adolescents with disabling mental disorders comprises a coordinated network of community-based, culturally adapted, individualized services and supports. Youths and their families participate at the center of a partnership with public and private organizations to tailor services that build on youths' strengths. Agencies that are brought together to wraparound services for youths include schools, police and probation departments, courts, recreation districts, sports programs, and housing authorities. Typically, the local mental health center has a designated team that is responsible for synchronizing the comprehensive services required by each young person. These services include:

- Supported education, including special education, teaching assistants in the classroom for one-on-one tutoring to supplement the teachers' efforts, and social workers who can show parents how to encourage and reinforce their child for making academic progress at school.
- Services such as medications, individual and group therapy, and social skills training that are offered by the mental health team.
- Residential services in the home or temporary and transitional placement in supervised living.
- Liaison with police, the courts, and probation department.

Wraparound services provide planned, scheduled, supervised, and supported living; training in activities of daily living; supported education; supported employment; and recreation. The key principle for this systemic approach to habilitation is *customizing individualized services consistent with normal community environments*. The services are created, delivered, and continuously monitored and updated to ensure that the youthful patients remain afloat in the community while slowly gaining the ability to ultimately transition as young adults to independent living.

As they demonstrate self-responsibility and progress in school and home, the youths are given more autonomy and choice in their goals and services. A defining feature of a wraparound system of care is that it is unconditional; if interventions are not achieving the person's goals, the team regroups to rethink the configuration of supports, services, and interventions to ensure success. In other words, students do not fail, but plans can fail and must be rewritten. The design of wraparound services is depicted in Figure 8.7 (Jones et al. 1984).

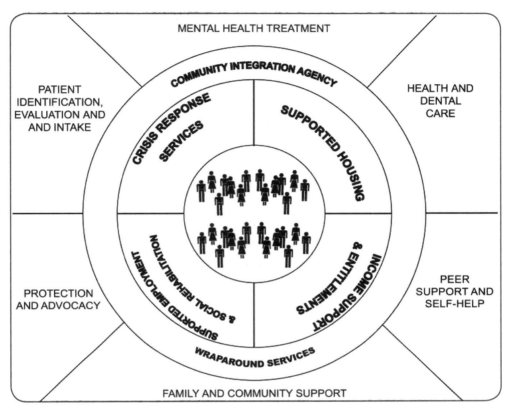

FIGURE 8.7 Design features of wraparound services. The distinctive feature of wraparound services is its locus in the patient's home or other naturalistic residence. An oversight community agency is earmarked to responsible for organizing, integrating, and delivering all needed services, which come not from a mental health consultation team, but from an array of community agencies that have the resources and expertise to deal with a spectrum of problems as they arise.

Community-based services with flexible levels of supervision and supports are provided by highly trained personnel as needed by the individual. The most severely impaired individuals can reside in a normal apartment only if they have supervision and support for up to 24 hours per day. The system of care arranges for an agency to assign live-in staff to ensure safety and supervision and to provide training in basic life and social skills. Opportunities, encouragement, and positive reinforcement are given for the youths' optimal use of those skills in their home environment. Evaluations of the past 15 years of systems of care revealed reductions in school absenteeism and dropouts, improvements in attendance and school grades, significant increases in employment for those past high school, reduced suicide attempts, fewer juvenile crimes and incarcerations, and fewer hospitalizations (Henggeler et al. 1998; Lonigan and Elbert 1998).

CLINICAL EXAMPLE

Joe was an 18-year-old high school senior when he developed a particularly malignant form of schizophrenia. While treatment stabilized his symptoms to some extent, he continued to hear voices that distracted him and interfered with his efforts to complete high school. Joe's personal goal was to be able to hold down a job and live on his own apart from his parents. He had always enjoyed horseback riding, an activity that was not adversely affected by his illness. The system of care responsible for his treatment developed a plan that enabled Joe to live at a dude ranch, where he was able to obtain remunerative work with horses, ride horses on his time off, eat with the staff, and have his own small apartment. He made friends, enjoyed his work, and obtained his GED with the assistance of a tutor. His medication needs and symptoms were evaluated and managed by a psychiatrist 500 miles away via telemedicine in conjunction with a family physician whose practice was near the dude ranch.

▶ Psychosocial Clubhouse

The psychosocial clubhouse provides opportunities for persons with mental illness to join together in a community of friends, called *members,* where decisions regarding social, vocational, housing, and other activities are made through mutual consent. A substantial proportion of members have concurrent substance abuse, and some have developmental disabilities. Referrals come from a variety of sources, including psychiatric inpatient facilities, homeless shelters, mental health centers, family members, and current members. Members are assisted by staff to articulate their own personal goals for community living, in the areas of work, recreation, social relations, and housing. The principal means by which members achieve their personal goals is by taking responsibility for running the various functions of the clubhouse society, including food services, clerical projects, janitorial work, recreational activities, and transitional employment. The self-help ideology is promoted by inviting members to participate in decision-making regarding the operations and ventures of the clubhouse organization, in fundraising, and as paid consumer-workers and aides (Hughes and Weinstein 2000).

Most clubhouses operate through peer support, with staff members serving as supervisors, facilitators, and administrators. Participatory democracy is encouraged through frequent community-wide meetings, positive and public praise for members' accomplishments, and a conscious effort to blur status barriers between those employed by the clubhouse as staff and the members who have mental illness. While each clubhouse hopes to motivate members to attend program activities through its upbeat and positive milieu, there is a modicum of group pressure for members to make voluntary choices.

The clubhouse model was intentionally conceived as a therapeutic community of persons with serious and disabling mental illness. Staff members were chosen for their personal qualities and informal ways of interacting with members to reduce stigma and hierarchical relationships. As the clubhouse approach has become more mainstream, its constituents around the country have become incorporated as nonprofit agencies with contracts from local mental health authorities. To qualify for funding, they have had to standardize and structure their intake, goal setting, treatment planning, and program evaluation. Most clubhouses now offer outreach and crisis intervention and employ psychiatrists to make diagnoses and prescribe psychotropic medications. Clubhouses are also incorporating evidence-based treatments developed by scientist-practitioners—supported employment, social skills training, and ACT. These trends are a positive move toward reciprocity with traditional psychiatric services that have begun to adopt the peer-support, self-help, and recovery ideology of clubhouses (Hughes and Weinstein 2000).

● EXAMPLE OF BEST PRACTICE

Thresholds is an exemplary clubhouse in Chicago offering recreational and social activities, housing, and vocational services to more than 2,600 members with serious mental illness each year. Most members have multiple previous hospitalizations, concurrent substance abuse, and psychotic disorders. Thresholds operates several clubhouses and 37 residences for 664 members, including group homes and apartments. More than 800 of the members work for pay in 1,172 job placements with 319 different employers, including 265 members who worked for Thresholds either in a sheltered clubhouse job or in one of the enterprises run by Thresholds. Rehospitalization of members stands around 20% per year (Dincin and Witheridge 1982). Discontinuation of medication is the most frequent cause of relapse and rehospitalization.

▶ Teamwork in Service Delivery

Mental health services are delivered by multidisciplinary teams that vary in composition and organization, work in a wide variety of settings, have divergent ideologies and missions, and use many different procedures. But the quality and impact of all teams are influenced by the same set of factors: staff competencies, cohesion, leadership, organizational communication, and interaction. Optimal integration and delivery of the full spectrum of services depend upon the blend of professional competencies of the team members and how the team goes about using these competencies. If systems of support services are the vehicles for treatment and rehabilitation, then teamwork is the vehicle's engine.

> "Teamwork permits common people to produce uncommon results"

Several characteristics of a multidisciplinary group of clinicians facilitate teamwork. First, effective teams must bring together people who possess the requisite expertise in diagnosis, psychopharmacology, functional assessment, treatment planning and evaluation, social skills training, family psychoeducation, supported employment, crisis intervention, and cognitive-behavioral therapy. Second, teams integrate the various areas of expertise at the level of service delivery. Methods for reliable and frequent intercommunication among clinicians are crucial for bringing the appropriate interventions into play at the proper time. To ensure high-quality interdisciplinary teamwork, it is useful for mental health teams to conduct their own self-evaluation of how they interact and collaborate. A sample from a self-assessment scale for multidisciplinary teamwork is shown in Table 8.3 (Fichtner et al. 2001).

Third, mechanisms for accountability in achieving favorable outcomes for patients must be established; for example, recognition and remuneration of staff members for their performance and quality of care, not for the hours they work or units of service provided. Finally, cultivating versatility among team members facilitates their delivery of flexible levels of intervention to meet the individualized and changing needs of patients. While responsibility for making clinical decisions is decentralized to team members, authority and accountability belong to the team leader for the team's organizational structure, scheduling of clinical assignments, ensuring cohesion, and conducting performance evaluations. Only when teams are freed from fossilized administrative policies will they be able to survive and thrive in an era of flux and challenges in the financing and delivery of services and priorities to clinical populations.

As the celebrated baseball coach Casey Stengel once said, "It's easy to get good players. Getting them to play together is the hard part." The concept of multidisciplinary teamwork is a vision in search of practical tools. Teamwork requires efficient modes of communication about patients' goals, progress, and problems; mechanisms for team members to discuss their concerns and differences of opinion regarding patient care; sharing of expertise; making and implementing decisions; and exchange of information with other providers and community agencies.

In the hubbub of busy clinical work and crises to manage, multidisciplinary teams often ignore the critical importance of active outreach to family members and nonprofessional staff who serve the residential needs of their patients. Failure to include these key reciprocal avenues of communication inevitably multiplies relapses and behavioral emergencies that cast a crisis mode over the functioning of the team. It is the responsibility of the team

---

● **TABLE 8.3**

Examples of items from a scale used by clinicians on multidisciplinary teams for self-assessment of team functioning

The team

» Members actively participated in the treatment-planning process, sharing ideas and suggestions.
» Considered motivating patients by identifying personally relevant goals of patients that were linked to the elements in the treatment plan.
» Considered cultural, ethnic, age, and gender issues in patient education and treatment planning.
» Represented various disciplines and contributed ideas and points of view that drew from their scope of practice, training, and experience.

The psychiatrist

» Elicited information from all members of the treatment team, synthesizing contributions for treatment planning.
» Explained diagnostic formulations and relevant pharmacotherapy to nonmedical members of the treatment team.
» Educated team members about medications, including their role in the biopsychosocial factors that influence patients' problems and facilitate therapeutic progress.
» Encouraged involvement of family members and other persons involved in the patient's natural support network.

The treatment plan team members

» Actively participated in eliciting assessment information from all those who know the patient—incorporating views of the various members of the team.
» Contributed ideas and points of view that are drawn from their respective disciplines' scope of practice, training and experience.
» Included the patient's problems, priorities, goals, needs, resources, strengths, and deficits in the treatment plan.
» Specified measurable and behaviorally defined goals that were regularly monitored with summaries and feedback to all members of the treatment team.

leader to convey priority to team members for their opening channels of interaction with families and residential care workers. Another principle for effective teamwork that requires visible and repeated leadership is "catching patients doing well." While accentuating the positive for patients' recovery can be done during scheduled contacts, going the extra mile with spontaneous phone calls can shift the focus of the team from problems and pathology to acknowledging patients' taking responsibility for themselves and enjoying their community participation. Ignoring this norm places the team in peril of picking up the pieces of patients' relapses and behavioral regressions.

NURTURING OF TEAMS BY ENLIGHTENED ADMINISTRATIVE LEADERSHIP

Even multidisciplinary teams with high levels of cohesion, motivation, and competencies will have their efforts undermined if functional and effective leadership is not forthcoming from the agency's top and middle managers and supervisors. To start with, it is vital for agency leadership to clearly articulate rehabilitation as its mission. Next, allocation of needed resources for evidence-based rehabilitation services puts the agency's "money where its mouth is" and conveys to clinicians that the agency is serious about rehabilitation for recovery. In addition to verbal and material support for rehabilitation, leadership at all levels needs personal and organizational skills. Action-oriented leadership "trickles down" to the members of the team, improving the team's functioning and the clinical impact of its efforts.

Leadership from the chief executive down to middle management can amplify the effectiveness of teams by insisting that clinicians give priority to the direct provision of services rather than time-consuming administrative activities such as attendance at lengthy staff meetings, pro forma charting, continuing education, and reports. When leaders emphasize clinical work, professional time and resources can be devoted to meeting the needs of patients. In addition, directors of mental health and other human service agencies must provide visible and vocal support to the enterprise of serving the most disabled clients. Endorsement of high-quality services involves more than announcements in agency newsletters or policies transmitted by email. "Managing by walking around" allows leaders to have personal contact with line-level clinicians and patients alike. Face-to-face encouragement of clinicians' efforts to meet new clinical demands and attain treatment goals reinforces their accomplishments.

CLINICAL LEADERSHIP OF MULTIDISCIPLINARY TEAMS

A capable and respected team leader is essential for personal support services of good quality. Teamwork may be best described as the functional collaboration, task clarification, communication, reciprocity, interdependence, and coordination through which teams successfully carry out their complex mission. On many multidisciplinary teams, role boundaries are blurred. This causes ambiguity in who is responsible for what, with whom, where, and when. The team leader is responsible for defining the distinct or overlapping roles for each of the team members. Leaders ensure that teamwork is fueled by collaboration, communication, reciprocity, interdependence, and coordination. Hierarchies for accountability are retained, but team leaders possess emotional intelligence that enables them to appreciate and work effectively with the relational aspects of getting the clinical work done.

Effective team leaders are good problem-solvers, but more importantly, they empower their team members—individually or in small groups—to solve problems facing the team. Capable leaders recognize the assets and limitations of each team member and play to people's strengths rather than insisting that everyone do the same thing and function interchangeably. Whether leaders are giving performance-enhancing feedback or listening carefully to worries, concerns, and annoyances, *communication skills* are the linchpin for success in mentoring, coaching, problem solving, and team building. Leaders do not have the loudest voice, but they have the readiest ear. Administrators manage programs, but team leaders empower people.

ROLE OF THE PSYCHIATRIST ON THE MULTIDISCIPLINARY TEAM

Because serious mental disorders are biomedical conditions that require accurate diagnosis, medicolegal decisions, pharmacological treatments, and documentation of services, the role of the psychiatrist is of special importance for a mental health team. Despite organized psychiatry's assertions of its unique value to multidisciplinary teams, this discipline has been marginalized and largely confined to conducting diagnostic evaluations and medication management sessions in most systems of care for the seriously mentally ill.

The lack of full participation and leadership by psychiatrists on treatment and rehabilitation teams has come about partly by default. One reason for the limited role of psychiatrists derives from the unattractiveness of careers in the public sector for psychiatrists. A vicious cycle has been established, since the enormous caseloads carried by the relatively few psychiatrists in any system of care further tarnish working conditions in the public sector and reduce the appeal of such work.

Another factor curbing leadership by psychiatrists stems from their training in academic hospitals and clinics, where they have only time-limited contacts with the seriously mentally ill. Treating patients during brief hospitalizations for acute relapses or for 15–20 minutes in outpatient medication management provides little opportunity to follow such patients over the long term, a prerequisite for appreciating their gradual improvement and recovery. These fleeting encounters, in which psychiatric resident and patient are like two ships passing in the night, deny residents important learning experiences for developing, maintaining, and enjoying supportive therapeutic relationships with the mentally disabled (Diamond et al. 1991).

Compounding the challenges of gaining personal satisfaction from getting to know the *person* behind the diagnosis and symptoms is the social distance between highly educated psychiatrists and a patient population that is often impoverished, inarticulate, and emotionally withdrawn. The emphasis on scientific medicine in educational venues, propelled by the sponsorship of pharmaceutical companies, gives short shrift to listening with care to a patient's human narrative. A psychiatric marketplace denoting *providers, consumers,* and *units of service* constrains patient–doctor communication, which is time-consuming but indispensable to the act of healing.

During their training, psychiatrists rarely learn skills for leading multidisciplinary teams. Nor do they get training in behavioral learning principles and psychosocial treatments that carry clinical relevance for patients receiving treatment and rehabilitation in the public mental health sector. Because psychiatrists are steeped in the authoritative functions of diagnosis, psychopathology, and psychopharmacology, they lack a recovery orientation, with its values and experience of collaborating with patients in setting personally relevant goals and selecting treatments to reach those goals. With their medical training, they focus on symptoms and sickness, not on functional abilities and recovery (Liberman et al. 2001).

Psychiatrists who work with persons with severe mental illness and who wish to contribute as key members or leaders of their teams must go beyond their prescription pads to acquire knowledge, attitudes, and skills congruent with contemporary practice guidelines for psychiatric rehabilitation (Kopelowicz and Liberman 2003).

BUILDING TEAMWORK THROUGH INTERACTIVE MENTORING AND PARTICIPATORY PLANNING

Effective teamwork is not taught in postgraduate training programs for mental health professionals, nor does it ordinarily flow from the natural personality attributes of individuals who choose to work on multidisciplinary teams. While outstanding team leaders with enthusiasm and a firm grasp on participatory problem solving can often build strong teams, educational and organizational strategies are needed by team members if their patients are to gain empowerment, self-responsibility, and illness self-management en route to recovery.

Training programs are designed to increase the knowledge and skills of team members, while organizational strategies foster administrative support, group cohesion, and decision making. But there is no point in strengthening teamwork and its support from policy makers, administrators, and supervisors without at the same time introducing evidence-based services that will improve clinical outcomes. Consultation and training must have as their goals increasing the efficacy of a team with its clientele. Thus, training and consultation from outside experts should be planned to have measurable effects on both the quality of treatment services and the morale and communication processes among team members. Good team *process* and *morale* is meaningless unless the team can also produce salutary clinical *outcomes*.

EDUCATIONAL TECHNIQUES

Once clinical staff, team leaders, administrators, and other stakeholders identify and agree on educational objectives and "buy into" a plan of action, the actual training phase can proceed. Bringing about change in the competencies of team members for improved clinical outcomes requires learning new treatment techniques. What is the best strategy to teach line-level staff how to competently deliver evidence-based services? Two guiding lights for optimal staff training are to 1) conduct the training in vivo in the clinical locales where the staff will be working with their patients and 2) use active-directive training techniques that yield *experiential learning*. Strategies for meeting the educational challenges facing consultant-trainers and clinical teams are listed in Table 8.4. The same continuing education approaches are relevant for all types and locations of treatment teams.

▌ Summary

Systems of care are *vehicles* for delivering services. Practitioners who provide services to persons with serious and disabling mental illnesses should not expect their patients and their social network to come to an office, clinic, mental health center, or psychosocial program. Given the nature of neuro-cognitive dysfunctions, social disabilities, and psychopathology associated with these disorders, practitioners increase the accessibility of their services by reaching out to their patients. This can be done by a variety of means—by home visits, community outreach, and agency-sponsored transportation, as well as through more technological modes of phone calls, e-mail, and tele-psychiatry.

● TABLE 8.4

Principles for training and consultation to strengthen multidisciplinary teamwork

- Obtain verbal and face-to-face mandates for change from top management. Mandates may involve changes in scheduling of staff and programs, changes in locations where services are offered, additional staffing, additional resources such as video equipment and computers, and incentives for patients' progress (Only tangible support from management will provide opportunities, encouragement, and reinforcement for desired improvements in the functioning of staff.)

- Use motivational interviewing to bring as many clinicians "on board" as possible with an understanding and support for the value of the changes to be made. (Why should staff make changes in their customary way of delivering services?)

- Identify advocates or "champions" for change who are eager and enthusiastic influential peers for spearheading participation in training and in becoming a "trainer of trainers." (Personal influence is the primary mediator of change in professional behavior.)

- Conduct training in the very clinical settings where the new treatment techniques will be used and with the very patient populations who are going to benefit from the techniques. (Credibility of trainers depends on demonstration of new treatment techniques with the patients at the host agency.)

- Require that consultants demonstrate the skills with real patients or in role-plays with staff taking the part of real clients. Credibility of training and of the techniques being trained is enhanced by showing how the methods can work with those patients whom the team or facility must serve. (Do as I say and do as I do.)

- Highlight how the new techniques have some similarity and derive from the same basic assumptions and ideology of techniques used by the team in the past. (Familiarity breeds acceptance for learning new methods.)

- Develop and offer "user-friendly" treatment techniques that do not require off-site training and education but, rather, can be provided by nonprofessionals as well as professionals. Not all staff have the personal or professional qualities to learn the innovative techniques. (Team members are always doing the best they can, so encourage staff members to do what they do best—accentuate the positive and de-emphasize the negative.)

- Build in competency or performance standards so supervisors, leaders, and managers can evaluate staff in their use of innovative and evidence-based methods and give positive and corrective feedback on a regular basis. (There's no point in investing in staff training unless the staff will be held responsible for using the know-how and skills that are taught.)

- Encourage and develop collegial support, peer learning, staff ideology, and strong leadership so that as clinical line staff begin to utilize innovations, continuation and growing competence will ensue.

- Encourage program implementation as a learning process with periodic reviews of staff competencies and client progress in using the new treatment program. As implementa-

(continued)

● TABLE 8.4 *(cont'd.)*

tion ensues, corrective feedback based on evaluation criteria and team meetings can further strengthen the team cohesion as well as the efficacy in using the new procedures. (Learning new knowledge and skills for a team is not just a means to an end but also an end itself.)

- Offer positive feedback and more formal recognition for the efforts of the team. Program maintenance requires considerable positive reinforcement from the team leader and top management. Recognition for the efficacy of new programs and services can vary from "clinician of the week" awards to descriptions of the program in an agency, department, or team newsletter. Periodic visits by the consultant-trainer are essential for program maintenance. (Consultants observe staff in action and provide encouragement and reinforcement for their improved functioning.)

However, only lip service will be delivered unless the system is capable and accountable for providing services in a flexible manner that is congruent with the type and phase of each person's disorder. Depending upon the person's functional and symptomatic status, practitioners on treatment and rehabilitation teams will vary the *comprehensiveness, specific biobehavioral modalities,* and *frequency* of service delivery. There are many different ways to organize and deliver comprehensive, coordinated, continuous, competent, and compassionate services:

- Personal support specialists, who coordinate and follow up on services they provide with collaborating professionals, other agencies, and the patient's natural support network
- Assertive community treatment
- Psychosocial clubhouse
- Integrated mental health care and related wraparound services

Establishing and sustaining teamwork in the provision of comprehensive and continuous services to seriously mentally disabled persons is arduous, with burnout of clinicians frequently occurring. Enthusiasm is essential for working with the mentally disabled and offering them evidence-based services. A passion for providing personal support services can be revived and sustained by consultation from external experts, initial and ongoing staff training, and staff retreats.

Collaborating with other mental health professionals in teamwork is not for the faint at heart. It requires a dual set of personal traits and professional competencies to engage in 1) good-quality communication, problem solving, coordination, and clinical decision making in conjunction with fellow clinicians; and 2) continuous, flexible, and evidence-based services that yield outcomes for improving patients' quality of life. Perhaps one of the most important attributes of effective practitioners and teams is *persistence*. There are few qualities so essential to success as the persistence demonstrated by clinicians who, among themselves, divide the work with the mentally disabled without letting patients fall through the cracks. Delivering recovery-oriented rehabilitation does not come quickly but is more likely when a mental health team hangs on after disappointments and frank failures. Effort only releases its rewards to the mentally disabled when practitioners refuse to quit.

▌ Key Points

- Specific modalities of rehabilitation—illness management, functional assessment, skills training, family services, and vocational rehabilitation—are delivered to patients and their families through a variety of clinical vehicles with different forms of organization, ideology, locus, and function.

- Clinical vehicles for rehabilitation include multidisciplinary treatment teams situated in community mental health centers, assertive community treatment teams that deliver services in vivo in the community settings where the patients spend their time, and psychosocial clubhouses that emphasize social, recreational, and vocational services.

- Integrated mental health programs represent innovations in service delivery. These offer comprehensive services, including supported housing and employment, within a specific facility via wraparound services in the community and through consultation-liaison with primary care providers and clinics.

- All vehicles for service delivery depend on multidisciplinary teamwork for their effectiveness. Teamwork is promoted by visible and tangible support for teams by middle and top administration, collaborative and assertive clinical leadership at the team level, integration of psychiatrists with the team's full range of clinical services, and practitioners who possess competencies to provide evidence-based services.

▶ Selected Readings

Bedell JR, Cohen NL, Sullivan A: Case management: the current best practices and the next generation of innovation. Community Ment Health J 36:179–194, 2000

Bond GR, Salyers MP: Prediction of outcome from the Dartmouth assertive community treatment fidelity scale. CNS Spectr 9:937–942, 2004

Bond GR, Drake RE, Mueser KT, et al: Assertive community treatment for the severely mentally ill. Disease Management for Health Outcomes 9:141–159, 2001

Burchard JD, Bruns EJ, Burchard SN: The wraparound approach, in Community Treatment for Youth: Evidence-Based Services for Severe Emotional and Behavioral Disorders. Edited by Burns B, Hoagwood K. New York, Oxford University Press, 2002, pp 357–392

Burns T: Community Mental Health Teams: A Guide to Current Practice. New York, Oxford University Press, 2004

Burns T, Firn M: Assertive Outreach in Mental Health: A Manual for Practitioners. New York, Oxford University Press, 2002

Carling PJ: Return to the Community: Building Support Systems for People With Psychiatric Disabilities. New York, Guilford, 1995

Corrigan PW, Liberman RP (eds): Behavior Therapy in Psychiatric Hospitals. New York, Springer, 1994

Corrigan PW, McCracken SG: Interactive Staff Training: Rehabilitation Teams That Work. New York, Plenum, 1997

Corrigan PW, McCracken SG: Training teams to deliver better psychiatric rehabilitation programs. Psychiatr Serv 50:43–45, 1999

Drake RE, Goldman HH, Leff HS, et al: Implementing evidence-based practice in routine mental health service settings. Psychiatr Serv 52:172–182, 2001

Falloon IRH, Fadden G: Integrated Mental Health Care: A Comprehensive Community-Based Approach. Cambridge, England, Cambridge University Press, 1993

Fichtner CG, Hardy D, Patel M, et al: A self-assessment program for multidisciplinary mental health teams. Psychiatr Serv 52:1352–1357, 2001

Gorey KM, Leslie DR, Morris T, et al: Effectiveness of case management with severely and persistently mentally ill people. Community Ment Health J 34:241–250, 1998

Liberman RP, Kopelowicz A: Teaching persons with severe mental disabilities to be their own case managers. Psychiatr Serv 53:1377–1379, 2002

Meredith LS, Mendel P, Pearson M, et al: Implementation and maintenance of quality improvement for treating depression in primary care. Psychiatr Serv 57:48–55, 2006

Mueser KT, Bond GR, Drake RE, et al: Models of community care for severe mental illness. Schizophr Bull 24:37–74, 1998

Pearce CL, Conger JA (eds): Shared Leadership: Reframing the Hows and Whys of Leadership. Thousand Oaks, CA, Sage, 2003

Phillips SD, Burns BJ, Edgar ER, et al: Moving assertive community treatment into standard practice. Psychiatr Serv 52:771–779, 2001

Rapp CA: The active ingredients of effective case management: a research synthesis. Community Ment Health J 34:363–380, 1998

Salyers MP, Masterton TW, Fekete DM, et al: Transferring clients from intensive case management: impact on client functioning. Am J Orthopsychiatry 68:233–245, 1998

Shepherd M, Strathdee G, Falloon IRH, et al: The management of psychiatric disorders in the community. J R Soc Med 83:219–228, 1990

Stein LI, Santos AB: Assertive Community Treatment of Persons With Severe Mental Illness. New York, WW Norton, 1998

Surber RW: Clinical Case Management: A Guide to Comprehensive Treatment of Serious Mental Illness. Thousand Oaks, CA, Sage Publications, 1994

Test MA: Training in community living, in Handbook of Psychiatric Rehabilitation. Edited by Liberman RP. Heights Needham, MA, Allyn & Bacon, 1992, pp 153–170

Unutzer J, Schoenbaum M, Druss BG, et al: Transforming mental health care at the interface with general medicine. Psychiatr Serv 57:37–47, 2006

Van Veldhuizen JR: FACT: a Dutch version of ACT. Community Ment Health J 43:421–433, 2007

Ziguras SJ, Stuart GW: A meta-analysis of the effectiveness of mental health case management over 20 years. Psychiatr Serv 51:1410–1421, 2000

▌ References

Austin N, Liberman RP, King LW, et al: A comparative evaluation of two day hospitals: goal attainment scaling of behavior therapy vs milieu therapy. J Nerv Ment Dis 163:253–262, 1976

Bond GR, Salyers MP: Prediction of outcome from the Dartmouthassertive community treatment fidelity scale. CNS Spectr 9:937–942, 2004

Chandler D, Meisel J, Hu T, et al: A capitated model for a cross-section of severely mentally ill clients. Community Ment Health J 34:13–26, 1998

Degruy FV: A note on the partnership between psychiatry and primary care. Am J Psychiatry 163:1487–1489, 2006

Diamond RJ, Stein LI, Susser E: Essential and nonessential roles for psychiatrists in community mental health centers. Hosp Community Psychiatry 42:187–189, 1991

Dincin J, Witheridge TF: Psychosocial rehabilitation as a deterrent to recidivism. Hosp Community Psychiatry 33:645–650, 1982

Falloon IRH, Fadden G: Integrated Mental Health Care: A Comprehensive Community-Based Approach. Cambridge, UK, Cambridge University Press, 1993

Fichtner CG, Hardy D, Patel M, et al: A self-assessment program for multidisciplinary mental health teams. Psychiatr Serv 52:1352–1357, 2001

Halpern J, Johnson MD, Miranda J, et al: The partners in care approach to ethics outcomes in quality improvement programs for depression. Psychiatr Serv 55:532–539,
2004

Henggeler SW, Schoenwald SK, Borduin CM, et al: Multisystemic Treatment of
Antisocial Behavior in Children and Adolescents. New York, Guilford, 1998

Hughes R, Weinstein D: Best Practices in Psychosocial Rehabilitation. Columbia,
MD, International Association of Psychosocial Rehabilitation Services, 2000

Jones ML, Hannah JK, Fawcett SB, et al: The independent living movement: a
model for community integration of persons with disabilities, in Programming
Effective Human Services. Edited by Christian WP, Hannah GT, Glahn TJ. New
York, Plenum, 1984, pp 315–336

Katon W, Robinson P, Von Korff M, et al: A multifaceted intervention to improve
treatment of depression in primary care. Arch Gen Psychiatry 53:924–932, 1996

Katon W, Russon J, Von Korff M, et al: Long-term effects of a collaborative care
intervention in persistently depressed primary care patients. J Gen Intern Med
17:741–748, 2002

Koegel LK, Koegel RL, Dunlap G (eds): Positive Behavioral Support, Including People
With Difficult Behavior in the Community. Baltimore, MD, Paul H Brookes,
1996

Kopelowicz A, Liberman RP: Integrating treatment with rehabilitation for persons
with major mental illnesses. Psychiatr Serv 54:1491–1498, 2003

Liberman RP, Kopelowicz A: Teaching persons with severe mental disabilities to be
their own case managers. Psychiatr Serv 53:1377–1379, 2002

Liberman RP, Hilty DM, Drake RE, et al: Requirements for multidisciplinary teamwork in psychiatric rehabilitation. Psychiatr Serv 52:1331–1342, 2001

Lonigan CJ, Elbert JC (eds): Special issue on empirically supported psychosocial
interventions for children. J Clin Child Psychol 27:138–226, 1998

Mueser KT, Bond GR: Psychosocial treatment approaches for schizophrenia. Curr
Opin Psychiatry 13:27–35, 2000

Mueser KT, Bond GR, Drake RE, et al: Models of community care for severe mental
illness. Schizophr Bull 24:37–74, 1998

Regier DA, Narrow WE, Rae DS, et al: The de-facto US mental health and addictive
disorders service system. Arch Gen Psychiatry 50:85–94, 1993

Salyers MP, Masterton TW, Fekete DM, et al: Transferring clients from intensive
case management: impact on client functioning. Am J Orthopsychiatry 68:233–
245, 1998

Stein LI, Santos AB: Assertive Community Treatment of Persons With Severe Mental Illness. New York, WW Norton, 1998

Strathdee G, Williams P: A survey of psychiatrists in primary care. J R Coll Gen
Pract 34:615–618, 1984

Test MA: Training in community living, in Handbook of Psychiatric Rehabilitation. Edited by Liberman RP. Needham Heights, MA, Allyn & Bacon, 1992, pp
153–170

Unutzer J, Schoenbaum M, Druss BG, et al: Transforming mental health care at the interface with general medicine. Psychiatr Serv 57:37–47, 2006

Van Veldhuizen JR: FACT: a Dutch version of ACT. Community Ment Health J 43:421–433, 2007

Weist MD, Lowie JA, Flaherty LT, et al: Collaboration among the education, mental health, and public health systems to promote youth mental health. Psychiatr Serv 52:1348–1351, 2001

Wells KB, Sherbourne CD, Schoenbaum M, et al: Impact of disseminating quality improvement programs for depression in managed primary care: a randomized controlled trial. JAMA 283:212–220, 2000

CHAPTER 9

Special Services for Special People

Special Services for Special People

If a man does not keep pace with his companions, perhaps it is because he hears a different drummer. Let him step to the music which he hears, however measured or far away.

R ECOVERY FROM severe mental illness is difficult to attain unless treatment and rehabilitation are individualized according to the unique needs of each patient. Especially challenging is meshing rehabilitation to the circumstances of special populations that differ from the more common mix of patients seen in customary treatment settings. In this chapter, we describe the services that are specially designed for patients whose characteristics set them apart from conventional groups. The special types of patients are:

- Patients from cultural and ethnic minorities.
- Dually diagnosed patients.
- Patients with treatment-refractory illness.
- Mentally ill offenders and patients with aggressive behavior.
- Older adults.

What makes these types of patients deserving of a separate chapter with a special focus? The kinds of patients we have selected for special attention have unusual problems that do not respond to customary treatments. Services that are helpful to them have been designed with particular features to meet their distinct needs. Practitioners who wish to serve effectively the needs of each group must have distinctive training, competencies, and experience. Finally, most of these categories of patients are located in unusual places that require clinicians to move out of the mainstream to serve them. "Different strokes for different folks" applies to the special needs of these special groups of patients.

A recurring theme heard from recovered individuals is the critical importance of their having encountered a practitioner who really made a difference for them. "Making a difference" for persons with unique cultures, age, gender, clinical characteristics, circumstances, and daily life experiences requires an informed, sensitive, empathic, and nonjudgmental connection between clinician and patient. Making that kind of special connection is not a simple matter, but we hope that its dimensions will be better understood by the time you complete this chapter.

▶ Rehabilitation of Persons of Diverse Cultural and Ethnic Backgrounds

CULTURAL AND ETHNIC DIVERSITY

The United States has always been identified by its dynamically changing culture, values, norms, and inventiveness. Assimilation is not a process of obscuring or eliminating the divergent cultures that have poured onto our shores, boundaries, and airports, but rather a confluence and synthesis from our long history of diversity. In the first decade of the twenty-first century, over 10% of the American population is foreign born, a proportion unequaled since the eighteenth century. A 2001 report of the Surgeon General of the United States, "Mental Health: Culture, Race, and Ethnicity," documented the disproportionately high burden of disability from mental illness among African Americans, Native Americans, Asian Americans and Pacific Islanders, and Hispanic Americans or Latinos (U.S. Surgeon General 2001). The higher burden stems from minorities having less access to care and having poorer-quality care than white Americans, rather than from their illnesses being inherently more severe or prevalent. Cultural differences between providers and patients also create barriers to treatment.

Cultural competence has become a defining feature of the ethos of mental health services. Stakeholders and policy makers have required mental health agencies to have practitioners on their staff who share the cultural and language backgrounds of minorities and offer them more hospitable accessibility. Rehabilitation must be adapted for many cultural and ethnic groups, but here we will draw from our experiences in California with Latinos, now the largest minority group in the United States.

LATINO CULTURE

At the outset, we must disabuse ourselves of the stereotypes that all Latinos have similar customs, attitudes, values, habits, and life views. There are as many different cultural patterns as there are Latinos from differing national origins: Mexicans, Dominicans, Puerto Ricans, Central Americans, South Americans, and Cubans. Even within a nationality, there are important differences between subgroups that must be taken into consideration when developing and implementing rehabilitation plans. For example, among recent Mexican immigrants, those from Yucatán are known to be very stoic, mild, pleasant, and able to handle pain, while those from Michoacán have a reputation of being very assertive and tough. Natives of Chiapas defend their rights and will never let the "White Mexicans" conquer them. Assimilated second- and third-generation Latinos are usually more similar to mainstream "Anglos" than to unacculturated Latinos. Many of these individuals are so integrated into the American culture that they no longer speak or understand Spanish.

Culture aside, practitioners should realize that individual differences within any one culture trump culture as a factor in conducting assessments, prescribing treatment, and evaluating progress. Patients from the same culture with different mental disorders or different personality traits should not have their treatment blurred or homogenized because they share the same culture and language. Latinos seeking mental health services are very different from one another in terms of their personal goals in life, family backgrounds, intellectual and cognitive capacities, and response to treatment. The basic principle of individualizing treatment must not be obscured by stereotypes or superficial characteristics such as skin color, language, or national origin. Some cultural features that need to be taken into consideration when evaluating and treating Latinos are listed in Table 9.1.

In adapting treatment programs from the mainstream, Anglo culture for use by Latinos with mental illness, attention needs to be paid to the nuances of language. For example, when the modules for training social and independent skills developed at the UCLA Psychiatric Rehabilitation Program were translated into Spanish, care was taken to select bilingual, indigenous mental health workers as participants on the translation team (Kopelowicz 1998). These indigenous editors were identified with different Latino nationalities. This enabled the translations to be congruent with the idioms of multiple cultures beyond the accuracy of their linguistic vernacular. The cultural adaptations that were made included using Spanish vocabulary at the elementary school level, considering the wide range of dialects and colloquialisms used by a variety of Latino subgroups, and forging a "universal Spanish" that would be comprehensible to all.

During implementation of the skills training modules, cultural considerations were incorporated into the training process. To allow for more spontaneity, clinicians, all of whom were indigenous and bilingual Latinos, began sessions by engaging in *plática,* or small talk. Also, group leaders

● **TABLE 9.1**

Features of Latino culture that are relevant to planning treatment and rehabilitation

FEATURE	DEFINITION
Nervios versus *locura*	*Nervios* refers to a general state of vulnerability to stress and to a syndrome brought on by adverse life events: trembling, crying, irritability, discomfort in the chest or head. *Locura* is a pejorative term for "crazy" and should not be used as a descriptor of a mental disorder.
Curanderismo	Use of traditional folk healers who attempt to restore emotional and physical balance by prayer, pledges to religious and supernatural forces, and rituals involving candles, artifacts, and herbal baths. *Curanderos* are often viewed as being chosen by God for their ability.
Independencia	In traditional Latino families, persons with disabilities do not have to work with the sole aim of making money to be valued by family and society. Physically and mentally disabled persons contribute to their family and community through a broad range of activities, such as cooking and cleaning, providing child care, giving time and attention to the needs of others, massaging another person, helping neighbors, and keeping others company when family members are working.
Machismo	*Machismo* has a positive connotation for the male as the provider for the family who is responsible for the welfare and honor of his family. Machismo also refers to the male's being sensitive and romantic with a keen sense of his own dignity. On the other hand, *machismo* describes the superiority of the male solely on the basis of gender—having power over women, not expected to share in domestic responsibilities, and expected to be sexually aggressive, strong, authoritarian, brave, and independent.
Marianismo	Women are viewed as spiritually superior to men and therefore capable of enduring all sufferings inflicted by men and adverse life events. The term *marianismo* implies the devotion women have to home and family. When women become mothers, they gain much more respect and hold a great deal of power despite being outwardly submissive.

engaged in appropriate self-disclosure to a) achieve *personalismo,* or a more personally related relationship with patients, and b) model appropriate ways to share problems and concerns that patients could learn and use when describing and applying newly learned skills in their everyday life.

Perhaps the most significant value of Latino cultures is *familismo*—family unity, well-being, and honor. More than 80% of Latinos with schizophrenia in the United States live with their families—a percentage almost twice that of Caucasians and African Americans. The emphasis is on the family group, not the individual as in mainstream culture, and on family commitment, obligation, and responsibility. Most Latino cultures have a deep sense of family loyalty, are reliant on extended family and social support networks, and emphasize mutual respect among family members. Family also provide a sense of community. Latino families tend to live near relatives and close friends, have frequent interactions, and exchange a wide range of goods and services that include child care, housing, food, and furniture.

It is with peril that mental health practitioners fail to recognize that in Latino cultures, *family comes first.* In a controlled clinical trial of family therapy for Latino patients with schizophrenia, substantial improvements and protection against relapse were found by providing the treatment in the home, where all relatives could participate.

TEACHING DISEASE MANAGEMENT TO LATINOS WITH SCHIZOPHRENIA: INVOLVING THE FAMILY

While all patients with serious mental disorders should have key family members involved in their treatment, such involvement is even more important in cultures where family contact and cohesiveness are lifelong and highly valued experiences. A successful demonstration can be seen in a family-aided educational program in disease management for Latinos with

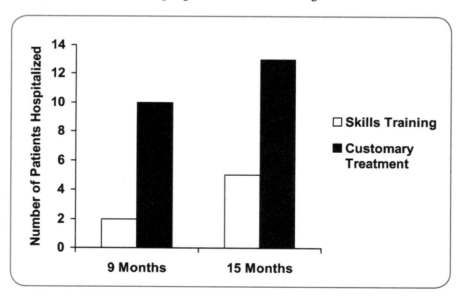

FIGURE 9.1 Adapting family-aided skills training in disease management for Latinos. This training was carried out in a community mental health center and markedly reduced rehospitalization rates. *Source.* Kopelwicz et al. 2003.

schizophrenia who were joined by their relatives (Kopelowicz et al. 2003). A community mental health center located in a section of Los Angeles heavily populated by first-generation Latinos invited families to participate in weekly education and briefings of the skills for managing medication and symptoms that their mentally ill relatives were learning separately in groups. Family members learned how to map these skills to the patients' home life by providing opportunities, encouragement, and positive feedback to patients for using what they had learned about disease management. The impact of this program at 9- and 15-month follow-up is shown in Figure 9.1. Compared with the patients randomly assigned to customary care, the patients who participated in disease management with family facilitation had significantly less hospitalization and lower levels of positive, negative, and total symptoms. They also used their skills in everyday life to achieve a higher level of functioning.

CLINICAL EXAMPLE

Francisco, a 41-year-old unacculturated Mexican American patient with schizophrenia, was brought to the mental health center by his wife and teenage sons for treatment of his long-standing schizophrenia. His family was invited to attend his treatment sessions for social support; they had made clear during his evaluation that his rudimentary grasp of English and being viewed as *loco* would embarrass him and destroy his pride. While the united front of his wife and children persuaded him to attend the clinic for treatment, he refused to take his antipsychotic medication when he found out that it was for "crazy" people. His florid psychosis and disability were becoming a serious family burden when the psychiatrist asked about the patient's health practices in Mexico.

It came to light that in Mexico, Francisco frequented *curanderos,* who function as folk healers for rural and traditional Mexicans. This gave his psychiatrist an opening for implementing a culturally relevant disease management intervention. He arranged for a joint treatment session at the mental health center with a *curandero*. At the treatment session, the *curandero* lit candles, used incense, and chanted prayers. In addition, the *curandero* made it clear to Francisco that his folk medicine would only be powerful if it was supplemented by daily use of medication. The psychiatrist also encouraged Francisco's wife and children to communicate their genuine feelings that medication would strengthen his *machismo* role in the family.

With authority figures he respected and his family lined up behind the value of medication, Francisco was persuaded to restart his antipsychotic drug. Long-term maintenance medication was achieved after the patient and his family conjointly completed rehabilitation programs on medication self-management and relapse prevention. Within 2 years, he was able to return to work in the construction trade and enjoy cordial relations with his family and friends—meeting the criteria for recovery.

Rather than insisting that patients from special cultures receive their treatment in usual mental health facilities, practitioners should build on the strengths of families, using community supports to bring about significant improvements in symptoms and functioning. In another study, low relapse rates were recorded when Latinos with schizophrenia were given family-focused services in their homes. An additional example comes from harnessing of the family and community to deal with a dilemma occasioned by a young Latino man with schizophrenia who absolutely refused to seek help from his local mental health center. The culturally competent therapist gathered 20 of his extended family in the patient's backyard to develop a treatment plan. The plan included his sister enlisting his aid as a babysitter; his brother arranging for him to be an equipment manager of a neighborhood soccer team; a prayer group at his church involving him in their meetings while excusing him to pace and talk to himself when these symptoms emerged; and a priest giving him a job as a gardener at the church. After 2 months, the young man agreed to accept injectable, long-acting antipsychotic medication because it was framed as a treatment for *nervios*—his restlessness, slowed activity, and difficulty concentrating.

▶ Rehabilitation of Persons With Co-occurring Mental Disorders

Epidemiological studies indicate that more than 40% of patients with one psychiatric disorder have two or more comorbid disorders. For example, patients with schizophrenia often have mood symptoms that fit the diagnostic categories of depression, obsessive-compulsive disorder, or social anxiety disorder. Figure 9.2 depicts the way that three different types of disorders—severe mental illness, substance abuse, and developmental disabilities—overlap with one another. Concurrent disorders complicate treatment and rehabilitation. The severity of illness—whether measured by symptoms or disability—is substantially greater among individuals with comorbidity,

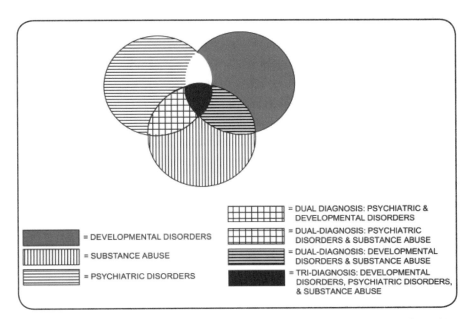

FIGURE 9.2 Graphic representation of co-occurring disorders among patients with psychiatric disorders, substance abuse, and developmental disabilities.

thereby posing a major challenge to designing and implementing psychosocial treatments. Especially daunting is the co-occurrence of substance abuse disorders with other psychiatric disorders, because those affected do poorly when their treatment is split and shared by separate agencies with separate responsibilities for either substance abuse or psychiatric disorders.

A general principle for rehabilitation of patients with comorbid disorders is the importance of integrated services in which clinicians are trained and competent in both disorders and work closely together. There are myriad types of comorbidities, but here we will describe rehabilitative interventions for three types of dual-diagnosis patients: substance-abusing persons with serious mental disorders, individuals with both developmental and mental disabilities, and persons with posttraumatic stress disorder (PTSD) and schizophrenia.

SUBSTANCE-ABUSING MENTALLY ILL PERSONS

The lifetime prevalence of substance abuse—including alcohol and illicit drugs—in the severely mentally ill is approximately 50% (Bartels et al. 1993). On the basis of epidemiological data, the federal government reported that at any one time, 4 million citizens have co-occurring serious mental disorder and substance abuse; 52% of these individuals received neither mental health nor substance abuse services (Substance Abuse and Mental Health

Services Administration 2002). In one study of consecutive admissions of schizophrenia patients to a large veterans hospital in Los Angeles, 34% were found to have cocaine in their urine (Shaner et al. 1993). Substance abuse has reached epidemic proportions among the severely mentally ill.

Integrated Treatment Approaches

While far from a panacea, services that are integrated, evidence-based, person-centered, and results-driven can make a dent in the therapeutic obstacles posed by substance-abusing mentally ill individuals. The key to integration is having the same treatment team address both disorders simultaneously. Of course, the clinicians on an integrated team must possess cumulatively the competencies that are required for effective delivery of each of the components that are brought together for integration. Table 9.2 lists evidence-based treatment elements that require competencies of the treatment team as a whole. Team members specialize in one or more of each of the practices. Optimal outcomes with dually diagnosed individuals result when the team collectively possesses the requisite elements and competencies that are then

---

● **TABLE 9.2**

Evidence-based practices that require competencies of team members for integrated treatment of dually diagnosed persons

1. Assertive outreach and engagement in the community
2. Motivational enhancement linked to the stages of treatment involvement
3. Integrated treatment program with the same team, with staff knowledgeable and capable of using interventions for both types of disorder (e.g., psychoactive medications and training in harm avoidance and relapse prevention)
4. Training in relapse prevention and harm avoidance, with flexibility and no extrusion from program for "slips" or relapses—Substance Abuse Management Module
5. Continuous case management by personal support specialists
6. Money management with representative payee
7. Close monitoring with urine tests
8. Safe, protected, and sober living residential environments
9. Vocational rehabilitation–supported employment such as Individual Support & Placement
10. Efforts for family reconciliation
11. Integration of 12-step program that accepts "double trudgers"
12. Spiritual opportunities with inspiration and dedication

adapted for local conditions. A major challenge to an integrated approach is adapting and melding evidence-based treatments that perform well for substance abuse with treatments that are efficacious for severe mental illness (Mueser et al. 2003). Perhaps the greatest challenge to staff members on integrated, dual-diagnosis teams is forming therapeutic relationships with patients having complex and provocative patterns of symptoms, addictions, and personality disorders.

For persons with schizophrenia and substance abuse, achieving and maintaining abstinence are complicated by deficits in motivation, insight, active participation, sustained attention, learning, memory, problem solving, decision making, and social ability. When embedded in an integrated treatment program, the best-validated services for the dually diagnosed take into account and accommodate for these deficits, as listed in Table 9.3. The benefits accruing to four cohorts of patients admitted during successive 6-month periods are shown in Figure 9.3 for an increasingly integrated program, in which evidence-based procedures were sequentially and cumulatively incorporated every 6 months (Ho et al. 1999). By the end of the 2 years, when the program was fully integrated, retention of patients in the program had more than doubled, the percent rehospitalized had fallen to below 25%, and sobriety had risen to more than 30%.

● **TABLE 9.3**

Empirically validated treatments for dually diagnosed patients

TREATMENT TECHNIQUE	PURPOSE
Integrated treatment services with the same treatment team trained in services applicable to both substance abuse and mental disorders	This basic principle ensures that comprehensive services are well coordinated, patients do not fall between the cracks of different agencies, participation meets requirements of continuity of care, patients with needs for maintenance psychotropic medications are not discriminated against by the abstinence ideology typically held by staff members of substance abuse agencies, and pharmacotherapy and psychosocial treatments are carried out with collaboration by the clinicians who are responsible for these different techniques. All treatments listed in this table are best provided within integrated treatment programs.
Motivational interviewing based on the stages of readiness for treatment	Motivates patients to participate in active treatment, goal setting, and contracting for urine screening tests and money management, including a representative payee.

(continued)

● **TABLE 9.3** *(cont'd.)*

TREATMENT TECHNIQUE	PURPOSE
Social skills training	Helps patients develop drug-refusal skills, make social contacts and relationships with clean and sober peers, and reconcile with families.
Education about mechanisms for substance abuse and dependence	Helps patients understand functions of abuse, addiction, triggers for abuse, cravings, withdrawal, and harmful consequences of abuse of alcohol and drugs.
Training in relapse prevention	Helps patients cope with triggers, craving, and high-risk situations; seek help from support persons; and interrupt periods of abuse before they become prolonged.
Supported employment	Helps patients recognize that work confers an identity, keeps them on a schedule, and provides satisfaction and self-efficacy. Work is a key element in providing motivation for remaining abstinent and having funds to engage in healthy pleasures and enduring relationships.
Family psychoeducation	Provides patients' families with information on drug and alcohol abuse and dependence as well as their role in facilitating abstinence. Family relationships are one of the most powerful incentives for remaining abstinent, as family ties can be ruptured by repeated or long-term drug or alcohol dependence or abuse.
Illness management, including money management and random urinalysis	Helps patients learn how to control their mental disorder with disease management procedures followed by use of a representative payee, and to gradually form an active partnership with clinicians in treatment.
Assertive community treatment consistent with stage of readiness for change, level of functioning, and independence and progress	Provides patients with mobile care, outreach, and availability around the clock as important means of containing relapses and adapting to clean and sober living.
Community reinforcement	Provides positive reinforcement to maintain ever-longer periods of sobriety, and uses various rewards relevant to each individual. Contingent reinforcement is also given to motivate active participation in treatment and abstinence.

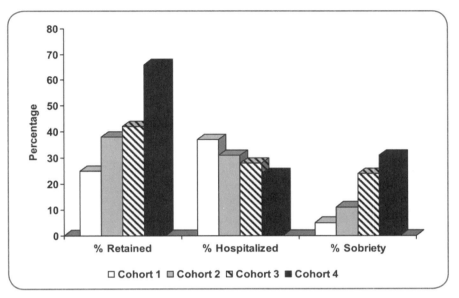

FIGURE 9.3 Sequential improvements in outcome, with incremental and cumulative addition of evidence-based services for the dually diagnosed. Patients were treated in an integrated dual-diagnosis treatment program with inpatient, day treatment, and outpatient continuity of care. *Source.* Data from Ho et al. 1999.

Substance Abuse Management Module

The Substance Abuse Management Module was designed to teach dually diagnosed patients the self-control skills required for relapse prevention and harm reduction within an integrated program for the dually diagnosed (Roberts et al. 1999). The basic concept of the module, around which the skills training is structured, is the *slippery slope from relapse to recovery.* Depicted in Figure 9.4, the slippery slope is a harm reduction model because it assumes that most individuals with a dual diagnosis will not achieve and retain sobriety indefinitely. The overarching goal of the module is to teach patients the skills for traction in climbing the slippery slope in order not only to reduce the likelihood of relapses but also to limit the duration and adverse consequences of a relapse if and when it occurs. Even when a patient progresses toward recovery, there is always the danger that events and experiences may result in the individual's sliding back down the slippery slope. This harm reduction strategy is called *damage control.*

The skills taught in the module aim to protect patients from the double jeopardy of relapse of substance abuse and mental illness:

- Making a "U-turn" requires the skills of moving away from whatever situation or stressor that is generating warning signs of a psychiatric

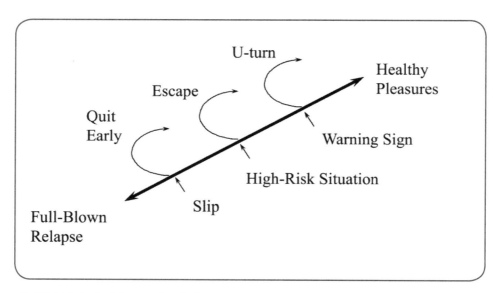

FIGURE 9.4 The "slippery slope" of relapse to abstinence for the dually diagnosed: the harm reduction model.

relapse or cravings that may herald a slip back into substance abuse. To provide a tangible memory aid for this skill, patients construct "emergency cards" that list the names and phone numbers of support persons—clean and sober individuals who have been recruited by the patients and who agree to be available when needed to help the patient make a "U turn."

- Beating a safe retreat helps patients to maintain self-control by escaping from high-risk situations that, unless avoided, can result in a slip. Patients practice this skill by conducting their own "fire drills," during which they engage in various escape behaviors from high-risk situations that might occur in the coming days, weeks, or months.

- Quitting as soon as possible after a slip is the appropriate coping response for avoiding a full-blown extended relapse. This skill contradicts the "abstinence violation effect." After a slip, most substance abusers will say to themselves, "Now I've blown it by using drugs/alcohol again, so I may as well keep using." Training in harm reduction contravenes this idea by replacing it with "I've slipped but only once/twice, and I can report this slip to one of my support people to get help to return to abstinence. By asking for help now, I can do damage control and hold on to my job, my money, and my family."

- Pursuing "healthy pleasures" that are alternatives to getting high and hanging out with drug and alcohol abusers reduces the dually diagnosed person's risk for relapse. Healthy pleasures can include any

● **TABLE 9.4**

Key concepts and skills of the Substance Abuse Management Module

SKILLS TAUGHT IN THE MODULE	MODULE CONCEPTS
If you slip, quit early and report it to a support person.	Practice damage control.
When someone offers drugs, say, "No."	Escape high-risk situations.
Don't get into situations where you can't say no.	Avoid high-risk situations.
Do things that are fun and healthy; persuade others to join in healthy pleasures; obtain a payee for learning money management skills.	Seek healthy pleasures.

enjoyable social or recreational activity in a setting where drugs and alcohol are not in evidence and in which the individual is accompanied by clean and sober friends or family members.

The sequence of key skills from the module (see Table 9.4) is printed on handouts and posters that compensate for patients' cognitive impairments in attention, learning, and memory.

LEARNING ACTIVITIES IN THE MODULE

The module learning activities have three components:

1. *Basic training* consists of eight 45-minute educational sessions designed to engage and motivate new patients while teaching relapse prevention principles. Each session is "stand-alone," so whenever patients complete the eight sessions with adequate participation signaling comprehension of the basic concepts, they graduate to the skills training component.

2. *Skills training* includes twenty-seven 45-minute sessions in which learning is ensured through videotape demonstrations of each of nine skills. The characters in the video graphically demonstrate the discrete, component behaviors of each skill with narration and visual aids that reduce the patients' cognitive impediments to learning. The

video segments for modeling the skills were made by actual dually diagnosed patients and therefore have great currency and credibility with participants. After watching the video, patients almost invariably make striking changes in their behavior, a credit to the power of social modeling and vicarious and procedural learning. The video, with questions and answers to document assimilation of the demonstrated skills, is followed by realistic role-plays taken from each patient's life. Patients are given homework assignments that are used as "grist for the therapeutic mill" during practice sessions.

3. *Practice sessions* are twice-weekly for patients at all stages of the module and for graduates who can come for maintenance, consolidation, and reinforcement of the skills. These sessions focus on applying the concepts and skills to individually relevant, real-life situations.

FROM GENERAL TO SPECIFIC SKILLS

Through videotape modeling and coaching in role-plays, the module provides very specific verbal and nonverbal behaviors as raw material for the skills. For example, the component skills of refusing drugs from a dealer include: avoid eye contact, keep moving, don't stop, don't engage in any conversation, repeatedly say no while shaking head "No!," wave hands and arms to signify "No, leave me alone," and throw to the ground any drug that the dealer places in your pocket.

MAINTAINING MOTIVATION

Clinicians have to establish and then maintain patients' motivation to continue through the arduous 6- to 9-month period of involvement in the Substance Abuse Management Module. Participation also needs to be sustained in other elements of an integrated program, such as attending 12-step support meetings, taking weekly urine tests, undertaking job searches, living in sober residences, and learning money management with the help of a representative payee. Five stages serve as the matrix for conceptualizing and succeeding in establishing and sustaining patients' motivation. The five-stage sequence is shown in Table 9.5.

It is important to realize that progress through stages of change is a dynamic process. Shifts and transitions in both directions occur over time, with each patient having a unique pattern that must be monitored with appropriate therapeutic responses. The processes involved in moving through the stages of motivation are not automatic or linear—to maintain

● TABLE 9.5

Stages of motivation for initiating and maintaining involvement in the Substance Abuse Management Module and integrated dual-diagnosis programs

MOTIVATIONAL STAGE	CLINICAL PROCESS AND FUNCTIONS
Precontemplation	Is in denial of problem(s) and is not thinking of treatment.
Contemplation	Acknowledges that a problem(s) exists and is thinking of seeking treatment. May be aware of the benefits of treatment and the adverse consequences of continuing substance abuse to himself/herself and the mental disorder.
Preparation	Plans to enter treatment in the near future—has obtained information about specific programs, obtained orientation, and discussed participation with friends and/or relatives. Recognizes that benefits outweigh costs for participation in program.
Action	Begins participation in treatment program and starts to make progress by learning and using skills in a natural environment, developing positive relationships with clinicians.
Maintenance	Continues to use skills learned during the program and to participate in self-help, psychiatric, and other maintenance services. Consolidates skills into personal lifestyle of sobriety with healthy pleasures. Adheres to prescribed maintenance psychotropic drugs.

their involvement, patients must obtain encouragement, reinforcement, and help with problem-solving from clinicians on their team.

The substantial learning and retention by dually diagnosed patients of the specific knowledge and skills taught by the module are illustrated in Figure 9.5. In addition, the patients exhibited significant increases in abstinence, decreases in psychiatric symptoms, and improvements in quality of life. All of these improvements were substantial and statistically significant. Finally, patients' relapse rates were more than halved—from 75% to 31%—in the 6-month period following completion of the module (Shaner et al. 2003). The module is a major element in a multifaceted, integrated program for the dually diagnosed at a large, urban veterans hospital where patients have psychotic disorders with cocaine, alcohol, and marijuana polysubstance abuse. Many of the patients in this program, when they continue as outpatients for 1 or more years, meet the criteria for recovery as described in Chapter 1.

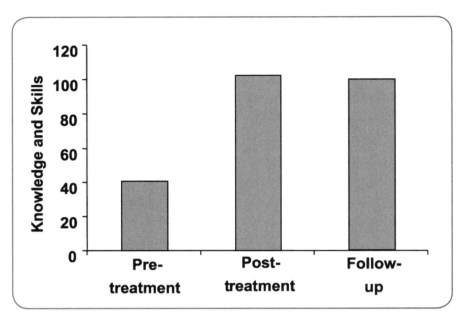

FIGURE 9.5 Learning relapse and harm reduction skills in the Substance Abuse Management Module. *Source.* Shaner et al. 2003.

DEVELOPMENTALLY DISABLED PERSONS WITH MENTAL ILLNESS

Developmentally disabled individuals are at higher risk for co-occurring mental disorders. Contributing to their higher risk are biological vulnerability and environmental stressors attendant on the 1) repeated failure experiences in learning and socializing, 2) stigmatizing effects of their odd appearance and behavior, and 3) impact of their challenging behavior on family members, caretakers, and the public. Their rate of psychiatric disorders is as much as five times greater than the rate in the population as a whole.

Evaluation and treatment of co-occurring psychotic, depressive, or anxiety symptoms with developmental disorders depend upon the verbal capacity of the individual. Verbally responsive patients can have their symptoms monitored by repeated administration of a rating scale as medication is given and titrated in dose. For more severely retarded individuals, evaluation requires repeated graphing of abnormal behaviors thought to reflect symptoms of a co-occurring mental disorder. The presumption of a mental disorder is supported if the provision of psychotropic medication returns the individual to a previous level of psychosocial functioning and withdrawal of medication leads to recrudescence of the inappropriate behavior. As in the case example on pp. 469–470, psychosis is identified by periodic behavioral regressions and emergence of aggressive and impulsive behavior in a person who is otherwise congenial and affectionate.

Behavior modification and supports, using positive programming, are very effective in teaching daily living skills and improving psychosocial functioning in persons with mental retardation and concurrent mental disorders. Supported employment and supported living have been notably successful with this population, enabling many individuals to live full lives in normal environments. For those who have psychotic symptoms, behavioral supports are combined with optimal medication regimens and behavior modification. A collaborative working relationship between psychiatrist and behavioral psychologist is essential for reducing distress, improving psychosocial functioning, and providing support and education to caregivers.

CLINICAL EXAMPLE

Selma, a 45-year-old customarily friendly woman with mild retardation, was referred because of command hallucinations associated with threats, property destruction, and physical aggression toward others: punching, biting, kicking, scratching, pinching, and pulling hair. After 23 years of institutionalization and 2 years of living in a group home, Selma moved into her own apartment with the aid of supported living services. She was on a maintenance regimen of clozapine and lithium, adjusted as needed by a psychiatrist who specialized in developmental disabilities. Despite the medication, approximately 20 episodes per week of aggressive behavior occurred. A behavior modification program was designed with Selma's participation.

The behavioral support plan began with her personal goals of continuing to live in her apartment with a roommate, learning how to cross the street independently, purchasing items in the neighborhood store, taking a beauty class, exercising, and taking a cooking class. Selma got a volunteer job at her church and at the Red Cross. She came to view her supported living staff as "family"—a feeling that was reciprocated by staff members. However, many of her assaults came out of the blue, preventing support staff from protecting themselves. A typical example was walking with a staff member and suddenly lashing out with a forceful punch to the face. After such events, Selma became upset, profusely apologized, and lamented responding to the "voice" that commanded her to hit. Clearly, the positive supports for her personal goals had to be supplemented with additional interventions.

With the supervision of a clinical psychologist, trained and certified in applied behavior analysis, a reinforcement program was instituted that provided an incentive to Selma to reduce the frequency and intensity of her aggression. For any hour during which she did not show aggression, threats, or property destruction, staff gave Selma positive social reinforcement. At the end of each day, staff gave stamps to Selma if she had had no episodes of aggression. When accumulated, stamps could be exchanged for a variety of pleasurable activities; for example, one of her favorites was going out to dinner with a staff member and her roommate with preparations that included getting her hair done, putting on makeup, and receiving a small gift. The reinforcement value of these earned activities was amplified by staff making them occasions for an enthusiastic "celebration of life."

Increasing numbers of stamps were given for consecutive days without aggression up to 6 days. If an incident occurred, Selma received no stamps for that day but was encouraged to resume her earnings the next day with upbeat expressions of confidence that she would be more successful in the ensuing days. Additional behavioral interventions included social skills training and in vivo desensitization in which Selma and staff role-played situations where she became frustrated but refrained from aggressive actions. After a year, Selma's aggressive outbursts were reduced from an average frequency of 20 per week to 1 per month. Her gaining self-control over her aggression permitted her to leave her apartment each day to do volunteer work at her church and the Red Cross and use her stamps to pay for cooking and exercise classes. Also, she took a beauty class, made purchases in neighborhood stores, and learned how to cross streets autonomously.

PERSONS WITH PSYCHOSIS AND POSTTRAUMATIC STRESS DISORDER

Because of their cognitive impairments, symptoms, passivity, and social disability, individuals with severe mental disorders are more likely to suffer physical and psychological trauma stemming from poverty; sexual, physical, and financial victimization; homelessness; and struggles over involuntary hospitalization, seclusion, and restraint. About 90% of the severely mentally ill have been exposed to trauma sometime during their lifetimes, and most have had multiple exposures. The prevalence of PTSD in severely mentally ill persons is approximately 25%, twice as high as in community samples.

In contrast to the effective cognitive-behavioral and pharmacological treatments for persons with singular PTSD, treatments for persons with PTSD and severe mental illness must be delivered within the context of comprehensive services and teamwork, which include active case management, with outreach as needed; illness self-management; medication management; social skills training; and integrated services when these dual disorders are complicated by a third, substance abuse and dependence.

Embedded in the comprehensive mental health services listed above are specific interventions designed for the needs of dually diagnosed persons with PTSD and severe mental illness. These include:

- Providing psychoeducation about both disorders, with inclusion of key family members and community caretakers.
- Teaching skills for coping with the anxiety and depressive symptoms that are inherent to PTSD; for example, breathing retraining, muscle relaxation, and social activation.
- Reframing PTSD symptoms as being treatable to induce realistic optimism for improvement.
- Building skills for problem solving and social and independent living to achieve higher levels of community functioning and adjustment.
- Using individual and group cognitive-behavioral therapy (CBT) in which gradual exposure to the trauma experience is introduced and arousal is increased and then diminished as continued exposure is maintained. Also, an alternative form of cognitive therapy elicits patients' beliefs about the meaning of the traumatic event and assists them in identifying maladaptive thoughts and patterns of emotions that have interfered with moving forward with a more constructive lifestyle.
- Recommending self-help support groups with peers, often facilitated by recovered individuals, whose credibility as leaders is enhanced by their also having suffered from PTSD.

Two myths that need to be exploded before psychiatric treatment and rehabilitation can be made broadly available to persons with co-occurring PTSD and severe mental illness are 1) patients with schizophrenia and related disorders are too fragile and vulnerable to psychotic exacerbations to benefit from the arousal induced by CBT; and 2) malingering or exaggerating symptoms of PTSD is motivated by the desire to obtain service-connected disability pensions by veterans.

Regarding the first myth, contrary to clinical concerns, there has been no documented evidence that persons with schizophrenia and PTSD experience exacerbations of psychotic symptoms when offered exposure therapies for their PTSD. Bursting the second myth, patients who were awarded

VA compensation for their PTSD did not reduce or terminate their mental health treatment after receiving their pensions; to the contrary, they not only remained involved but actually participated in twice as much treatment subsequent to settling their claims for service-connected disability. This suggests that patients with PTSD seek and use mental health services commensurate with the symptoms and disability that prompted their claims for pensions.

▶ Persons With Treatment-Refractory Mental Disorders

Despite the best combined efforts made with drug and psychosocial therapies, there are large numbers of seriously mentally ill patients whose symptoms and social functioning respond suboptimally or not at all. Forty percent of outpatients with schizophrenia cannot be stabilized at low levels of symptomatology, and 20% have a refractory illness, even when they have been treated with adequate doses and durations of antipsychotic medications and have been compliant with their regimens. Many patients with bipolar and major depressive disorders experience enduring social and occupational disability because of persisting or recurrent symptoms as well as cognitive, motivational, and functional impairments.

Psychosocial interventions, whether intentional or naturalistic, are always concomitants of drug therapy; therefore, treatment-refractoriness should be conceptualized as failure to show clinical improvement, in response to not only medication but also concomitant psychosocial treatment. An often decisive influence on patients' symptoms and social functioning is the quality of their daily living environment (Brenner et al. 1990). We focus here on psychosocial therapy, including patients' living environments, in describing strategies for the rehabilitation of persons with treatment-refractory schizophrenia. The same strategies, with minor modifications, are also effective with individuals having other disorders that are resistant to customary treatments.

What, then, are the specialized psychosocial services that can complement pharmacotherapy in treating persons with refractory schizophrenia? The two evidence-based psychosocial treatments for this population are both derivatives of learning theory: reinforcement therapy and CBT. The commonalities of these therapeutic approaches may help to explain their efficacy.

Common elements in reinforcement therapy and CBT require practitioners to:

- Follow specific protocols and manuals consisting of structured, consistent, planned, and scheduled interventions; their effectiveness depends on how faithful the clinician is in following the principles and procedures delineated in the manuals.
- Use lengthy and intensive periods of treatment with repetition until behavioral criteria are achieved, followed by gradual fading of the interventions and behavioral assignments to allow patients to implement the skills they have learned in their everyday life. Intermittent reinforcement, follow-up booster sessions, and continuing case management are important for long-term benefits and generalization.
- Provide frequent positive reinforcement for even small amounts of improvement. Clinicians must avoid having their focus "seduced" by complaints, symptoms, anger, regression, and other behavioral problems presented by the patient. Instead, the intrepid therapist, who is determined to open the lock that restricts participation in community life, responds with genuine enthusiasm for small signs of improvement. The importance of the therapeutic relationship is no more apparent than here.
- Compensate for or reduce neurocognitive and symptomatic impairments that otherwise would impede learning.
- Connect treatment settings with naturalistic living environments for generalization of improvements. Generalization is promoted when family, friends, and mental health professionals provide opportunities, encouragement, and reinforcement to the patient for using the skills learned in treatment. Eventually, durability of improvement is promoted by the patient's increased self-confidence and natural reinforcement from the community.

REINFORCEMENT THERAPY

The basic element in reinforcement therapy, also termed *contingency management, credit incentive system, social learning,* or *token economy,* is a motivational system that organizes the environment to provide extra incentives for adaptive behavior, thereby compensating for the negative symptoms and cognitive impairments of persons who have been largely unresponsive to treatment. This is accomplished through the systematic and consistent use of credit cards, money, tokens, coupons, points, or other visual feedback that is amplified by concomitant praise. Tangible and social reinforcement are given to patients contingent upon their exhibiting the social, instrumental, and verbal behaviors that will enable them to function at a higher level, with less professional supervision and with a better quality of life. The motivational efficacy of the reinforcers depends on their being exchangeable for a wide range of valued rewards, privileges, and incentives.

Reinforcement therapy can be effectively used in a wide range of treatment settings—inpatient units, residential treatment and rehabilitation facilities, day hospitals, psychosocial rehabilitation or clubhouse programs, patients' homes, and natural community environments. For example, improvements ensue from "behavioral contracts" wherein patients are paid small amounts of money or coupons for free movies, restaurant meals, and CDs in exchange for doing volunteer work, attending classes, refraining from inappropriate behavior, and adhering to medication regimens.

The first step in designing a token economy is identifying the specific behaviors to be increased or decreased in frequency or intensity. For example, self-care and appropriate social participation in therapeutic activities would be targets for positive reinforcement, whereas aggressive and intrusive behaviors might result in token fines or differential reinforcement of other behaviors. Differential reinforcement is a particularly powerful technique, as staff ignore inappropriate behavior but rapidly respond to any sign of alternative, appropriate behavior, whatever it may be. Because social attention reinforces inappropriate or "psychotic" behavior, when staff members shift their attentiveness and tangible reinforcers to appropriate behavior, change occurs rapidly and often dramatically.

The system requires highly specific behavioral descriptions so that all staff members will deliver contingent reinforcement in the same way and patients will experience the fairness of the program through its consistency. For example, one patient with treatment-refractory illness received bonuses in his money management program for increased travel on local buses to places where he participated in social and recreational activities. After identification of the target behaviors, contingencies for the delivery of the tokens are created that will govern the consequences of the target behaviors. Contingencies describe *if-then* rules connecting the target behavior with reinforcers. Patients are encouraged to collaborate on developing specific contingencies for token reinforcement of a wide variety of behaviors, which can be individualized depending upon the patient's deficits, strengths, and goals. In selecting behaviors targeted for reinforcement, it is vital from an ethical and therapeutic point of view that the behaviors be consistent with those required for patients to reach a better quality of life in the community.

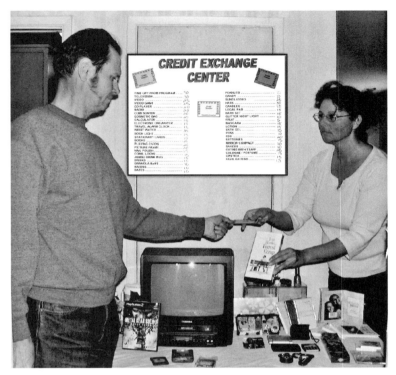

FIGURE 9.6 Patient exchanging credits for reinforcers such as television rental, snacks, and time off from the treatment program.

Almost all psychiatric inpatient units utilize a "level system" that links the functional level of patients with their degree of supervision, freedom of action, choices, and privileges. But creating a learning environment that can overcome the cognitive deficits of patients with treatment-refractory disorders is much more challenging. The complement of ward staff must be organized to deliver frequent and individualized rewards contingent upon well-specified, observed adaptive behavior. In Figure 9.6, a patient attending a community mental health center is shown exchanging points from his credit card for snacks, rental of a portable television, and a day off from his program.

At the Camarillo State Hospital in California, a reinforcement therapy program operated continuously for 26 years for the most cognitively and symptomatically impaired persons throughout the state. All had disorders that were treatment-refractory despite repeated trials of different psychoactive medications and psychosocial treatments. An integrated pharmacological and behavioral program of interventions was guided by daily and weekly ratings of participation in activities of daily living, participation in hospital and community-based jobs, social skills training, and recreational groups.

• TABLE 9.6

Clinical problems of patients with treatment-refractory illnesses showing improvement of 50% or more with reinforcement therapy at Camarillo (California) State Hospital

Screaming and tantrums	Incoherent speech and mutism
Poor work and leisure skills	Inactivity and amotivation
Delusional speech	Persistent suicidality
Hallucinations	Morbid obesity
Social isolation	Polydipsia
Assault, verbal aggression, and property destruction	Incontinence
Stereotypic and bizarre movements and posturing	

Ratings were also made of the severity of psychiatric symptoms, polydipsia, self-stimulation, and aggressive, self-injurious, and bizarre behaviors that prevented these individuals from re-entering community life. As shown in Table 9.6, a wide array of positive and negative symptoms, psychosocial deficits, and bizarre and intolerable behaviors were successfully modified. More than 75% of the patients were sufficiently improved for discharge into the community, where case managers helped them maintain their gains for many years (Glynn et al. 1994). The efficacy of reinforcement therapy or the token economy is among the most frequently replicated findings in the treatment of disabled psychiatric patients with treatment-refractory disorders, with more than 100 studies showing the efficacy and effectiveness of these approaches throughout North America and Europe (for reviews, see Glynn 1990; Kazdin 1985).

In one randomized, controlled study, 97% of patients with treatment-refractory schizophrenia who received reinforcement therapy were successfully discharged from long-term hospitalization, followed by 15 months or longer of community tenure (Paul and Lentz 1977).

The effectiveness of reinforcement therapy is derived in large part from the positive attention, communication, and recognition—praise and warm and friendly conversational exchanges—given verbally and nonverbally by staff in the process of disbursing points, credits, or tokens for improved functioning. *Social reinforcement* is the most powerful motivation for therapeutic purposes. Moreover, it is portable, free, and an effective component in all modalities mediated by interpersonal therapeutic transactions.

● EXAMPLE OF BEST PRACTICE

Patients who had been hospitalized for many years in New York state hospitals because of treatment-refractory disorders were transferred to the 30-bed Second Chance program, where they participated in a milieu organized around the principles and practice of reinforcement therapy. Patients received daily ratings and points or tokens on 10 criteria for appearance and grooming, room cleanliness, behavior at meals, participation in groups, and socially appropriate behavior. Points were exchanged for each patient's level of on-ward and off-ward privileges. Patients received weekly printouts of their own report of points earned, which informed them of their progress and of areas in which further change was needed. In addition to the point and token systems, the unit offered a full range of skills training, cognitive rehabilitation, and recreational groups.

Large improvements were noted in almost every area relevant to successful tenure in the community. Upon arrival, the patients had been in state hospitals an average of 7 years; in the Second Chance program, 77% of the participants were discharged into the community after an average of 145 days. In conjunction with frequent, planned, and scheduled skills training, cognitive rehabilitation, and recreational activities, reinforcement therapy reduced episodes of seclusion and restraint from 17.9 incidents per month to 2 incidents.

TARGETED BEHAVIOR THERAPY

Not every psychiatric facility can gather the considerable resources, expertise, and organizational wallop required to create an effective social learning program for inpatients or day treatment patients. There are, however, more focal behavior therapy techniques that have made their mark on specifically targeted psychotic symptoms that have been refractory to previous treatments:

- *Attention-focusing therapy* has been shown to be effective in counteracting poverty of speech for incoherent patients with schizophrenia as well as improving sustained attention to permit learning of social skills.
- *Habit reversal treatment* has been repeatedly shown to be effective in reducing dystonias, chronic tics, and Tourette's disorder.
- *Social skills training* has been shown to be effective in reducing negative symptoms that were unresponsive to medications. Since

negative symptoms are defined by lack of communication, emotional expressiveness, and social involvement, social skills training is tailor-made for teaching interpersonal behaviors that can displace negative symptoms.

- *Required relaxation* can be effective for out-of-control behaviors such as agitation, shouting, screaming, head banging, self-injurious behavior, and aggression.
- *Shifting patients' attention to external stimuli* can reduce or eliminate auditory hallucinations.

While many persons with unwanted, refractory hallucinations gain surcease by listening to music—especially music that is piped directly into the ear with headphones—an even more effective technique is to engage the patient in actively participating in an ongoing conversation. This works extremely well if the conversational partner repeatedly prompts the patient to maintain eye contact with the partner and to respond frequently to the partner's questions. Another example using attentional shifting occurs when the patient with frequent hallucinations is instructed to sing or hum a song. Patients who use their vocal activity for humming or singing popular songs and music may temporarily displace hallucinations by 60% or more, bringing this intrusive symptom under their control.

These behavioral interventions may be operating therapeutically by diverting the patient's attention from "inner speech" that presumably derives from abnormalities in the neural networks that are associated with speech and hearing; in other words, auto-stimulation of these brain networks may be responsible for the generation of "voices." This suggests that external stimuli—such as engaged conversation, reading out loud, music, and singing or humming—may activate and occupy that part of the brain responsible for hearing inner speech, thereby displacing the abnormal activity in that region.

TREATMENT MALL

A recent innovation for state hospitals and other long-stay residential treatment programs is the *treatment mall.* In the traditional form and structure of these institutions, therapeutic and recreational activities were held on the ward, with the result that each inpatient unit served as a self-contained hospital within a hospital. To better prepare patients for community life and to get patients off their custodially oriented wards, the Middletown Psychiatric

Center in New York created a treatment mall. The mall is a centralized center for rehabilitation that enables patients to leave their wards and go to a location that is designed like a community-based shopping mall. Here, "one-stop shopping" for rehabilitation services is available morning and afternoon for patients. Consistent with consumer empowerment, patients participate in decisions regarding the focus and functions of each "shop" within the mall.

The centerpiece of the mall services is a series of skill-building modules that are patterned after the evidence-based modules of the UCLA Psychiatric Rehabilitation Program. An academic model is used in some hospitals, with core and elective "courses" during each of three semesters in a year. Topics include illness management, communication skills, anger management, computer skills, basic math and English, exercise and other wellness activities, substance abuse management, anxiety management, and ways to look and feel better. Patients with cognitive deficits that interfere with learning are able to participate in cognitive remediation. Progress notes are written on "crack-and-peel" adhesive paper that is sent to the patient's ward team and placed in the chart with feedback to patients that provides opportunities for positive reinforcement. Over 25 hospitals have adopted the treatment mall as the primary locale for psychiatric rehabilitation.

COGNITIVE-BEHAVIORAL THERAPY

The same technique used for CBT of depressive and anxiety disorders has been adapted for treatment of hallucinations and delusions that have not responded adequately to antipsychotic medication. Cognitive therapy for schizophrenia originated from the assumption that patients with dysfunctional belief systems and distortions underlying hallucinations and delusions refractory to medications can learn to identify these thought patterns and test their validity through behavioral assignments. The cognitive approach rests on a trusting therapeutic relationship in which the clinician maintains a nonconfrontational, accepting attitude toward the patient's delusions and hallucinations, then tactfully probes and explores the evidence supporting such beliefs. Finally, alternative reasons for the delusions and hallucinations are tactfully probed, explored, and examined with Socratic questioning for their explanatory value. Alternative explanations for hallucinations, for example, are considered for their satisfactoriness in describing the causes of "voices." One patient came to the conclusion that it was abnormal hyperexcitability and over-stimulation of the auditory cortex that were responsible for his "voices."

Sample procedures from CBT for patients with psychotic symptoms are:

- Validate the patient's experience but not his/her interpretation of the symptom: "You are actually hearing voices. It's not your imagination, and you are not crazy. Did you know that most people in the world hear a voice or voices at times?"
- Employ collaborative empiricism and guided discovery: "You and I will work together to learn more about your voices, what they mean, and what you can do to get some relief from them."
- Identify beliefs underpinning the hallucinations: "As we discuss the voices, they seem to have as their intent bringing harm to you; also, to demean, weaken, influence, manipulate, attack, and insult you."
- Gently question the patient's interpretation of the voices: "Are you certain that the voices you are hearing are people wanting to do you harm? Do you know those people and where they live? It is possible that people are saying these bad things about you, so let's consider that as well as other explanations. Can you think of any other reason why you are hearing these voices; for example, where and how do we hear each other talk? When I speak to you, just like now, what happens to the sounds of my voice after they are picked up by your ears?"
- Question the reality of the patient's paranoid attributions of voices to other people by asking questions that require the patient to give more specific information about the putative people who are tormenting him/her: "Can you tell me more about the people who are insulting you and putting you down? Exactly how do they sound? Can you give me an example? How old are these people? How did they get to know you? Why would they want to hassle you? What right do they have to insult you and make you feel afraid? How would they know so much about you, your home, and your possessions? If these people are talking to you from far away, how are you able to hear them? What other explanation might account for your hearing the voices? Let's just for a moment assume that the voices are not coming from other people. If the voices are not spoken by other people, what's another way that you might hear them?"
- Together with the patient, discuss alternatives for understanding the voices: "Have you ever heard your own thoughts out loud inside your head? When you were afraid of something, did you ever talk to yourself silently to get control of the situation? I hear voices sometimes, like my father who is dead—I hear him tell me things that he used to say."
- Show the patient a picture or a model of the brain and explain how the brain might produce voices that are heard by the patient: "Let me show you the part of the brain called the auditory cortex. This is the part of the brain that allows us to hear. If that part of the brain is destroyed by a

stroke, we might not be able to hear at all. What do you think you might hear if that part of your brain is hyperactive, hyperexcitable? If that part of your brain is overactive and gets stimulated by a brain chemical that is necessary for passing signals from one nerve cell to another, is it possible that it could be sending signals to you that are the same as the signals you get when it is stimulated by my voice right now?"

There are several alternative, rational explanations for hallucinations that can supplant the patient's irrational belief that other people from the external, "real" world are communicating with him/her:

1. Hearing voices that threaten to rob, exploit, or hurt the patient may be legitimate concerns and fears that the patient has about his/her tenuous and vulnerable living arrangements and ability to defend himself/herself and his/her property.
2. Rosalie's voices insisted that she was a bad person and would be hurt and punished. She gained control over these hallucinations by a combination of positive, coping self-statements ("I'm a good person. My family loves me, God loves me, and I don't have to be any different") and acceptance ("Everyone has bad experiences like this, so I'm going to ride the wave. I know that they never last more than 20 minutes and always go away"). The key element in CBT is for the patient to arrive at a new formulation of the source and significance of the hallucinations and then gain self-control over them.

While psychoeducation regarding our scientific knowledge of hallucinations is part of the technique, it is essential for the patient to view the new explanation as more convincing, to give up the incorrect attributions, and to engage in behavioral experiments that will confirm the alternative normalizing beliefs as time passes. This approach to therapy has resulted in modest but statistically significant reductions in the frequency and intensity of hallucinations and the severity of dysphoric reactions to them. Some studies have found a reduction of approximately 25% in psychotic symptoms, with improvements in insight and depression (Kingdon and Turkington 2005). Usually treatment sessions with the patient are given 3 hours per week. Involving the family or other caregivers in the training is important to get the benefits of the therapy to spread to the patient's everyday life at home and in the community.

It is not surprising that the patients who are most likely to respond to CBT are intelligent, cognitively flexible, and able to engage in verbal interchange and reasoning. This treatment relies on establishing rapport with the patient. Enlisting sufficient cooperation for time-consuming intellectual exercises requires confidence and comfort with the therapist. In using CBT for psychotic symptoms, the practitioner often accompanies the patient into the latter's natural environments for instigating and completing behavioral assignments aimed at disconfirming the patient's unrealistic explanations of the symptoms. Even when CBT produces improvement in hallucinations, most patients continue to be disabled by negative symptoms of schizophrenia. Social skills training may be useful in combination with CBT for facilitating change in the cognitive and behavioral realms associated with positive and negative symptoms of schizophrenia.

In the following case example, we will see assessment and treatment integrated with a *focus* on bringing Dorothy's psychotic symptoms under control while instigating and teaching prosocial behavior. The *multimodal* rehabilitation program for Dorothy included targeted behavior therapy, CBT, and social skills training. The *locus* of treatment was her home.

CLINICAL EXAMPLE

Dorothy developed schizophrenia while she was in college. Her career aspirations to become a veterinarian were aborted by persistent tormenting auditory hallucinations and persecutory delusions that often led to screaming fits as a means of escaping her misery. The screaming episodes increased in frequency over the next 4 years, presumably because of the concern and reassurance that they produced in her parents. When sympathetic expressions are given contingent on psychotic behavior, the latter receives positive reinforcement that has the inadvertent effect of increasing the symptoms. Compounding Dorothy's wretchedness was the loss of her pet dog and cat, who were given to a family friend because they were frightened by her screaming. Her voices threatened her with the plague and told her that she was going to be tortured because of her being responsible for thousands of pet dogs and cats being euthanized in animal shelters. Dorothy constantly sought reassurance from her parents, begging them to call animal shelters to tell them that she was opposed to euthanasia for abandoned pets.

Many times each day, usually in response to her voices, Dorothy would become agitated and have a screaming episode, each of which could last up to 10 minutes. Her parents were concerned about her safety and the tolerance of neighbors for the screaming that sounded threatening and dangerous. Several times, neighbors called the police to investigate the screaming. When she screamed, Dorothy's facial muscles and veins would bulge and her face would flush, reflecting a high degree of arousal. Numerous efforts to treat Dorothy's psychosis and bursts of screaming were made, including consultations with several national experts in pharmacological treatment of schizophrenia. All medications and their combination, including clozapine, had little effect on her symptoms or screaming. Several times she joined psychosocial rehabilitation clubs and day treatment programs, but the other members and staff were unable to tolerate her screaming.

Because Dorothy's screaming jeopardized her tenure in the community, a psychologist who was competent in behavior therapy was consulted. He made a home visit and, with everyone's agreement, decided to focus initially on teaching her to gain control over the screaming fits. Required relaxation was selected as the intervention. The psychologist discussed the treatment with Dorothy and her parents until they understood its rationale. The key element in required relaxation is reduction of high levels of emotional and autonomic arousal, which in this case was feeding Dorothy's screaming outbursts and also exacerbating her hallucinations. The technique was demonstrated initially when Dorothy was calm, and she said it felt good to be in control of her tension and fear. She was embarrassed by her episodes of screaming and dismayed that they prevented her from leaving the home for more than a few hours.

A week later, the behavior therapist spent 2 days with Dorothy and her parents in their home. When she began pacing and talking to herself loudly and angrily—warning signs of impending screaming—the therapist engaged her in the required relaxation. The technique consisted of easing her into a relaxed, prone position on the carpet and calming her with repeated instructions to relax and imagine a pleasant scene and listening to gentle music. After 5 minutes of sustained relaxation, she was able to rise and return to her customary activities, such as reading, watching television, conversing with her parents, or doing some gardening. Dorothy's striking response to required relaxation is depicted graphically in Figure 9.7. Prior to the required relaxation, the episodes of screaming averaged 32 per week but rapidly diminished to nil with the intervention. Dorothy was able to use relaxation on her own, which had the additional benefit of giving her a greater sense of self-control, empowerment, and responsibility for her own well-being. She integrated relaxation into her everyday routine, using it twice daily instead of waiting for the escalation of tension, hallucinations, and loud speech.

Although her symptoms were attenuated somewhat, Dorothy continued to suffer from her persisting hallucinations and the persecutory delusions they fostered. She stated that the voices and her talking out loud to them meant that she was crazy and made people think she was goofy and stupid. Thus, Dorothy was motivated to work with her therapist to

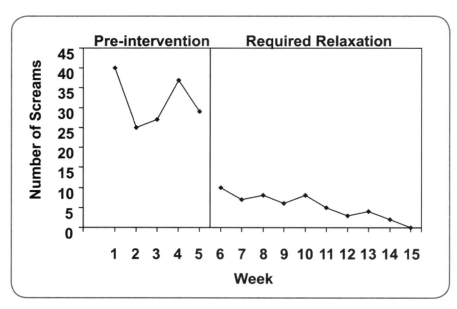

FIGURE 9.7 Effect of required relaxation on agitation in a patient with treatment refractory schizophrenia and hallucinations. *Source.* Redrawn from Liberman et al. 1994.

consider alternative explanations for her voices. She was assured that she did indeed hear the voices and was shown a model of the brain with the different regions clearly demarcated. As an intelligent person, she was able to understand how the auditory cortex and its associations might be generating abnormal amounts of neurotransmitters and electrical activity that could be producing the voices she heard.

She was gently encouraged by her therapist to compare the evidence for explaining the voices: people external to her versus excessive excitability of certain brain regions. She did behavioral experiments such as asking her parents and others if they could hear the voices and using the Internet to discover technologies that could project sound through space and buildings. She also watched documentary videos that described the functions of the brain and how these went awry in schizophrenia. Her parents, who were long-standing members of the National Alliance on Mental Illness (NAMI), introduced her to peers who had recovered from schizophrenia. These peers invited her to attend their NAMI Peer-to-Peer and In Our Own Voice educational seminars. There she interacted with others whose hallucinations and persecutory ideas had resolved with treatment. She gradually placed more credence on the "hypersensitivity" of her brain being responsible for her hallucinations and delusions. The hallucinations and delusions didn't disappear, but she was no longer distressed by them. When her voices intervened, she learned to say to herself, "It's my hypersensitive brain; I'm not insane."

As she gained more self-control and took more responsibility for her illness, her previous interests in caring for animals returned. Her beloved pets were returned to her, which buoyed her morale and gave her much pleasure. Now that she was able to make forays on her own outside her home, the behavior therapist referred her to a social skills training group at the local mental health center. She articulated her personal goal as a desire to become a veterinarian. Rather than despoil her cherished dream, the skills trainer used it as motivation for her to take steps that would move her in that direction. In the skills training group she practiced making phone calls to veterinarians and animal shelters to find part-time volunteer work, then role-playing volunteer job interviews. After several false starts, she obtained a 3-hour-per-day volunteer job with a pet grooming shop where the owner took a liking to her and gave her positive reinforcement for her work. At this time, she has agreed to participate in the mental health center's supported employment program, with the goal being to find remunerative work involving pets.

▶ Rehabilitation of Mentally Ill Offenders

By default, jails, prisons, and forensic hospitals house increasing numbers of severely mentally ill individuals as a result of deinstitutionalization, homelessness, restricted policies for involuntary hospitalization, and criminalization of the mentally ill. Patients who, in former years, would have had their needs met by state hospitals are now incarcerated by the criminal justice system as treatment of last resort. Individuals are arrested most often for behaviors that the community finds intolerable, such as vagrancy, public urination and defecation, loitering, trespassing, petty theft and shoplifting, threatening and aggressive behavior, and substance abuse. Epidemiological studies have revealed that upward of 20% of individuals in county jails and state and federal prisons suffer from serious mental disorders. With more than 3,000 mentally ill inmates, the Los Angeles County Jail may be the largest psychiatric institution in the country.

The emphasis in almost all of these restrictive settings is on security, supervision, and safety, with little more than psychiatric evaluations, psychotropic medications, and custodial services available to the inmates. Rehabilitation is almost nonexistent, with the exception of sparse work details, educational classes, group "talk therapy," crafts and hobbies, and recreation. There have been some notable pioneering efforts to establish psychosocial rehabilitation in prison and forensic settings that have struggled to coexist with the prevailing punitive and custodial ideology held by security staff and administration as well as the general public.

Establishing and sustaining a therapeutic climate and milieu have been challenging, requiring compromises with overarching security for prevention of aggressive behavior and escapes. Therefore, successful implementation of rehabilitation in restrictive settings depends upon the selection, training, and supervising of staff, with the responsible program innovators offering considerable in vivo demonstrations of treatment procedures. Attitudinal obstacles, such as the belief that the mentally ill are preordained to chronicity and disability, can be overcome by compelling demonstrations of patients acquiring adaptive skills and prosocial behavior. A good example of the learning capacity of mentally ill offenders is their demonstrating that they understand the charges filed against them and the nature of court proceedings for their competency hearings.

TRAINING IN SOCIAL SKILLS AND DISEASE MANAGEMENT

Because of their user-friendliness and ease of implementation, the modules of the UCLA Social and Independent Living Skills Program—described in Chapters 3 ("Illness Management") and 5 ("Social Skills Training")—have been introduced in prisons and forensic hospitals in Canada and the United States. The California Department of Mental Health established a psychiatric rehabilitation program at the Vacaville State Prison in which mentally ill inmate-patients progressed through three levels of decreasing security as they revealed increasing skills in social and independent living. By the time they reached the third, day treatment level, they had completed training in basic communication skills, had practiced them with the mental health and security staff, and were stable enough to sleep in a dormitory and attend vocational rehabilitation and recreational activities off their unit. The remainder of the rehabilitation program consisted of their participating in modules for teaching disease management, recreation for leisure, and community re-entry skills.

Replicating this skills training program at a correctional facility in North Carolina, two master's-level behavior specialists supervised by a clinical psychologist led four modules: Medication Management, Symptom Management, Recreation for Leisure, and Basic Conversation Skills. Inmate-patients attended two module groups per day, 4 days per week for 1.5 hours per module. Each group comprised 7–10 inmate-patients. Over a 10-year period, 700 inmate-patients from the North Carolina prison system participated in the program, with 81% of them improving sufficiently to be paroled or transferred to prison outpatient units for aftercare (MacKain and Messer

2004). As an indication of the relevance of skills training technology for mentally ill offenders, clinicians from all United States federal prisons were trained to use the modules for social and independent living skills.

SOCIAL LEARNING PROGRAMS

Using the same behavioral principles and incentive systems as described earlier in this chapter for patients with treatment-refractory disorders, social learning programs have been mounted in several forensic facilities. The effectiveness of the social learning program at the maximum-security Fulton State Hospital in Missouri was documented by a 92% reduction in aggressive behavior from a stable, 3-month baseline. Total appropriate behavior of patients almost doubled from their entering the program to 1 year later. As an intermediate step between completion of the inpatient social learning program and successful reintegration into community life, patients lived in a group home within the security of the hospital grounds, where behavioral techniques were continued with more intermittent reinforcement and lower levels of supervision and monitoring (Menditto et al. 1994).

Skills training shifted to an emphasis on patients' applying their interpersonal dexterity to employment situations that were available with supports in the community. Sixty-four percent of the forensic patients entering the group home phase were successful in transitioning to community life. These individuals reported significant increases in their satisfaction with the quality of their lives, optimism about living independently, and hope for the future. Their progress toward recovery also was reflected by their engagement in functional activities during tenures of 7 or more years in the community with no instances of rearrest. Teaching social skills and reinforcing the full range of adaptive behaviors on a regular schedule displace the kinds of offensive and inappropriate behavior that often result in the criminalization of the mentally ill.

MANAGEMENT OF AGGRESSIVE BEHAVIOR

Aggression toward self and others and property destruction are criteria for involuntary hospitalization as well as for arrest, detention, and referral to high-security forensic facilities, jails, and prisons. Frequently, these behaviors continue to occur during incarceration, resulting in severe punishment in correctional settings and excessive use of seclusion and restraint in psychiatric hospitals.

Medications have been used as chemical restraint with little benefit on aggressive behavior, unless the behavior is a direct consequence of untreated psychotic or mood disorders. The Civil Rights Division of the U.S. Department of Justice frequently files legal complaints against hospitals and prisons that fail to develop alternatives to punishment in dealing with aggressive and destructive behavior of the mentally ill.

While most institutions have policies and procedures for *managing and terminating episodes* of hostile, aggressive, and destructive behavior, these rarely include rehabilitation approaches. A basic principle of rehabilitation is to *teach skills and offer supportive programs that lead to adaptive and functional social and instrumental role behavior.* The procedures described in the rest of this section will provide an overview of effective CBTs for aggressive, destructive, and threatening behaviors. However, it must be understood that reducing or eliminating the offending aggression is only the first step in rehabilitation. Once the anger, aggression, or destructive behavior has been brought under control, all the modes of skill building and social supports described at length in this book must be offered to empower the individual to communicate for meeting his/her needs and take advantage of social and occupational opportunities.

Anger Management

Useful for both preventing and treating violent behavior, anger management techniques are used by clinicians to lead the aggressor through a series of collaborative steps that involve cognitive and behavioral interventions:

- Identify the triggers for violence in the person–environment interaction: frustrations, annoyances and grievances, and insults and assaults by another.
- Illuminate the thoughts and emotions elicited by the triggering event: is the event interpreted as a provocation, threat, debasement, fear, anxiety and arousal, or anger?
- Determine whether the interpretations and reactions are realistic or based on misperceptions, misinterpretations, and overarousal.
- Identify alternative interpretations and explanations for the event when justified.
- Generate various options for behavioral coping responses that may avoid or minimize an aggressive act: withdrawal and avoidance, request for help from staff, use of calming self-talk, and self-induced relaxation.

In working with persons who are chronically angry and at risk for aggression, a sequence of treatment phases are used that involve cognitive restructuring, skill acquisition, and application training. The skill acquisition phase involves the patient in an active process to learn new cognitive and behavioral coping responses as well as develop better ways to manage stress and arousal. The therapist models and demonstrates the coping skills and has the patient rehearse the behavior with coaching and positive feedback.

CLINICAL EXAMPLE

Gene, a 32-year-old man with paranoid schizophrenia complicated by substance abuse, was incarcerated for aggravated assault with a knife. Both before and after imprisonment, he was irritable and quarrelsome, and his behavior often escalated into loud arguments followed by aggression. Because antipsychotic medication failed to reduce his aggression, Gene was referred to an anger management therapist. The therapist reviewed with Gene recent episodes when he had become angry. Some of the events were provoked by other inmates. Most of the episodes, however, were examples of Gene's misinterpreting the gaze, comments, or interactions as threats, insults, or teasing.

In the skill acquisition phase, Gene observed a series of photos and videotape vignettes in which subjects displayed various emotional expressions, including anger, sadness, disgust, and surprise. After correctly identifying the emotions associated with each portrayal, Gene and his therapist reviewed recent situations in which Gene had detected these emotions in those with whom he was conversing and interacting. Next, Gene was urged to consider alternative explanations for the verbal and nonverbal behavior of others that he was misinterpreting. Gene practiced situations where he got aroused and annoyed by something said to him but caught himself by asking, "What else might explain the other person's comments, tone of voice, and facial expression?"

In addition to repeatedly practicing these drills of accurate social perception, Gene and his therapist collaborated on developing behavioral coping skills that would be more effective in handling such situations. These coping skills included being assertive, asking the other person for clarification of what he was thinking and feeling, calmly expressing how he felt, and beating a hasty but judicious retreat to avoid an escalating situation. Gene's frequency of aggressive acts gradually fell from three a week to one every 2 months. In addition, the severity of his isolated episodes of aggression was much attenuated by his use of anger management.

Finally, training the patient to apply anger management in everyday situations consists of the therapist guiding the patient through provocative but safe and secure situations in which the newly acquired coping skills can be used. This final phase is also defined as *stress inoculation.*

Psychosocial Treatment in Lieu of Seclusion and Restraint

The use of physical control for aggressive, self-injurious, or destructive behavior must weigh the rights and safety of the individual against the safety of others—staff and fellow patients. While the courts have sanctioned the physical confinement of persons who are behaving dangerously, many psychiatric facilities limit or prohibit the use of seclusion and restraint. When these methods are used to excess, the federal courts, Justice Department, and patient advocacy organizations challenge the procedures as cruel and unusual punishment. Excessive use of seclusion and restraint may also reflect the failure of the institution to implement positive practices and psychosocial rehabilitation. In addition, many staff members prefer not to use physical control.

In this section, we present an overview of behavioral interventions that can reduce the need for seclusion and restraint. Aggressive, self-injurious, and destructive behaviors represent a "locked gate" that prevents an individual from returning to the community. A recovery-oriented approach to rehabilitation gives leeway to temporarily controlling therapies as a means to the ultimate goal of eliminating behaviors that the community will not tolerate. The evaluation and treatment procedures described in this section facilitate community reintegration of patients without resorting to the draconian methods of seclusion and restraint.

Before selecting an intervention, a practitioner using the framework of behavior analysis inquires, "What is causing the aggressive behavior, and how can it be changed?" Behavior analysis comprises the steps described in Table 9.7. The behavioral interventions that are effective alternatives to restrictive interventions such as seclusion and restraint are defined in Table 9.8.

The triggers of aggressive behavior are usually awkward and ineffective efforts by patients to obtain some need or request and the consequent frustration and anger. Staff members' typical responses to a patient's aggression involve struggling to restrain the aggressive individual, thereby inadvertently reinforcing the very behavior they intended to control. Loss of privileges, social isolation, and other adverse consequences of the destructive behavior more effectively convey to the patient the personal costs of his/her aggression without the use of physical punishment. Once the destructive behavior is controlled, social skills training can teach the patient to obtain a more positive response from others through appropriate interaction.

● TABLE 9.7

Stepwise behavior analysis of aggression

1. Identify antecedents of aggression or of stimuli correlated with the behavior's onset. An example is when a patient becomes frustrated and angry when staff members refuse his unreasonable requests.

2. Specify the aggressive behavior in operational terms so that all will agree when it occurs (e.g., shouting threats and expletives with fists clenched, angry facial expression and shoving or hitting).

3. Note the immediate consequences of the aggression that may be inadvertently maintaining it. Staff members can congregate in show of force and speak to patient in soft tone of voice, reassuring him that he will be all right if he de-escalates by sitting down and relaxing.

4. Inventory the patient's social, personal, and cognitive strengths and deficits and conduct a survey of personally relevant reinforcers for the patient. Reinforce the patient's positive qualities, using reinforcers that are appropriate to his values and preferences while ignoring provocative behavior.

5. Identify alternative ways of reducing anger and aggression in the current and future episode. Implement positive programming, differential reinforcement for behavior other than threats and anger, and social skills training to improve the patient's ability to express his frustration in words and to ask staff members to explain how and when he can have his request honored.

● TABLE 9.8

Examples of behavioral interventions for reducing aggressive and destructive behavior in children, adolescents, and adults

Positive programming	Planned and scheduled activities that are pitched to successfully engage the patient in appropriate behavior can displace frustration, angry interactions, and various types of aggression. Abundant reinforcement should be given to the patient for interacting appropriately in the activity.
Differential reinforcement of alternative, competing, and other behaviors	Staff gives social and tangible reinforcement to the patient for any behavior or interactions that are *not aggressive* or preludes to aggression. In practice, reinforcement is delivered after a specific interval has passed without aggression—for example, a person with frequent aggression might be on an every 15-minute schedule for reinforcement, with the time between reinforcements gradually lengthened as the frequency of aggression declines.

(continued)

● **TABLE 9.8** (*cont'd.*)

Stimulus control	A special location or signal is established for engaging in abusive, threatening, or obscene talking, and the patient is instructed to go to that location when such behavior occurs. The person can remain in the designated area for as long as the provocative behavior continues. The individual is typically ignored during this time, but as soon as the intolerable behavior ceases, the patient returns to the planned and scheduled activities, during which social interaction takes place and abundant reinforcement is given for appropriate behavior. In this technique, the special location becomes the stimulus for inappropriate behavior, and the environment in the rest of the unit or classroom gradually loses its stimulus value for the unacceptable behavior. A feasible and effective stimulus control procedure is called *time out from reinforcement,* in which the stimulus is a chair situated at the end of a corridor facing the wall. Patients can use this procedure for self-control and "cooling off" by taking a time-out when experiencing anger, arousal, or frustration. On a psychiatric unit for aggressive patients, this stimulus-control procedure was successful in reducing and eliminating violent behavior in 74% of the patients.
Contingent observation	Patients who demonstrate anger, verbal abuse, or destructive acts are instructed to sit quietly for a predefined period on the perimeter of a group activity. They watch peers and staff interact in appropriate ways and benefit from vicarious learning.
Overcorrection and teaching interaction	This technique combines instructional control with social skills training. When a patient is assaultive or destructive of property, he/she is instructed to make amends in an excessive, or overcorrecting, manner. In the case of breaking a chair, the patient is given some duct tape and is required to patch and fix the chair and also polish or dust all of the other chairs in the area. Then, the patient meets with a clinician, who asks the patient to identify the reasons for his/her destructive behavior. A behavioral analysis of the situation is done in a collaborative manner: antecedents and consequences of the aggression are examined for their role in the untoward event.

These treatment techniques for mentally ill offenders have been applied in community aftercare and parole programs as well as in forensic hospitals and prisons. Their effects are amplified by *conditional release or contingent parole* policies. Under these policies, seriously mentally ill inmates from prisons or forensic mental health institutions are discharged to the community at the end of their sentences or when psychiatrically rehabilitated and safe for community re-entry, but with several conditions. They must attend aftercare treatment programs one or more times each week, participate actively and not passively, demonstrate progress in achieving their personal goals for rehabilitation, and submit to random urine checks for use of illicit substances. Depending upon the contingencies embedded in the policy and state law, failure to meet the established conditions in the aftercare program can result in immediate return to the forensic facility. Conditional release has cut in half recidivism rates for mentally ill offenders in California.

The recovery of a person with schizophrenia or another disabling mental disorder is clearly impeded when that person displays bizarre behavior in response to hallucinations and delusions. Aggression, polydipsia, incontinence, abusive language, or screaming also marks the person as socially undesirable and will be stigmatizing. Rehabilitation, in conjunction with appropriate types and doses of psychotropic medication, can help the individual expand his/her repertoire of adaptive behavior that will displace antisocial acts. From that point, the recovery process can unfold with educational and supportive approaches, including the learning of disease management, social and independent living skills, and family problem solving; supported employment; housing; and continuing services from assertive community treatment teams.

▌ Rehabilitation of Older Adults

Challenging mental health care systems, the rapidly growing population of mentally ill older persons comprises the most disabled, vulnerable, dependent, doubly stigmatized, and underserved of patients with psychiatric disorders. Aging persons with serious mental illness have considerable problems with the behaviors essential for independent functioning: compliance with medication, access to physicians, money management, shopping, food preparation, nutrition, use of transportation, doing laundry, housework, care of their personal possessions, socialization, use of the telephone, and even the most basic activities of daily living such as ambulating, showering, and grooming. The impact of functional disability on quality of life is worsened by the geographical dispersion of family members and the resulting loss of supportive and caring relationships. Rehabilitation services that have documented effectiveness for preserving and remediating physical and psychosocial functioning are listed in Table 9.9.

Application of the rehabilitation services identified in Table 9.9 by a residential facility for elders with psychotic disorders complicated by medical problems and dementia resulted in salutary changes, as shown in Figure 9.8 (Patterson 1992). The rehabilitation services were introduced sequentially at different points in time after differing durations of baselines for three cohorts of patients. Monthly measurements were graphed for the mean number of 1) adaptive social activities engaged in by the residents and 2) restraints and extra medications for agitation. The dramatic effects of the implementation of rehabilitation were accompanied by substantial and significant improvements in independent functioning, domestic activity, socialization, and self-direction as measured by the Adaptive Behavior Scale.

Older adults with serious mental illness commonly have multiple medical problems compounded by poor general health that adds to their overall disability and increases the likelihood of their being placed in nursing homes or other supervised care. Therefore, rehabilitation services for older adults must cross the boundaries between psychiatric and medical care, an effort that requires outreach to other agencies, interagency agreements, communication, and joint planning and coordination. Collaborative care that integrates mental health and medical treatments is rational and congruent with the well-established chronicity of both types of disorders and their consequent needs for long-term continuity of services as an essential part of recovery. Diabetes, chronic lung disease, hypertension, and multiple sclerosis, as well as schizophrenia, recurrent depressions, and bipolar disorder, are enduring conditions that require indefinite, flexible levels of intervention that includes both medication and psychosocial services.

One such demonstration was carried out in New England, where community health nurses without formal psychiatric training completed a course on using social skills training (Bartels et al. 2004). They applied this approach to groups of elderly schizophrenia patients who met in the common rooms of their assisted living facility. The goals of the skills training were identified through ecological surveys of the needs of the elderly individuals, including situations pinpointed by the individuals themselves. Many of the interpersonal situations that were troublesome for the elders involved self-management of medications, illness management, and securing dignified and adequate medical and social services for which they lacked requisite community skills. Elders were randomly assigned to receive customary services or psychiatric and health rehabilitation services that encompassed a full range of capacities

● TABLE 9.9

Rehabilitation services of special value to elderly persons with mental disabilities

- Social, psychiatric, and medical services that are supportively "wrapped around" the elderly, many of whom are cognitively impaired and physically infirm

- Interventions that improve activity levels for elderly mentally ill living in residential facilities, including
  » Scheduling activities, including "tea time" chats with staff
  » Opening the kitchen for snacks as needed
  » Providing open access to the nursing office
  » Arranging community outings with destination shopping, restaurant, and other recreational activities
  » Using interior design to facilitate small group interaction

- Training and personal supports in disease management for elders
  » Is imperative, especially in providing motivation and prompting, monitoring, and reinforcing reliable adherence to multiple medical regimens.
  » Streamlines medical and psychiatric regimens and reaches out to medical professionals providing services to the elderly, resulting in fewer adverse drug interactions and improved coordination and outcomes.

- Interventions that minimize the effects of mobility problems
  » Physical and occupational therapy, training in activities of daily living, supported living, and consultation with and provision of psychoeducation to families and staff of assisted living facilities and nursing homes
  » Attention to the emotional and financial burdens of family members who carry most of the burden of care for elders with mental disorders, which will reduce strain on the family and, in turn, stress on the patient

- Collaboration that involves positioning a psychiatric nurse in primary care clinics and practices for consultation on elderly depressed outpatients
  » Enables nurses to integrate mental health treatments with treatments for medical problems.
  » Reduces stigma and markedly improves outcomes.
  » Enables patients to get all needs in "one-stop shopping."

- Adaptation of rehabilitation to the limitations of the elderly, including
  » An activity contingency plan with separate lists of pleasant events, adjusted for participation with varying energy levels, pain, weather, social contacts, finances, access for persons with canes and wheelchairs, and transportation
  » Adjustments to compensate for visual, hearing, and cognitive impairments
  » Use of large-print handouts, multimedia formats, well-lit room with limited background noise, and repetition (e.g., through use of audiotape or videotape at home), which improves participation of elders

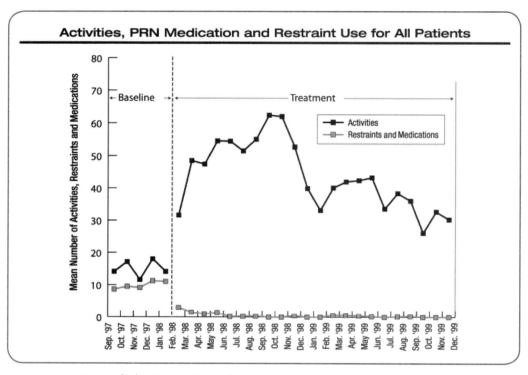

FIGURE 9.8 Increased adaptive activities and reduced restraints and medication after introduction of multimodal rehabilitation for elderly patients with psychosis and co-occurring medical problems and dementia in a residential setting. *Source.* Redrawn from Patterson 1992.

related to the independent functioning of the participants. The design of this systemic approach to rehabilitation of older adults is depicted in Figure 9.9.

Individuals who received skills training plus conventional health management services showed substantial and significantly greater improvements in independent living skills than those receiving nursing and medical services alone. Areas of community functioning that showed the greatest improvement for those receiving skills training were social mixing, care for possessions, personal appearance and hygiene, food preparation, and health management. The value of the integrated intervention was heightened because its effectiveness was achieved by practical nurses and bachelor's-level case workers who provided both skills training and health management. Successful cross-training of nursing personnel and paraprofessionals indicates that the integrated program may be realistically transported to other communities where similar personnel are available.

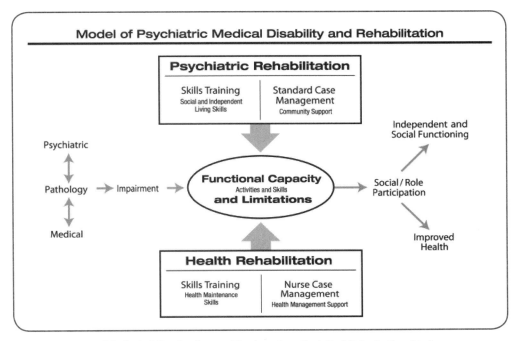

FIGURE 9.9 Model of rehabilitation for psychiatric and medical disabilities in the elderly.

▶ Special Services for the Problems of Other Groups of Special People

There are other unique populations of the severely mentally ill of which space constraints dictate only brief mention. These include adolescents, including those in transition to adulthood; young patients with the recent onset of a severe mental disorder; women; the homeless; persons living in impoverished and crime-ridden inner cities as well as in geographically remote rural areas; and patients with concurrent medical disorders such as morbid obesity, diabetes, hypertension and other cardiovascular disease, and HIV/AIDS. Treatment and rehabilitation strategies, services, and modalities have been developed to meet at least some of the clinical requirements and disability status of these subgroups of the severely mentally ill (see pp. 498–499).

The prospects for recovery are particularly bright for young persons with the recent onset of a serious mental disorder. The time and effort required to identify the early signs of schizophrenia and other chronic disorders are repaid many times over by the favorable response of this population to treatments specially designed and delivered for early intervention. These young individuals have a head start on the recovery marathon because their symptom remission more readily occurs. Furthermore, their impairments and disabilities have not yet become chronic and are therefore more malleable through rehabilitation.

For this reason, increasing attention has been given to developing innovative approaches for patients with the recent onset of a mental disorder. For example, efforts are under way in Scandinavia, Australia, Canada, and the United States to identify individuals with early signs of their disorder so that treatment can be initiated before disability ensues. A major challenge to early intervention is the denial of illness by young patients whose efforts to flee the stigma of mental illness often take the form of "flight into health" and nonadherence with medication. Motivational interviewing and conjoint psychoeducation with family members can create an enduring therapeutic alliance that often counters treatment refusal. With the hope of preventing schizophrenia, several groups are attempting to provide biobehavioral interventions at an even earlier prodromal phase of schizophrenia. It is too early to come to conclusions about the value of these approaches; however, they have inspired considerable interest among professionals and hope among patients and their families.

SPECIAL POPULATION	SPECIAL TREATMENT
Persons with recent-onset schizophrenia	Linking treatment to patients' personal goals and including family members and patients as part of the treatment team.
	Psychoeducation for patients and families, and motivational enhancement to highlight personal salience of antipsychotic medication. Social skills training, supported education, and employment as keys for friendship and "getting a life."
Youths transitioning to adulthood	Residential treatment using social learning principles with social skills training and wraparound educational, vocational, and housing services. Motivational enhancement for reliable use of maintenance psychotropic medications.
Persons with borderline personality disorder	Behavioral family therapy to facilitate progress to self-support and independent living.
	Motivational enhancement to engage in treatment, followed by training in emotional regulation using techniques of mindfulness, relaxation, and meditation.
	Learning to accept disturbing thoughts, anger, and frustration rather than acting out impulsively and self-destructively in response to them.
	Social skills training to improve and gain satisfaction from interpersonal relationships.

Women	Teaching about interactions between medications and female hormones, pregnancy, and postpartum depression. Teaching personal safety and coping skills to abused women recovering from trauma. Teaching parenting skills for mothers with serious mental disorders.
Homeless mentally ill persons	Using tangible reinforcers—food, clothing, shelter, showers, and financial entitlements—to facilitate engagement in treatment.
	A longitudinal, trusting relationship with an outreach worker who is empathic for concerns of the homeless for autonomy, privacy, and freedom of movement. Rehabilitation can only be effective after appropriate and stable housing has been achieved.
Mentally ill persons in crime-ridden areas	Teaching patients "street smarts" to maintain safety, prevent stigma, and avoid conflicts with gang members, drug pushers, and police.
	Using the Substance Abuse Management Module for teaching drug refusal, harm avoidance, and "healthy" pleasures.

▶ Summary

The concepts, principles, and practices of biopsychosocial rehabilitation are equally applicable to all patients with disabling mental disorders, including the full range of special populations: persons from minority cultures, individuals with dual diagnoses, persons with treatment-refractory illness, mentally ill offenders, aggressive individuals, persons with borderline personality disorder, and older and very young persons. Rehabilitation *practices* need to be adapted to the special characteristics of clinical state, developmental level, lifestyle, culture, level of functioning, and treatment setting. We are all challenged to learn how to develop trusting, working relationships with individuals from very different backgrounds and with very different perspectives on mental illness than ourselves. When practitioners are informed and competent in relating and collaborating with persons with diverse backgrounds, treatment is more effective and recovery from symptoms and disability is a realistic goal.

For patients from special populations to achieve their personal goals, there must be a systemwide approach for organizing novel services with strong administrative support. Practitioners are forewarned about entering unfamiliar waters without the strong, visible, and continuing mandate from top and middle management. Resources, recruitment of clinicians experienced with the special population, and inclusion of the stakeholders from that population are all prerequisites of successful program development. For example, developing a dual-diagnosis treatment program or one devoted to the mental health and medical needs of the elderly necessitates having an experienced and supportive program manager whose administrative leadership provides an open door for solving problems that inevitably involve both clinical and human resources. The program manager or designated rehabilitation coordinator must be given authority to monitor the program and use whatever personnel interventions may be necessary to assure quality improvement and regular scheduling and implementation of rehabilitation services.

All successful treatments pegged to patient groups that have distinctive needs are characterized by creativity in organizing resources and innovativeness in adapting and refocusing existing treatments. Effective services for special populations often depend on flexibility, active outreach, and consultation and liaison with other health and social entities to work out shared responsibilities for treatment and supports. Having paid respects to the importance of tailoring treatments for populations with unique characteristics, I must also stress that *people from different backgrounds and life experiences are much more alike than different.* Therefore, planning rehabilitation for special populations requires tweaking but not wholesale changing of treatments that have been empirically validated with more commonly encountered patients.

We must beware of the pitfalls that come from condescension or other stereotypes toward persons with special characteristics and make every effort to elicit their sometimes idiosyncratic personal goals and preferences for treatment. Like more conventional patients, persons with special forms of mental disabilities should be engaged to whatever degree possible in a collaborative treatment process. Tailoring treatment to the special characteristics of the patient requires unique balances between teaching skills and providing environmental supports. For example, elderly patients and patients with treatment-refractory schizophrenia have a greater need for "wraparound" services than for skills training. It is not reasonable to expect individuals who are physically and cognitively impaired to learn or relearn the full range of skills required for complete autonomy. However, even persons with lifelong mental disorders have every reason to expect to improve with rehabilitation and achieve some level of recovery from their illness and disability if they receive long-term continuous, comprehensive, coordinated, collaborative, consumer-oriented, and competent care.

❱ Key Points

- The kaleidoscopic diversity of mental disorders does not always lend itself to diagnosis-specific treatments. For special groups of patients, the criterion-based diagnostic categories and standard treatments do not do justice to their clinical needs. In particular, specially crafted and adapted treatments are essential for older adults, aggressive persons, and mentally disordered offenders, as well as for individuals from distinctive cultures and those with dual diagnoses and treatment-refractory disorders.

- Treatments and services have been designed and effectively applied to these special categories of patients whose unique characteristics demand approaches that are congruent with their needs and complexities.

- Even within the special populations, individual differences among the patients are far more important than the common characteristics that they share. Thus, the imperative of individualizing treatment trumps clumping each cultural and clinically unique group and painting them with the same indiscriminate brush.

- Among the varied ethnic, racial, and cultural groups of patients, Latinos deserve attention because of their disproportionately great and rapidly growing representation in the United States. Culturally competent treatment includes such considerations as integrating families in services, destigmatizing mental illness by referring to it as *nervios* (medically based) rather than *locura* (crazy), and understanding that cohesiveness of families preempts independent living.

- An evidence-based example of a treatment that meets the expectations and norms of Latinos is the use of skills training for illness management in which family members are intrinsic to the treatment enterprise. Treatments should be congruent with the level of acculturation and specific ethnic regions in Latin America from which patients emigrated.

- Services that are integrated, evidence-based, person-centered, and results-driven can make a dent in the therapeutic obstacles posed by substance-abusing mentally ill individuals. Effective elements of service include motivational enhancement, teaching skills for harm reduction and relapse prevention, money management through representative payees, random urine tests, vocational rehabilitation, and spiritual and religious supports.

- The Substance Abuse Management Module teaches patients to climb the "slippery slope" from relapse to recovery, focusing on a variety of skills, money management, and community supports.

- Patients whose illness has been refractory to customary biobehavioral services require more intensive, incremental, and long-term psychosocial approaches with a reliance on cognitive-behavioral therapy, contingent reinforcement programs targeted at behaviors that interfere with community functioning, reinforcement sampling, and clozapine.

- Mentally ill offenders, all too often relegated to institutions where safety, security, and supervision outweigh rehabilitation, benefit from illness management and learning skills that promote community adjustment and "street smarts." Contingent release programs with involuntary outpatient services reduce the likelihood of recidivism.

- Aggressive patients benefit from immersion in planned and scheduled treatments that teach them appropriate social interactions and social problem solving. Teaching skills that enable individuals to communicate appropriately for achieving their needs is central to anger management; the teaching interaction, differential reinforcement for nonaggressive behaviors, and time out from reinforcement have an evidence base to their use.

- Older adults with serious mental illness commonly have multiple medical problems that are compounded by poor general health, which adds to their overall disability. Rehabilitation services must cross the boundaries between psychiatric and medical care, utilizing evidence-based practices that are adapted to the elderly and feasible when used in collaboration with medical and social service agencies. Although treatment requires more repetition to overcome cognitive deficits, there is solid evidence that seniors can and do respond to the same treatments that are effective for younger patients.

▶ Selected Readings

Cohen CI (ed): Schizophrenia Into Later Life: Treatment, Research, and Policy. Washington, DC, American Psychiatric Publishing, 2003

Corrigan PW, Mueser KT: Behavior therapy for aggressive psychiatric patients, in Understanding and Treating Violent Psychiatric Patients. Edited by Crowner ML. Washington, DC, American Psychiatric Press, 2000, pp 69–85

Hoagwood K, Burns BJ, Kiser L, et al: Evidence-based practice in child and adolescent mental health services. Psychiatr Serv 52:1179–1189, 2001

Huff RM, Kline MV (eds): Promoting Health in Multicultural Populations: A Handbook for Practitioners. Thousand Oaks, CA, Sage Publications, 1999

Janicki MP, Ansello EF: Community Supports for Aging Adults With Lifelong Disabilities. Baltimore, MD, Paul H Brookes, 2000

Kingdon DG, Turkington D: Cognitive Therapy of Schizophrenia. New York, Guilford, 2005

Koegel LK, Koegel RL, Dunlap G (eds): Positive Behavioral Support: Including People With Difficult Behavior in the Community. Baltimore, MD, Paul H Brookes, 1996

Kopelowicz A: Adapting social skills training for Latinos with schizophrenia. Int Rev Psychiatry 10:47–50, 1998

Kopelowicz A, Zarate R, Gonzalez-Smith V, et al: Disease management in Latinos with schizophrenia: a family-assisted, skills training approach. Schizophr Bull 29:211–227, 2003

LaVigna GW, Christian L, Willis TJ: Developing behavioral services to meet defined standards within a national system of specialist education services. Pediatr Rehabil 8:144–155, 2005

Liberman RP: Biobehavioral treatment and rehabilitation for older adults with schizophrenia, in Schizophrenia Into Later Life. Edited by Cohen CI. Washington, DC, American Psychiatric Publishing, 2003, pp 223–250

Liberman RP, Wong SE: Behavior analysis and therapy procedures as alternatives to seclusion and restraint, in The Psychiatric Uses of Seclusion and Restraint. Edited by Tardiff K. Washington, DC, American Psychiatric Press, 1984, pp 35–68

Linehan MM: Skills Training Manual for Treating Borderline Personality Disorder. New York, Guilford, 1993

Lopez SR, Kopelowicz A, Canive J: Strategies in developing culturally congruent family interventions for schizophrenia: the case of Hispanics, in Family Interventions in Mental Illness: International Perspectives. Edited by Lefley HP, Johnson DL. London, Praeger, 2002, pp 61–92

Meyers RJ, Miller WR: A Community Reinforcement Approach to Addiction Treatment. New York, Cambridge University Press, 2002

Mueser KT, Noordsy DL, Drake RE, et al: Integrated Treatment for Dual Disorders. New York, Guilford, 2003

Mueser KT, Rosenberg SD, Jankowski MK, et al: A cognitive-behavioral treatment program for posttraumatic stress disorder in severe mental illness. American Journal of Psychiatric Rehabilitation 7:107–146, 2004

Osher F, Steadman H, Barr H: A best practice approach to community re-entry from jails for inmates with co-occurring mental and substance abuse disorders. Crime Delinq 49:79–96, 2003

Patterson RL: Psychogeriatric rehabilitation, in Handbook of Psychiatric Rehabilitation. Edited by Liberman RP. New York, Macmillan, 1992, pp 276–289

Paul GL, Lentz R: Psychosocial Treatment of Chronic Mental Patients: Milieu Versus Social-Learning Programs. Cambridge, MA, Harvard University Press, 1977

Rosenberg SD, Mueser KT, Friedman MJ, et al: Developing effective treatments for posttraumatic disorders among people with severe mental illness. Psychiatr Serv 52:1453–1461, 2001

Substance Abuse and Mental Health Services Administration: Report to Congress on the Prevention and Treatment of Co-occurring Substance Abuse Disorders and Mental Disorders. Rockville, MD, U.S. Department of Health and Human Services, November 2002. Available at: http://www.samhsa.gov/reports/congress2002/index.html. Accessed May 28, 2007.

Sue DW, Sue D: Counseling the Culturally Diverse: Theory and Practice. New York, Wiley, 2003

U.S. Surgeon General: Mental Health: Culture, Race, and Ethnicity (SMA-01-3613). A Report of the Surgeon General. Rockville, MD, U.S. Department of Health and Human Services, 2001. Available at: http://download.ncadi.samhsa.gov/ken/pdf/SMA-01-3613/sma-01-3613A.pdf. Accessed May 28, 2007.

Welsh A, Ogloff J: The development of a prison-based program for offenders with mental illness. International Journal of Forensic Mental Health 2:59–71, 2003

Wong SE, Slama KM, Liberman RP: Behavioral analysis and therapy for aggressive psychiatric and developmentally disabled patients, in Clinical Treatment of the Violent Person. Edited by Roth LH. New York, Guilford, 1987, pp 20–53

▶ References

Bartels SJ, Teague GB, Drake RE, et al: Substance abuse in schizophrenia: service utilization and costs. J Nerv Ment Dis 181:31–37, 1993

Bartels SJ, Forester B, Mueser KT, et al: Enhanced skills training and health care management for older persons with severe mental illness. Community Ment Health J 40:75–90, 2004

Brenner HD, Dencker SJ, Goldstein MJ, et al: Defining treatment refractoriness in schizophrenia. Schizophr Bull 16:551–561, 1990

Glynn SM: Token economy approaches for psychiatric patients: progress and pitfalls over 25 years. Behav Modif 14:383–407, 1990

Glynn SM, Liberman RP, Bowen L, et al: The Clinical Research Unit at Camarillo State Hospital, in Behavior Therapy in Psychiatric Hospitals. Edited by Corrigan PW, Liberman RP. New York, Springer, 1994, pp 39–60

Ho AP, Tsuang JW, Liberman RP, et al: Achieving effective treatment of patients with chronic psychotic illness and comorbid substance dependence. Am J Psychiatry 156:1765–1770, 1999

Kazdin AE: The token economy, in Evaluating Behavior Therapy Outcome. Edited by Turner R, Asher LM. New York, Springer, 1985, pp 225–253

Kingdon DG, Turkington D: Cognitive Therapy of Schizophrenia. New York, Guilford, 2005

Kopelowicz A: Adapting social skills training for Latinos with schizophrenia. Int Rev Psychiatry 10:47–50, 1998

Kopelowicz A, Zarate R, Gonzalez-Smith V, et al: Disease management in Latinos with schizophrenia: a family-assisted, skills training approach. Schizophr Bull 29:211–227, 2003

Liberman RP, Van Putten T, Marshall BD, et al: Optimal drug and behavior therapy for treatment refractory schizophrenic patients. Am J Psychiatry 151:756–759, 1994

MacKain SJ, Messer CE: Ending the inmate shuffle: an intermediate care program for inmates with a chronic mental illness. Journal of Forensic Psychology Practice 4:87–100, 2004

Menditto AA, Valdes LA, Beck NC: Implementing a comprehensive social learning program within the forensic psychiatric service of Fulton State Hospital, in Behavior Therapy in Psychiatric Hospitals. Edited by Corrigan PW, Liberman RP. New York, Springer, 1994, pp 61–78

Mueser KT, Noordsy DL, Drake RE, et al: Integrated Treatment for Dual Disorders. New York, Guilford, 2003

Patterson RL: Psychogeriatric rehabilitation, in Handbook of Psychiatric Rehabilitation. Edited by Liberman RP. Needham, MA, Allyn & Bacon, 1992, pp 276–289

Paul GL, Lentz R: Psychosocial Treatment of Chronic Mental Patients: Milieu Versus Social-Learning Programs. Cambridge, MA, Harvard University Press, 1977

Roberts L, Shaner A, Eckman TA: Overcoming Addictions: Skills Training for People With Substance Abuse and Schizophrenia. New York, WW Norton, 1999

Shaner A, Khalsa ME, Roberts L, et al: Unrecognized cocaine use among schizophrenic patients. Am J Psychiatry 150:758–762, 1993

Shaner A, Eckman T, Roberts LJ, et al: Feasibility of a skills training approach to reduce substance dependence among individuals with schizophrenia. Psychiatr Serv 54:1287–1289, 2003

Substance Abuse and Mental Health Services Administration: Report to Congress on the Prevention and Treatment of Co-occurring Substance Abuse Disorders and Mental Disorders. Rockville, MD, U.S. Department of Health and Human Services, November 2002. Available at: http://www.samhsa.gov/reports/congress2002/index.html. Accessed May 28, 2007.

U.S. Surgeon General: Mental Health: Culture, Race, and Ethnicity (SMA-01-3613). A Report of the Surgeon General. Rockville, MD, U.S. Department of Health and Human Services, 2001. Available at: http://download.ncadi.samhsa.gov/ken/pdf/SMA-01-3613/sma-01-3613A.pdf. Accessed May 28, 2007.

CHAPTER 10

New Developments for Rehabilitation and Recovery

10

New Developments for Rehabilitation and Recovery

Skate to where the puck is going to be, not where it was.

WAYNE GRETZKY

NEW DEVELOPMENTS in psychiatric rehabilitation abound, and each innovation brings more of the mentally ill into the fold of recovery. Those of us who have labored in rehabilitation have seen our field yield services that have improved the lives of thousands of our patients and fertilized the emerging recovery movement. A new paradigm of *recovery* has been introduced into mental health; persons who have serious and disabling mental disorders can recover from their illnesses and live reasonably normal lives with other citizens in the community.

Psychiatric rehabilitation is generating evidence-based services that have expanded clinical treatment and gained validation through professionally endorsed practice guidelines, expert consensus, and best practices. Research is translating principles and technologies from behavioral and cognitive sciences into current clinical use. As a result, disability is gradually loosening its grip on ever-growing numbers of patients. There is no better way to combat the stigma of mental illness than to demonstrate that recovery is a predictable and common outcome related to the effectiveness of treatment and rehabilitation. To push stigma into the historical trash bin of past prejudices and discrimination, recovery will have to be unmistakably real, visible to patients, family members, practitioners, policy makers, legislators, the media, and the general population.

Recovery does not occur naturally; it requires a concerted effort on the part of patients, families, and professionals. Recovery is both an ongoing experiential lifestyle and objective benchmarks reflecting symptom remission, improved social and vocational functioning, and expansion of persons' social and independent living skills. As best practices of rehabilitation are more broadly disseminated and utilized by mental health practitioners, significant improvements can be expected in attitudes and actions that promote empowerment, self-responsibility, hope, and fulfillment. But recovery is a two-way street; experiencing greater hope for the future, responsibility for taking charge of one's life, and empowerment motivates patients to participate more actively in best practices and evidence-based services. Recovery cannot be expected to somehow rise to the surface from good intentions, an optimistic ideology, and the power of positive thinking. However, by combining efficacious rehabilitation technology with personal acceptance and positive self-reinforcement of one's gradual improvement in quality of life, recovery can be accelerated.

> "Man cannot discover new oceans unless he has the courage to lose sight of the shore."
> ANDRÉ GIDE (1869–1951)

A full-service partnership among professionals, patients, and professionals can produce a synergy for promoting recovery. Working together, we can pool our varied perspectives and create strategic modes of rehabilitation that are comprehensive, continuous, coordinated, consistent, competency-based, collaborative, consumer-based, and compassionate. Seriously mentally ill persons and their families should be vigorous participants in setting their own personal goals for treatment that will, if attained, enable them to reach and sustain recovery.

❿ Rehabilitation Tomorrow

While rehabilitation of the mentally ill has made major strides, there is still far to go. There are too many mentally disabled persons who receive no treatment or rehabilitation. How can we open the doors of rehabilitation to them and their families? The vast majority of our colleagues in mental health neither have heard of evidence-based practices nor are capable of using them with fidelity. What can we do to disseminate best practices to practitioners beyond the inadequate printed or spoken word? With high hopes bred by the recovery movement, our constituencies will expect more from us—better treatments, more enduring outcomes, and greater numbers of patients taking their place as functional citizens integrated in our communities. Looking ahead into a future that will be shaped by our work, we must make some choices. If we are to help our patients move forward toward normalization and community integration, we have to decide which "bridges to cross and which ones to burn."

The brain is the organ of interest for those of us who practice psychiatric rehabilitation and for our patients and their loved ones. As researchers learn more about the specific mechanisms that govern the functioning of the brain, novel pharmacological, cognitive, and behavioral treatments will make inroads on the neurobehavioral and social processes that impede functional and personally meaningful recovery.

In this chapter, we focus on new directions for psychiatric rehabilitation:

- Cognitive rehabilitation
- Extending the reach of rehabilitation with technology
- Prevention of mental disability
- Integrated vision and mission for recovery

▶ Cognitive Rehabilitation

Because cognitive functioning is directly linked to the ability of persons with mental disabilities to learn from their daily life experiences and make good use of them, new methods for improving cognition should also increase the possibilities for recovery. Is there evidence from basic neuroscience research to encourage new developments for cognitive rehabilitation?

PLASTICITY OF THE BRAIN: BASIS FOR COGNITIVE REHABILITATION

The plasticity of the brain is the rationale for cognitive rehabilitation. There is enormous functional flexibility in the 100 billion neurons of the brain, each of which makes an average of 1,000 connections with others, for some 100 trillion interconnections. Even when the brain's integrity has been compromised by illness or injury, the brain can compensate for the lost neuronal circuits and enable the individual to remain functional. In late adolescence and adulthood, the period of high risk for the onset of serious mental disorders, neuronal growth and development continue, with dendritic and axonal sprouting, modifications of receptor density, and alterations in white matter of the brain. Enriched environments and life experiences likewise can increase reserve brain capacity.

A nervous system injury, like a stroke, induces expression of both growth-promoting and growth-inhibiting genes that together determine the location and degree of reconnections around the dead cells to restore more function. But these neuronal mechanisms in the brain need to be activated and stimulated by behaviorally oriented treatments. For example, residual weakness and disuse of an arm, hand, or leg from a stroke can be treated effectively with physical therapies that elicit repeated behavioral responses aimed at challenging the brain to form new circuits.

In the case of stroke rehabilitation, physical therapists immobilize the patient's arm and hand that remain normal, forcing the individual to repeatedly utilize the weak arm and hand to perform a variety of tasks: unlocking a door, picking up small paper clips, pushing miniature cars around a track, and manipulating utensils. Programs that employ intensive retraining of stricken muscles and the nerves that control them can restore walking, climbing stairs, and talking in stroke victims during lengthy physical and speech therapy. Speech therapy for stroke victims, which also depends on the principle of repetition, requires the individual to repeatedly form sounds and then words. This enables many individuals to speak again with coherence.

COGNITIVE FUNCTIONING IN RECOVERY FROM SERIOUS MENTAL DISEASE

A key cognitive deficit in schizophrenia and other serious mental disorders involves working memory. Working memory is important for effective social or occupational role functioning, enabling individuals to hold more than one piece of information in their minds at the same time. When we make a phone call, enter our workplace, or go into a store to shop, we rely on our working memory. For example, when making a phone call, we have to keep in mind the phone number, what we want to say and convey, how we might respond if we get the person or a voice mail message, what we will do if the person we are calling is not available to speak, and how we will communicate our needs to the person if we encounter disinterest or a negative reply.

Working memory depends upon normal functioning of the prefrontal cortex, the most human of our brain areas, and its connections to other brain regions. Persons with schizophrenia show little or no activation in the prefrontal cortex when challenged by a working memory task. Functional recovery for persons with severe and persistent schizophrenia depends upon treatment that will improve or compensate for cognitive deficits, such as working memory. Recovery is slowed if cognitive deficits are permitted to impair psychosocial functioning, which, in turn, impedes attainment of personal goals and desired social roles.

Figure 10.1 compares key cognitive functions of persons who have recovered from schizophrenia, persons who have not recovered from schizophrenia, and normally functioning individuals (Kopelowicz et al. 2005). In every category of cognition but one, the recovered patients were functioning as well as the normally functioning control subjects; on the other hand, the nonrecovered patients were significantly below normal in

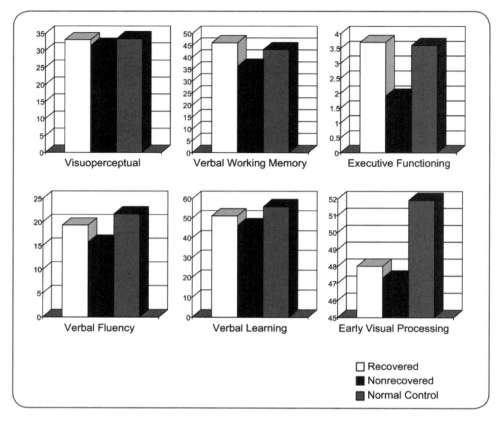

FIGURE 10.1 Neurocognitive functioning of recovered and nonrecovered persons with schizophrenia and normally functioning control subjects. *Source.* Data from Kopelowicz et al. 2005.

functioning. The one impairment that persisted in differentiating recovered patients from control subjects was early visual processing, which has been hypothesized as an enduring phenotypic "marker" of the genetic predisposition to schizophrenia. These findings suggest that many of the cognitive functions essential for recovery from schizophrenia are potentially malleable and open to remedial interventions.

Promising new treatments for improving areas of the brain responsible for cognitive and emotional functioning have been documented in the pharmacological and behavioral treatment of schizophrenia, obsessive-compulsive disorder, and major depression (Baxter et al. 1992; Hogarty et al. 2004; Spaulding et al. 1999). Patients with these disorders suffer from impairments in various types of memory, verbal learning, attention, reaction time, judgment, decision making, problem solving, and social perception. All of these impairments can interfere with learning skills and a person's ability to perform social and vocational roles.

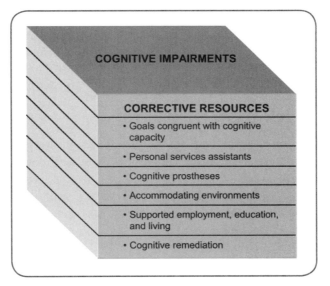

FIGURE 10.2 Correctives for cognitive impairments.

Evidence-based drug and psychosocial treatments that eliminate or ameliorate the symptoms of depression and obsessive-compulsive disorder have been shown to normalize brain areas associated with the symptoms (Brody et al. 1999; Schwartz et al. 1996). Since these symptoms and associated cognitive deficits interfere with learning, individuals with residual disabilities who benefited from such treatments enter social and vocational rehabilitation at higher platforms of readiness for training. Enhanced learning capacity also would be expected to result in faster and more substantial rehabilitation.

Two general treatment strategies for cognitive rehabilitation have been designed and tested for their efficacy in ameliorating cognitive deficits in schizophrenia and other major mental disorders. *Restorative* approaches improve cognitive functions by targeting deficits directly through either pharmacological or behavioral interventions. In contrast to restorative techniques, *compensatory* techniques aim to improve functioning by recruiting relatively intact cognitive processes to fulfill the role of impaired processes or by using prosthetic aids and social supports to compensate for the loss of function. These alternative interventions are now being translated from basic biological cognitive neuroscience and behavioral research into clinical practice. *Cognitive rehabilitation* is the term that encompasses both direct remediation approaches and compensatory approaches.

Examples of cognitive rehabilitation are shown in Figure 10.2. Setting treatment goals that do not burden a patient's cognitive capacities is a compensatory approach that can be exemplified by encouraging a patient with poor verbal learning and memory to select an occupation that requires physical and mechanical tasks and is consistent with the patient's abilities. Personal support specialists can work around cognitive deficits by providing assistance for those community activities that challenge the patient's cognitive deficits. Thus, for a patient with considerable impairment in working memory, the personal support specialist might accompany the patient to the Social Security office to inquire about a complicated change in benefits. Examples of cognitive prostheses that can compensate for memory lapses are marked calendars posted in a prominent place and reminder phone calls or postcards for appointments.

An accommodating environment might be a sound-attenuated work cubicle or quiet location that enables a distractible individual to maintain a focus of attention sufficient to perform in a job. Clinicians providing supported employment and education regularly take into account an individual's cognitive impairments and strengths in matching person to job or educational courses. Examples of restorative and compensatory modalities for cognitive rehabilitation are shown in Table 10.1.

● **TABLE 10.1**

Examples of restorative and compensatory approaches for cognitive rehabilitation

MODALITY	SPECIFIC TECHNIQUE	REHABILITATIVE EXAMPLE
Remedial or restorative		
Psychosocial	Attention shaping	Increased sustained attention for participation in social skills training group
Psychosocial	Cognitive remediation	Computer training of basic cognitive skills
Pharmacological	D-Cycloserine	Improved verbal and spatial learning and memory
Compensatory		
Psychosocial	Errorless learning	Modeling, task analysis, shaping, in vivo practice
Psychosocial	Cognitive adaptive therapy	Matching cognitive deficits with environmental reminders, cues, prompts, signs, and posters

As these new areas of research mature and show positive effects on patients' cognitive capacities, it should be possible to improve learning, memory, sustained attention, judgment, decision making, initiative, and problem solving. If these cognitive functions improve, they could conceivably translate into better psychosocial functioning of individuals and recovery. Two types of experimental treatment and research are *neurocognitive pharmacology* and *cognitive remediation*.

NEUROCOGNITIVE PHARMACOLOGY

Findings of therapeutic interest for neurocognitive pharmacology came from a study of cognitive functioning in hospitalized, severely disabled, long-stay patients whose schizophrenia was refractory to customary treatments. They received optimal doses of either the atypical antipsychotic drug risperidone or a traditional drug, haloperidol. Significant improvements for risperidone, but not haloperidol, were found in verbal working memory, problem solving, reaction time, and accurate perception of expressions of emotion (Green et al. 1997). Improvements in cognition as a result of risperidone and other novel antipsychotic drugs have been explained by their effects on the dopamine, serotonin, and other neurotransmitter systems in activating three brain regions that are instrumental for performing cognitive tasks: dorsolateral prefrontal cortex, parietal cortex, and supplementary motor area. The comparative neurocognitive effects of risperidone and haloperidol are depicted in Figure 10.3. The neurocognitive effects of antipsychotic drugs are mixed, with some studies showing beneficial pharmacotherapeutic impact, while others are equivocal at best. These differences in findings may be more apparent than real. The studies have been methodologically disparate, with different doses of medications, different cognitive tests, lack of controls on the mode of administration of the tests, patients at varying phases of their disorder, differences in age and sex of patients among the studies, and varying methods of recruitment of patients (Mishara and Goldberg 2004; Woodward et al. 2005).

Novel drugs that can repair or compensate for the brain abnormalities in schizophrenia and other serious mental disorders are now under development. D-Cycloserine, an antibiotic originally developed for tuberculosis, has been shown to accelerate recovery from panic and agoraphobia during cognitive-behavioral therapy. This agent also remediates deficits in verbal and spatial learning and memory. When this drug is given together with rehabilitative interventions that require learning and memory, patients with a variety of mental disorders show accelerated therapeutic responses to

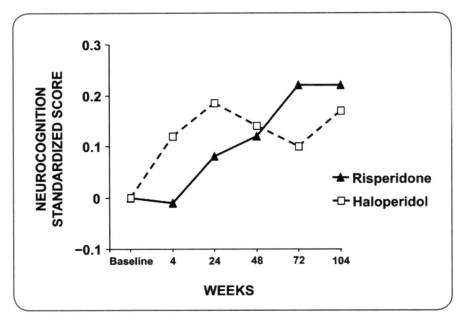

FIGURE 10.3 Neurocognitive effects of risperidone versus haloperidol in persons with treatment-refractory schizophrenia. *Source.* Data from Green 1999.

psychosocial rehabilitation. D-Cycloserine, along with D-serine and glycine, which enhance *N*-methyl-D-aspartate (NMDA) receptor function and neurotransmission, has therapeutic potential in improving negative symptoms and cognitive deficits of schizophrenia. If drugs can improve cognition, it is likely that patients receiving such drugs will gain advantages when they subsequently participate in social and vocational activities that otherwise would burden and strain patients' cognitive capacities.

It is well known that smoking is endemic in persons with schizophrenia, presumably because nicotine reduces the concentration of neuroleptic drugs in the blood and brain, thereby reducing unpleasant side effects. However, it has been more recently demonstrated that nicotine exerts powerful, direct neurocognitive effects in persons with schizophrenia. Nicotine improves attentional and working memory deficits in schizophrenia, whereas abstinence worsens these two cognitive capacities. Thus, it appears likely that schizophrenia patients may self-administer nicotine through cigarette smoking to remediate cognitive deficits. Investigators are now designing drugs that produce nicotine-like cognitive remediation without the addictive and pathological effects of nicotine and cigarettes. Caffeine is another drug that, when ingested in modest doses, improves alertness, attentiveness, and memory. If pharmacological agents can improve brain activity, can we use psychosocial interventions to *train the brain*?

COGNITIVE REMEDIATION

Training the brain is one of the most promising new directions for rehabilitation. If basic brain mechanisms essential for learning, memory, attention, initiative, problem solving, and emotional responsiveness can be normalized using behavioral and educational techniques, the number of patients who gain the potential for recovery from schizophrenia and other severe disorders will be multiplied. The use of the computer, with its vast programming capabilities for repetitive drills and exercises to remediate cognition, is depicted in Figure 10.4.

In a series of studies with schizophrenia patients by investigators and collaborators at the UCLA Clinical Research Center for Schizophrenia and Psychiatric Rehabilitation, social perception, memory, sustained attention, and more complex executive functions such as problem solving have been normalized by behavioral therapies such as cueing, repeated practice, and contingent positive reinforcement (Green 1999; Green et al. 1990; Silverstein et al. 2001; Spaulding et al. 1999; Van der Gaag et al. 2002). The substantial improvements in executive functions and sustained attention resulting from cognitive remediation, with functioning and attention reaching normal levels, are shown in Figure 10.5.

These methods also can lead to improved social and vocational functioning relevant to everyday life, as is shown in Figure 10.6. In this research, patients with schizophrenia were randomly assigned to receive supportive

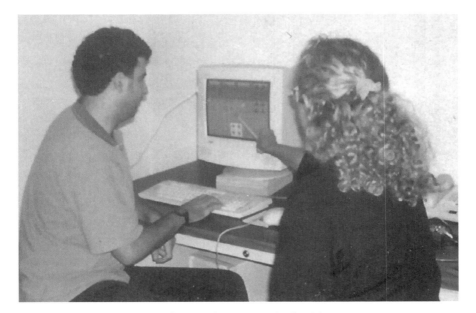

FIGURE 10.4 Cognitive remediation using computerized training.

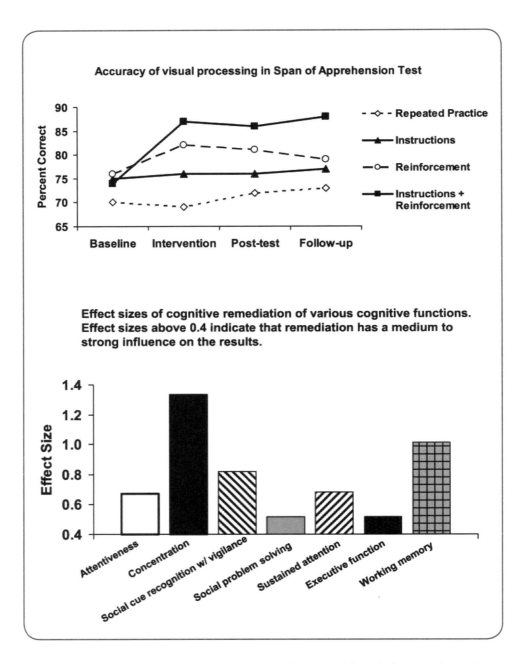

FIGURE 10.5 Cognitive remediation of Span of Apprehension Task (SPAN) of sustained attention and other neurocognitive capacities in persons with schizophrenia. Instructions and positive reinforcement of the SPAN result in levels of sustained attention within the normal range. Effect sizes for other cognitive functions that are above 0.4 indicate that the remediation has a medium to strong influence on the improvement in performance. Training the brain to improve cognitive functioning includes specific instructions and positive reinforcement contingent upon correct performance on cognitive tasks *Source.* Data from Kern et al. 1995 and Twamley et al. 2003.

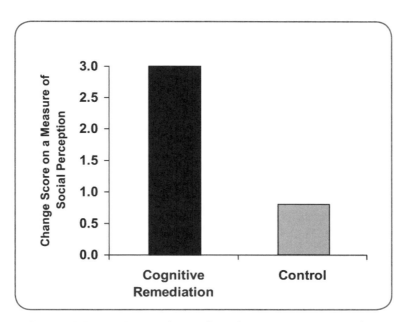

FIGURE 10.6 Cognitive remediation of social perception in persons with schizophrenia improves the accuracy of their interpreting verbal and nonverbal aspects of communications from others during conversations. *Source.* Data from Van der Gaag et al. 2002.

therapies or 22 sessions of training in accurate perception of the emotions of others in the laboratory, where they learned to filter relevant from irrelevant stimuli, practice various facial expressions, and role-play recent experiences in recognizing emotions of others and responding appropriately. The training also included recalling memories of past events that aided the individual in understanding the cues, context, norms, and rules for appropriate behavior in social situations. A third focus of training was to understand the meaning of facial expressions through rapid recognition of the emotions of people in social situations. Results of the study showed a significant beneficial effect of training on social perception, bringing the patients who received the training close to the normal range (Van der Gaag et al. 2002). Prospective, follow-up studies have revealed that accurate perception of emotions in others is an important predictor of social and vocational functioning.

Recent demonstrations of the beneficial effects of cognitive remediation with schizophrenia patients are harbingers of future progress in social and vocational rehabilitation. Three well-controlled studies used cognitive remediation to achieve improvements in 1) *sustained attention* associated with basic conversation skills, 2) *working memory* and hours worked on a job per week, and 3) *verbal and working memory, cognitive flexibility,* and *social cognition* and their effects on social adjustment (Bell et al. 2001; Hogarty et al. 2004; Silverstein and Wilkniss 2004). The considerable improvement in neurocognition resulting from the varied remedial strategies used in these studies portends favorably for novel therapeutic approaches that will hasten recovery in cognitively impaired individuals.

Attention Training

Reinforcing sustained attention was highly effective in enabling patients to achieve longer periods of active involvement and participation in a group for training conversation skills. Therapists provided "shaping tokens" and praise contingent on incrementally longer periods of sustained attention in highly distractible, disorganized, long-stay hospitalized patients. Patients were given tokens, exchangeable for a variety of desired commodities, each time they exceeded their previously ascertained duration of focusing their attention on the therapist. Patients increased their sustained attention from an average of less than 2 minutes to an average of 45 minutes. As sustained attention increased to normal levels, tokens and praise were given more sparsely (Silverstein et al. 2001). In Figure 10.7, a therapist is giving a token to a patient in a conversational skills group contingent upon that patient's increased duration of sustained attention to the trainer.

Patients concomitantly participated in a 90-minute group for learning conversation skills. Their spontaneously initiated, coherent, and relevant speech was measured in this skills training module. As can be seen from the results shown in Figure 10.8 for one of the patients, sustained attention rose from 10 to 55 minutes and appropriate speech increased from zero to approximately five spontaneously initiated comments. Patients who did not receive the shaping tokens and praise showed no increase in their socially directed attention (Silverstein and Wilkniss 2004). This method of training the brain's attentional capacity, now replicated in California, New York, Illinois, Missouri, and Nebraska, documents the specific clinical benefits of cognitive remediation for social conversation.

Cognitive Enhancement for Work and Social Functioning

Another study shows the benefits of cognitive remediation on the work capacity of outpatients with schizophrenia. All 145 patients participated in a transitional employment program, holding down jobs in various depart-

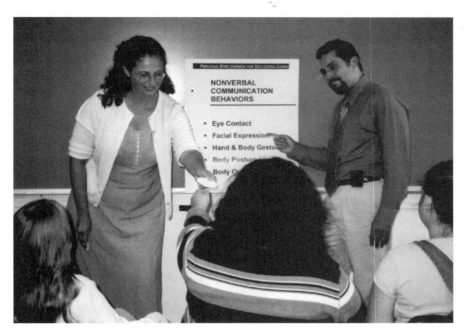

FIGURE 10.7 Attention-shaping is shown taking place in an ongoing session of conversational skills training. A co-therapist is handing a token to a patient who has just met her criterion duration of sustained attention to the trainer. At the same time, praise is given to her for meeting her goal. A poster listing the nonverbal skills being taught in the conversational skills group is used to orient patients and amplify the learning process.

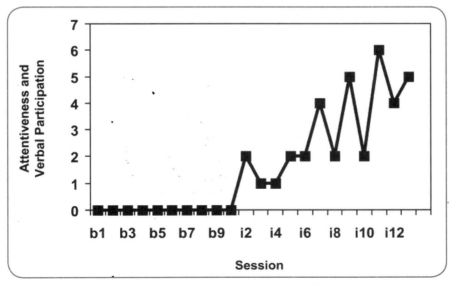

FIGURE 10.8 Remediating sustained attention in a patient with treatment-refractory schizophrenia with behavior shaping. *Source.* Data from Silverstein et al. 2001.

ments of a medical center that paid $3.40 per hour for 15–20 hours per week. In addition to work assignments, patients in the cognitive training program were given 5 hours of computer-mediated training of attention, memory, and cognitive flexibility per week for 6 months. They also received daily feedback on their attentiveness and memory during work and a weekly social skills training group. Fifty-two percent of the patients who got the computer-based memory training normalized their performance on memory tasks, a finding that lends further weight to the malleability of the brain and the feasibility of recovery from schizophrenia.

The patients in this program had their hours worked recorded for 12 months. Patients in the cognitive training program worked an average of 11 hours per week. This was significantly greater than the 7 hours per week worked by their counterparts who participated only in transitional employment. In grasping the significance of cognitive remediation for schizophrenia, a key lesson to be learned is the importance of intensity and duration of training if clinically significant improvements are to be expected (Bell et al. 2001).

In another program with a longer duration of treatment, a different form of cognitive enhancement was conducted with outpatients receiving a variety of antipsychotic medications. As in the other projects, the treatment derives from the assumption that neuroplasticity enables the brain to respond to systematic training of cognitive functions deemed important for social functioning and recovery (Hogarty et al. 2004). The researchers randomly assigned 121 patients to either cognitive enhancement plus enriched supportive therapy or enriched supportive therapy alone. Cognitive enhancement included 75 hours of computer-assisted training in attention, memory, and problem solving combined with 1.5 hours per week of exercises in social perception and interaction. The latter encompassed skills taught in the Basic Conversation Skills Module: recognizing social norms, identifying "go" and "no go" signals from one's conversational partner for timing one's conversational openers, enhancing motivation and learning topics for starting conversations, balancing active listening and self-disclosure, maintaining flexibility of problem solving in communicating effectively with others, and extending conversation skills into everyday social contacts. Treatment lasted for 2 years (Hogarty et al. 2004).

As depicted in Figure 10.9, the patients who received cognitive enhancement showed substantially more improvements on a composite measure of neurocognition, which included verbal memory, working memory, problem solving, executive functions, psychomotor speed, and vigilance. Greater improvements also were experienced in speed of information processing, cognitive style, social cognition, and social adjustment. Consumer satisfac-

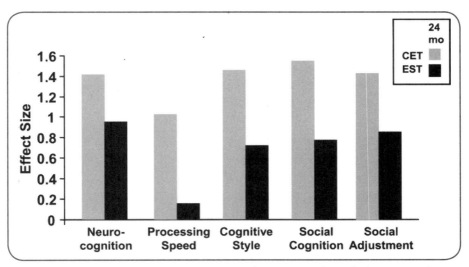

FIGURE 10.9 Improved performance in cognitive functioning and social adjustment with cognitive enhancement therapy for schizophrenia patients. CET = cognitive enhancement therapy; EST = enriched supportive therapy. *Source.* Data from Hogarty et al. 2004.

tion with cognitive enhancement therapy was very high, as witnessed by 87% of participating patients stating that the treatment was enjoyable and helped them achieve a better quality of life (Hogarty et al. 2004).

As computers become more creatively programmed, portable, and integrated with telephone, video, and voice for interactive communication, the field of cognitive remediation will concomitantly expand in utility and impact in ways that presently we can only imagine. Advances in cognitive remediation will also come from the close interrelationships among cognition, emotion, and motivation. It is becoming clear that greater efficacy is found from forms of cognitive remediation that are intrinsically motivating to the patient. That is, the participants must see the computer training of cognitive functions as relevant to their own personal goals in life. Connecting cognitive remediation to motivational enhancement has been successfully done; for example, when individuals realize that improved learning and memory will quicken their obtaining a desired job, they spend more time and work harder on their remediation tasks.

COMPENSATING FOR COGNITIVE DEFICITS: ERRORLESS LEARNING AND COGNITIVE ADAPTIVE TRAINING

Consistent with the plasticity of the brain, it has been known for some time that human beings can compensate for lost sensory and cognitive functions by using alternative, reserve brain capacities. Whether psychosocial functioning is improved by interventions that act directly or indirectly to overcome cognitive deficits, the bottom line for advocates of recovery is improved personal competencies that enhance prospects for work, friendship, and community participation.

There are two new compensatory techniques that override the many cognitive disabilities associated with schizophrenia and other serious mental disorders: errorless learning and cognitive adaptive training.

Errorless Learning

Errorless learning minimizes the demands on a mentally ill person's already burdened and deficient explicit memory that requires conscious and effortful processing of verbal information. Errorless learning makes use of implicit or procedural learning and memory, which are intact in persons with schizophrenia and related disorders. Implicit learning and memory rely on automatic cognitive processing that is fueled by overlearned, heavily practiced, and spontaneous behavioral skills. Examples of procedural memory are driving a car, riding a bike, skiing, greeting someone, and saying "thank you" or "sorry." In all these examples, requisite behaviors are carried out with little or no conscious thinking. Once social and instrumental abilities are mastered through errorless learning, they can remain in a person's behavioral repertoire durably and without expending the less available, verbally mediated memory.

In errorless learning, the interpersonal or vocational activities that the individual must learn for improving his/her social adjustment first are broken down through a task analysis into very simple steps. To enable the patient to learn a skill without committing errors, the therapist, teacher, or job coach utilizes guided instruction, modeling or demonstrations, coaching, practice, positive feedback, and repetition of the correct responses with close supervision throughout. The patient and therapist then proceed stepwise to more difficult task elements. One work task required patients with schizophrenia and schizoaffective disorder to sort business records alphabetically by name of customer, then city of address, and finally type of product purchased. A second work task required individuals to assemble a toilet tank mechanism. These two work tasks had been validated by community employers and vocational counselors as equivalent to those expected from entry-level employees. As shown in Figure 10.10, patients who participated in the errorless learning procedure were significantly more accurate in the respective tasks than their counterparts who received more conventional training (Kern et al. 2002).

Errorless learning can also be applied to rehabilitation of deficits in social

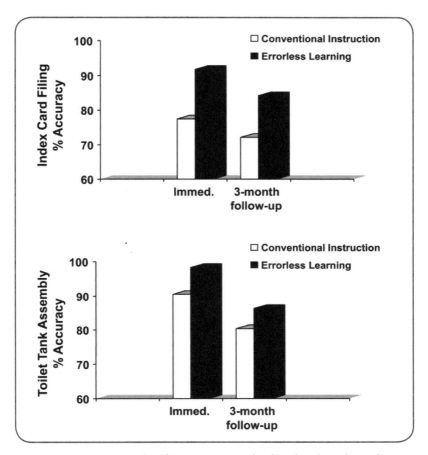

FIGURE 10.10 Improved performance on entry-level work tasks with errorless learning for patients with schizophrenia or schizoaffective disorder. *Source.* Data from Kern et al. 2002.

skills, an area of considerable awkwardness for persons with serious and disabling mental disorders. In a study conducted with 60 clinically stable outpatients with schizophrenia, patients were randomly assigned to either errorless learning of social problem-solving skills or another approach to social problem solving, in which no errorless learning principles were used. As noted in Figure 10.11, the patients who received errorless learning significantly improved their social problem-solving skills that required dealing with novel problems not encountered by the patients during their training. The patients in the contrast group did not show significant improvement in social problem solving (Kern et al. 2005). Errorless learning principles have also been applied to transitional employment, psychogenic polydipsia, basic conversation skills, money management, and self-care skills such as personal hygiene and maintaining one's personal possessions.

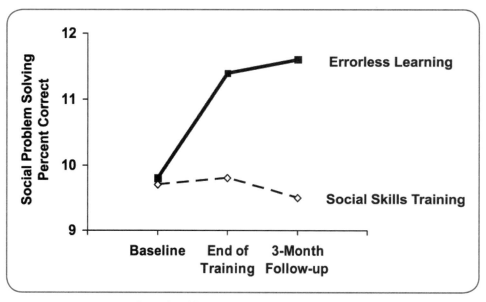

FIGURE 10.11 Improved social problem solving with errorless learning for patients with schizophrenia or schizoaffective disorder. *Source.* Data from Kern et al. 2005.

Cognitive Adaptive Training

Cognitive adaptive training utilizes environmental cues and prompts to compensate for deficits in memory and problem solving. Signs, labels, checklists, alarms, signaling devices, and electronic communication such as cell phones, beepers, pagers, and electronic alarms built into the caps of medication bottles are utilized to provide reminders for essential activities of daily living, medication use, attendance at treatment appointments, and work. The prescription for the types of cognitive adaptive training that any one patient may need derives from assessments of the patient's 1) level of memory, attention, apathy, problem solving, initiative, and goal-directed activity; 2) functional needs; and 3) home or work environment. The clinician makes a home visit to identify safety hazards; to organize clothing, dressing, and personal hygiene sites; and to determine the location of medication so that reminders, posters, and other cueing devices may be strategically placed (Velligan et al. 2000).

The overall therapeutic purpose of cognitive adaptive training is to improve and sustain the adjustment and quality of life of individuals living in the community. When the training is successful, individuals whose learning, memory, and problem-solving abilities are compromised by cognitive deficits can meet expected norms for self-care, money management, room and apartment maintenance, and appointments (Velligan et al. 2000).

CLINICAL EXAMPLE

Michael lived in an apartment but was always on the verge of relapsing and being hospitalized because of forgetting to take his evening medication. He also was overweight with marginal hyperglycemia. He would eat dinner at 5 P.M., fall asleep watching television, and awaken in the middle of the night and snack from the refrigerator. His sleepiness, superimposed upon his memory deficits, interfered with his medication compliance. A personal support specialist surveyed his apartment and, with Michael's concurrence, installed an electric alarm clock with the alarm set for 7:30 P.M. each evening, the time that Michael customarily dozed off. Michael agreed to respond to the alarm by taking his meds, after which he turned off the alarm. A sign with large print stating, "SET ALARM 7:30 P.M." and "NO NITE SNACKS," was taped to the refrigerator door. The sign also held cartoons of an obese person carrying a huge amount of snacks and a person entering a psychiatric hospital. These simple cues were successful in improving the regularity of his use of medication and led to significant weight reduction.

Extending the Reach of Rehabilitation With Technology

Computers, video feedback, telepsychiatry, mobile phones, beepers, and wireless, handheld devices are to psychiatric rehabilitation what technologies such as angioplasty, endoscopy, joint replacements, heart–lung machines, and arthroscopy are to medicine. Electronic technology can be useful for both extending and amplifying treatments beyond the limitations of face-to-face contacts. Many mental health centers and hospitals have computers, but they are reserved for use of the staff. Similarly, clinical facilities are often equipped with video and monitors with DVD or VCR players, but these devices are usually restricted to continuing education programs for employees.

Computers and video are no longer costly, they are easy to use, and patients find them engaging and motivating. In fact, in their everyday lives, patients spend a lot more time watching television and surfing the Web than they do talking about solving their problems. Telephones are an untapped resource for two-way communications with patients for problem solving, encouragement of community-based assignments, and reminders. Voice mail can be used to positively reinforce patients' progress. The therapeutic

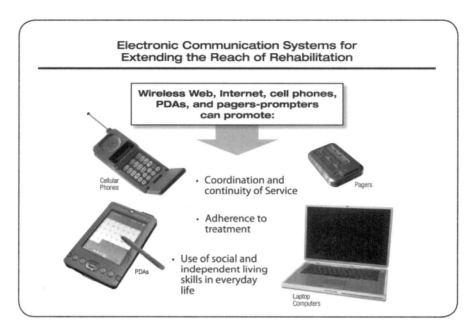

FIGURE 10.12 Electronic communication systems for extending the reach of rehabilitation.

alliance is strengthened when patients hear their clinicians' voices, knowing that their message will be listened and responded to. Telephones are well established as a means of improving adherence with appointments, treatment assignments, continuity of care, and effectiveness of cognitive-behavior therapy; unfortunately, phones are rarely used for the purpose by mental health centers or clinics (Mohr et al. 2005). In the future, it will be cost-effective for mental health programs to distribute cell phones to their clientele and encourage clinical contacts to be made on the phone as well as in person. Electronic devices that can stretch the patient–practitioner relationship beyond the consulting office are depicted in Figure 10.12.

Several applications of computers in the service of diagnosis, assessment, psychosocial treatment, and rehabilitation have shown promise and will almost certainly become more widespread in the future. Computerized treatment for depressive and anxiety disorders has been shown to be both efficacious and cost-effective, even when administered in general practices with supervision by a nurse (Carlbring et al. 2006; Marks et al. 2003; McCrone et al. 2004; Proudfoot et al. 2004; Spek et al. 2007). Patients report improved quality of life and satisfaction with use of computer-assisted treatment. The medical history and current symptoms, physical examination findings, and laboratory test results can be entered into a computer programmed with artificial intelligence to yield differential diagnoses. Created by the cumulative knowledge base of panels of specialists, the expert system specifies the treatments that can be expected to be effective based upon each patient's diagnostic profile.

In the case of neurorehabilitation of poststroke patients, the brain's ability to rebuild itself and learn new tasks relies upon long-term, time-consuming exercises. Technological innovations have led to robot-assisted rehabilitation. Robots are computers programmed to provide support and movement in treadmill training and manipulate weakened arms in constraint-induced therapy. This saves the costly time of physical therapists and relieves them of what otherwise would be monotonous exercises. Robots and computers never get bored. Learning motor skills needed for walking and using one's arms is accompanied by positive changes in brain physiology and structure as documented by functional magnetic resonance imaging. Rehabilitation aims to make those changes lasting improvements.

Computer-assisted cognitive-behavioral therapies for mood, psychotic, anxiety, eating, and dissociative disorders have been shown to be as effective as and more efficient than treatments delivered solely by face-to-face contact with therapists. Applications can be as varied as:

- Handheld computers to remind, encourage, and reinforce generalization of treatment through completion of homework assignments.
- Computer-driven interactional procedures for learning how to successfully navigate the varied and often stressful pathways of community life—using a videodisc with touch-screen choices, multimedia file handlers, and instructional design software.
- Virtual reality, by which the patient is thrust into simulations of his/her problem situations armed with coping and problem-solving skills.
- Desktop computers programmed for cognitive remediation.

For patients who have severe disturbances of interpersonal communication and information processing, interaction with a computer can be less socially overstimulating and anxiety-provoking than treatment with a live therapist or in a group. In one experimental project, patients answered questions related to their rehabilitation that were presented on a computer screen after being given samples of appropriate ways of responding to the situations. Topics included the patient's individualized treatment plan and goals, current functioning, criteria for discharge, insight into illness, medication issues, and identification of treatment team members and their roles. Those patients who had the benefit of interacting with the visual presentations exhibited significantly better learning and understanding than those who received education on the issues in a group setting.

Computer-driven interactive videodisc programs can capitalize on procedural, implicit modes of vicarious and observational learning that are relatively intact in the seriously mentally ill. The participant identifies with a role model who is shown on video traversing challenging situations of community life. One such interactive videodisc learning program, "How to Get Out and Stay Out: The Story of Cathy," accurately depicts a prototypical patient dealing with real-life problems during her first day after discharge from the hospital (Olevitch and Hagan 1991). For example, the video shows Cathy buying items in a store, taking a walk alone in a park, preparing a meal, and having trouble sleeping. After each scene, the patient-learner can choose from among several alternative coping responses and is given feedback on his/her choices by watching how Cathy handled the situation. After the program was administered to patients, evaluation revealed improved scores on a wellness rating scale and unambiguous evidence that the patient-viewers maintained a high level of attentiveness and interest in the videodisc sessions.

While computer-driven programs are no substitute for the therapeutic relationship, there are a number of potential advantages of embedding psychosocial treatment and rehabilitation in a computer matrix. These advantages apply to a wide variety of programs, including enhancing medication adherence, teaching vocational and basic education skills, and providing training for development of more complex social skills. A microprocessor, the Med-eMonitor, is capable of cueing the taking of medication and warning patients when they are taking the wrong medication or taking it at the wrong time. It also records side effect complaints and, through remote signaling, alerts treatment staff of patients' failures to take medication as prescribed. Staff can then contact the patient by phone and assist him/her in problem solving with regard to changing types and doses of medication. Automated electronic devices such as the Med-eMonitor have the potential for improving the self-management by patients in disease management.

The NeuroPage is an interactive, proactive mnemonic system for persons with memory problems. It combines computer and paging technology to enable patients with memory and scheduling problems to receive reminders or cues 24 hours a day, wherever they may be. Advantages of computer-assisted rehabilitation are listed in Table 10.2.

The Internet provides an opportunity for practitioners to provide psychoeducation and encourage self-help support for patients and their families. Video-streaming adds another dimension to the instructional capacity of the Internet. A private, secure educational Web site with family-to-family chat capabilities has been shown to be well accepted by families, effective in teaching relevant information about schizophrenia, and successful in

● **TABLE 10.2**

Advantages of computer-assisted treatment and rehabilitation

● ●

- Slow learners can acquire knowledge and skills better through tireless repetition that might burden a live therapist with boredom.
- Patients with information-processing problems are offered one piece at a time for social learning.
- Patients can proceed through training programs at their own speed.
- Training is more consistent, with higher fidelity to criteria of quality.
- Access to therapy is extended because patients can participate from home or other locales more conveniently than they can when traveling to a clinic or hospital.
- Motivational enhancement is built into the computer programs such that patients can receive reliably and abundantly delivered, contingent positive reinforcement.
- Computer-assisted treatment can be readily integrated with existing treatment programs.
- Visual displays can compensate for deficits that patients have in verbal and working memory and sustained attention, yielding improved results for patient education and social skills training.
- Treatment and rehabilitation result in time savings for already scarce, professionally prepared clinicians.

enhancing families' coping with the burden of illness. Video-streaming and mini-lectures on the management of schizophrenia were offered by experts on various topics of interest to the families. Online discussions of the information, as well as shared problems and coping methods, were facilitated by psychiatrists and psychologists. Consumer satisfaction was substantial. Many families lived too far from the mental health agency, so the chat room was their major access to education and stress management (Glynn et al. 2006). Gaining acceptance for computer-assisted treatment and rehabilitation will not be an easy task. As shown in Figure 10.13, issues of privacy and the human desires for a personal, face-to-face, healing relationship are obstacles that will have to be surmounted. With webcams now linked to computers, on-line "house calls" that permit doctor and patient to see each other as they communicate via the Internet are now being implemented in various medical specialties.

Other examples of Internet-based cognitive-behavioral therapy for patients with depressive and anxiety disorders have brought about significant improvement of symptoms and improved quality of life (Carlbring et al. 2006; Marks et al. 2003). The new Internet technology includes modules for

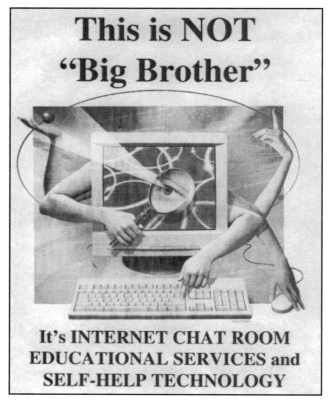

FIGURE 10.13
Role of Internet technology in rehabilitation. Internet technology can be put in the service of a more cost-effective rehabilitation if protection of privacy can be assured and some measure of real-life contact with mental health professionals is provided.

teaching patients goal setting, pleasant events, behavioral activation, cognitive restructuring, sleep and physical health, and relapse prevention. Because upward of 30% of individuals with schizophrenia and related disorders suffer from concurrent anxiety and depressive disorders, adapting these forms of Internet-mediated treatment has potential utility in psychotic disorders. It is often the case that anxiety and depression experienced by persons with schizophrenia are more disabling than psychotic symptoms; thus, cognitive-behavioral therapy delivered via the Internet can be seen as a rehabilitative intervention that goes beyond solely symptom relief.

A current drawback to Internet-based therapies is the difficulty in sustaining participation when the "draw" of personal contact with a clinician is not available. It is preferable to use Internet and other computer applications as ways to assist and supplement "live" interactions with practitioners, not supplant face-to-face treatment. If the practitioner has even a brief or intermittent therapeutic relationship with the patient, benefits and credibility from the Internet rise. In Table 10.3, applications and advantages are listed for telephone communication, telepsychiatry, and video-assisted rehabilitation.

● TABLE 10.3

Rehabilitation applications for telephone, telepsychiatry, and video-assisted technology

APPLICATION	ADVANTAGES
Telephone	
Supportive and behavior therapies	Are cost-effective; reduce therapist time
Prompt reinforcement of social contacts	Amplifies patient–practitioner relationship
In vivo and homework assignments	Counteract social isolation and boredom
Reliable use of medication	Enhances self-responsibility and hope
Cell phone text messaging	Plays role in relapse prevention, crisis intervention
Problem solving at a distance	Maintains continuity across space and time
Telepsychiatry	
Diagnosis, functional assessment	Is reliable, cost-effective
Psychoeducation	Makes available experts with credibility
Social skills training using modeling and coaching	Permits use of live models and recovered clients
Video-assisted treatment	
Vicarious, observational learning	Allows variety of social models to choose from
Reinforcement of social skills and problem solving	Serves as component of skills training modules
Observational learning of emotional expressiveness	• Treatment of negative symptoms
Video feedback of role-play performance	• Multiple reinforcement by group members
Self as model by watching video feedback	• Enhanced learning

▌ Prevention of Mental Disability

The continuum of prevention to rehabilitation is being looked at with fresh eyes. Now that the field of psychiatric rehabilitation has made significant inroads in reducing disability among those who have known the misery of serious and persisting mental disorders, interest is being shown in the prevention of disability. If treatment techniques have proved effective in the rehabilitation of the mentally disabled, why not adapt those same treatments for preventing disability in the first place? Interventions for prevention or treatment of disability are based on similar concepts of causality, such as the *vulnerability-stress-protective factors model of psychopathology* and the effects of these factors as they influence *impairments,*

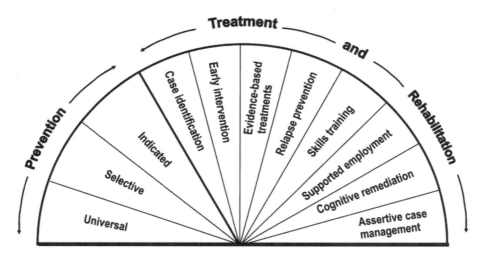

FIGURE 10.14 Continuum of prevention to treatment and rehabilitation.

abilities, and *social participation.* Therefore, it is reasonable to expect that an effective intervention for treating an already developed mental disorder also may be effective in preventing the disorder in individuals who are at high risk.

The continuum from prevention to rehabilitation is displayed in Figure 10.14. There are no significant boundaries between prevention and treatment and between treatment and rehabilitation. Within the imperative continuity-of-care principle, treatment and rehabilitation are fluid and overlapping in terms of their modalities and services. It is not desirable to conduct pharmacological treatment in a psychosocial vacuum, and almost all seriously mentally ill patients who receive psychosocial services also receive medications. Preventive interventions in psychiatry, as well as in other fields of medicine, utilize pharmacological and psychosocial modalities similar to those familiar to clinicians in treatment and rehabilitation.

Among the treatments that have reduced the symptoms and suffering of schizophrenia, antipsychotic drugs have been at the forefront. It is not surprising, therefore, that attempts would be made to use antipsychotic drugs to block or attenuate the development of schizophrenia by dispensing them to young people who are at high risk for developing the illness. One high-risk group, children of a parent with schizophrenia, could be a target for prevention, but only 10%–15% of such offspring would be expected to develop the disorder. Another high-risk group has been identified and targeted for preventive intervention. These are young people in their teenage years who are experiencing prodromal symptoms of psychosis, similar to the warning signs of relapse described in Chapter 3 ("Illness Management").

PREVENTIVE INTERVENTION WITH LOW-DOSE ANTIPSYCHOTIC DRUGS

In studies conducted in Australia, Canada, Europe, and New England, treatment research teams cast a wide net in their communities to identify youngsters who were exhibiting prodromal symptoms of psychosis (McGlashan et al. 2006; McGorry et al. 2002). Among the symptoms were problems concentrating, unusual ideas and fantasies, daydreaming that interferes with school performance, loss of interest in previously enjoyable activities, and lack of initiative. The youngsters were randomly assigned to receive low-dose antipsychotic medication plus stress management for 6 months or 1 year versus just placebo, followed by a second year of conventional services as needed. Results have been modest at best and discouraging at worst. At the end of the second year, there were no differences in the rate of developing psychosis between the groups. Moreover, the rates of dropout and nonadherence to antipsychotic medication were very high, partly due to unpleasant side effects of the medications (McGlashan et al. 2006). These initial studies are important because they show that efforts at preventive intervention can be undertaken, but their tepid results point future prevention researchers in the direction of nonpharmacological interventions or a combined pharmacological and psychosocial program of prevention.

There is good reason to expect better prevention outcomes from an intervention strategy that combines low-dose medication with a regimen of comprehensive, evidence-based psychosocial treatments. As described in Chapter 3, many young persons with the recent onset of schizophrenia make excellent symptomatic and functional recoveries when they are engaged in a positive and active therapeutic alliance with personally meaningful goals and a systematic and well-coordinated array of evidence-based psychosocial treatments. If a similar approach were made available to young persons *at risk* for schizophrenia with comprehensive, coordinated, collaborative, and competency-based services, it is likely that better results in prevention would ensue than have been reported up to now. This broader strategy for preventive intervention was recommended by this author in the report of the Institute of Medicine on reducing risks for mental disorders (Institute of Medicine 1994).

An essential principle in offering services to youngsters who have not met criteria for a mental disorder—and their families—is adapting interventions to the personally relevant goals of the recipient individuals as well as to their developmental and cultural status. For example, holding the program's services in a nonmedical and nonpsychiatric setting—such as a storefront, school, or church—will reduce the stigmatizing barriers to engagement and ongoing participation. The first generation of prevention efforts has been plagued by dropout and irregular attendance. By including activities that are normative and consistent with the recreational values of the youngsters, program services will be seen as fun rather than as burdensome or boring. Involving peers in the services who can be role models for stress management, good family relations, and social skills will reduce the age barriers between participants and therapists.

PSYCHOSOCIAL PREVENTIVE INTERVENTION

Youngsters with schizotypal personality traits are another high-risk population for the development of schizophrenia and other disabling mental disorders. Evidence from family studies, neurocognitive assessments, brain imaging, and psychopathology suggest that schizotypal traits may be behavioral phenotypic indicators for genetic vulnerability to schizophrenia. One large study found a significantly greater rate of psychotic disorders developing in persons who had had high levels of schizotypy 10 years before they entered college (Machon et al. 1995). But even without clear proof of the relationship between schizotypal traits and the development of psychotic disorders, individuals with schizotypal personality disorder have distressing symptoms, cognitive impairments, and disability in the areas of school, work, and social relations.

We undertook a controlled treatment trial of social skills training with high school students who scored in the upper decile on schizotypal traits with two aims: 1) to evaluate the feasibility of engaging schizotypal high school students in a course of eight weekly sessions of social skills training; and 2) to determine if the training would have salutary effects on cognitive impairments such as perceptual aberration, other schizotypal symptoms, and social competence. The main topics and skills covered during the training were basic conversation skills, assertiveness skills, and problem-solving skills. Specific interpersonal situations that were problematic for each student were identified and used for the social modeling, role-played practice, and homework assignments; thus, the training was individualized by the personal goals of each student. Examples of skills that were selected are:

- Asking a peer to the senior prom.
- Interviewing for a job.
- Discussing a disciplinary action with the vice principal.
- Making a presentation in class on the value of a volunteer job.
- Responding to teasing by other students.

- Using empathic communication with parents and siblings to strengthen family relationships.

Results were encouraging. Students participated actively in all sessions, expressed appreciation for being able to discuss problems they were having, and reported acquiring skills that helped them to overcome the problems. Attendance was excellent and attrition was nil. Compared with a control group, the students who participated in social skills training showed significant increases in their social competence and significant reductions in schizotypal disorganization, social anxiety, lack of friends, constricted affect, and suspiciousness (Liberman and Robertson 2005). Follow-up assessment 1 year later revealed even greater reductions in schizotypal traits and maintenance of the improvements in social competence. Prevention of psychiatric disability from schizotypal personality disorder, as well as of psychiatric disorders themselves, may emerge from future extensions of this research.

▶ An Integrated Vision and Mission for Recovery

In this chapter we outlined three promising innovations in psychiatric rehabilitation. As improved rehabilitation services are crafted by future generations of scientist-practitioners, the goal of recovery will gain a functional foundation with stronger support for our patients' experience of hope, empowerment, responsibility, and a meaningful life. Ultimately, the promise of recovery must be anchored in *eliminating or minimizing intrusive symptoms* and in *achieving a functional life* among nondisabled people in the community. "Form follows function" means that the road to recovery will take many different forms—in terms of each individual's subjective experiences and type of functional life.

The recovery movement is riding a crest wave of popularity that has captivated political leaders, administrators, self-help and peer-support organizers, practitioners, researchers, family members, and patients. Psychiatric rehabilitation and its practitioners will be taxed like never before to fulfill expanding expectations for recovery. Make no mistake: recovery is a hard row to hoe. A better future for our patients will not come from self-congratulatory applause for the ascendance of the recovery vision if we fail to meet the clinical challenges that arise from this optimistic vision.

The current enthusiasm for recovery can be a window of opportunity for rehabilitation if we raise the bar of expectations for ourselves as practitioners. Or it could be yet another disappointment born of ideological zealotry outrunning clinical realities. We cannot afford another collapse of public confidence similar to that which followed disenchantment with psychoanalysis, deinstitutionalization, and community mental health. One way for rehabilitation practitioners to obtain (not fulfill) better outcomes (not results) is through performance-based funding for services rendered. When payment of professional fees becomes contingent upon demonstrable progress of patients toward recovery, there will be a rush of practitioners to adopt evidence-based innovations. This contingent reinforcement approach is emerging as a viable policy in general medicine and has been shown to be effective in performance-based funding for agencies providing vocational rehabilitation (Gates et al. 2005).

It is timely for psychiatric rehabilitation to claim its importance in the field of mental health and to even the playing field with psychopharmacology. The enormous investment in developing, studying, and marketing "novel" pharmacological agents for the seriously mentally ill has paid off handsomely for the pharmaceutical companies. Unfortunately, the pharmacological bandwagon has left our patients with a bevy of new drugs having little in the way of efficacy beyond what was available 20 years ago, but with a broader range of perilous side effects.

Are we ready to work ever harder to gain better results from our current resources, personnel, organizations, and treatments? Can we accept the public spotlight on the reality of recovery as measured by more of our patients returning into normal community life? An affirmative response requires us to integrate principles of psychiatric rehabilitation with all that we have learned from evidence-based treatments, clinical experience, and partnerships with other stakeholders in the mental health arena. In particular, we should not shrink from integrating consumers—patients and family members—into our everyday work in rehabilitation.

INTEGRATING CONSUMERS INTO REHABILITATION

Greater involvement of patients and families in the design and implementation of innovations for rehabilitation should be welcomed. Our field will profit from different perspectives and ideological traditions that are constructively conjoined for a synthesis of interests, ideas, and services. Until recently, self-help organizations have been peripheral in mental health systems of care. Fortunately, the past 20 years has seen a positive turnaround, with self-help organizations gaining visibility and becoming a constructive force in rehabilitation. Consumer organizations have given the greatest impetus to the recovery movement.

Within the self-help community, the terms *patient* and *client* are viewed as demeaning and stigmatizing because they have been associated tradition-ally with passivity and powerlessness in the clinical encounter. *Consumer, member,* and *person with a mental disorder* are preferred because they convey a more egalitarian, participatory role. Consumers have made many contri-butions to service delivery: peer support and counseling; consumer repre-sentation on national, state, and local advisory boards for mental health; consumer participation as paid workers in mental health organizations; political and mental health advocacy; participation on local and na-tional research committees; consumer-run businesses and money-making enter-prises for employment of the mentally ill; educational programs; social clubs; and acceptance of persons with mental disorders regardless of the severity of the illness or disability.

There are three forms of peer support among persons with severe mental illness: 1) mutual support groups, which may or may not include profes-sional facilitators; 2) consumer-run services; and 3) employment by mental health agencies of patients who have made good recoveries from their illnesses. Evaluation of mutual support groups has documented improve-ment of symptoms, enlargement of social networks, and better quality of life. However, these results are only suggestive, since they emanate from uncontrolled studies and it is well known that patients who are already on a trajectory of recovery are the ones who usually join self-help groups.

Consumer-run services fall into two categories: 1) firms that contract with local mental health agencies to provide support, spur advocacy to bet-ter services, and destigmatize mental illness; and 2) self-help organizations that provide drop-in, recreational, and self-help services and consumer-run companies that sell services and products such as janitorial services, gar-dening and landscaping services, catering, and restaurants. These programs have shown their feasibility and, most importantly, destigmatize mental illness by demonstrating the self-support capacity of the mentally ill as citi-zens within their community.

Given the limited human resources with professional training for serving the multifarious needs of the mentally and developmentally disabled, the availability of recovered patients as salaried and supervised workers in deliv-ering appropriately delimited services is a path into the future for rehabilita-tion services. The major self-help organizations are listed in Table 10.4.

We are already seeing consumer organizations being embraced by the mental health professions, state and local mental health agencies, and aca-demic departments of psychiatry, psychology, and social work. Working together has produced a synergy in forging new priorities and improving the quality of mental health services. For example, the National Alliance

> ● **TABLE 10.4**
>
> **Self-help organizations**
>
> - Anxiety Disorders Association of America (www.adaa.org)
> - Compeer (www.compeer.org)
> - Consumer Organization and Networking Technical Assistance Center (CONTAC) (www.contac.org)
> - Depression and Bipolar Support Alliance (www.dbsalliance.org)
> - GROW in America (888-741-4769; www.growinamerica.org)
> - Mental Health America (formerly National Mental Health Association) (www.nmha.org)
> - Mental Health Recovery (www.mentalhealthrecovery.com)
> - Mental Illness Education Project, Inc. (www.miepvideos.org)
> - NARSAD (National Alliance for Research on Schizophrenia and Depression) (www.narsad.org)
> - National Alliance on Mental Illness (NAMI) (www.nami.org)
> - National Empowerment Center (www.power2u.org)
> - National Mental Health Consumers' Self-Help Clearinghouse (www.mhselfhelp.org)
> - National Mental Health Information Center (www.mentalhealth.samhsa.gov)
> - National Schizophrenia Foundation
> - Obsessive Compulsive Foundation (www.ocfoundation.org)
> - Project Return Peer Support Network: The Next Step (888-242-2522, 323-346-0960; www.mhala.org/project-return.htm)
> - Recovery Inc. (www.recovery-inc.com)
> - Schizophrenics Anonymous (www.sanonymous.org)
> - U.S. Psychiatric Rehabilitation Association (USPRA) (www.uspra.org)

on Mental Illness (NAMI) has successfully advocated for state governments to support the costs of more expensive, new drugs for patients with serious mental illness as well as the implementation of evidence-based services such as assertive community treatment and supported employment. NAMI issues periodic state-by-state "report cards" on the quality of the states' mental health services. This independent evaluation motivates state legislatures to appropriate more funds for mental health. In California, consumer organizations spearheaded the passage of a statewide initiative, the Mental Health Services Act, that increases the amount of money available for mental health services through a 1% tax on personal income above $1 million.

Despite the great progress made by NAMI and other consumer organizations, there are still stigmatizing currents that keep consumers from sailing into clear water of normality. Laws and policies against voting by the mentally ill, common in many states, constitute a fence that has been erected against the full participation of the mentally ill as citizens of their communities. However, an alliance of consumer groups with psychiatrists and the American Bar Association will recommend that mentally ill patients be prevented from voting only if they cannot indicate, with or without help, a specific desire to participate in the voting process. Mentally ill individuals tend to vote if they wish to vote and demonstrate comprehension of the purpose and consequences of elections.

In the future, we shall see even closer collaboration between mental health professionals and consumers. As more individuals with severe mental disorders recover, they will form a reservoir of mental health workers with credibility for those who are mentally disabled and searching for role models in their quest for recovery. To promote integration, common goals, and collaboration in the mental health workplace, professionals and consumers serving as peer supporters will have to learn to view themselves and each other in a mutually respectful light.

For peer supporters to make a contribution to rehabilitation services and obtain satisfaction from their work, it is absolutely essential that they participate in the development and specification of their job descriptions and performance standards. The rest of the treatment and rehabilitation team should also participate in this process so there is a consensus from the start regarding their role, relationship to professional staff, and supervision. Accommodations and working relationships between professionals and peer supporters will occur naturally during their work together. One increasingly popular mode of service provided by consumers has been outreach to the homeless and other patients who are difficult to engage in mental health services. Reluctant patients who fear treatment, stigma, and hospitalization are often more responsive to consumers like themselves, feeling less defensive and benefiting from the natural and spontaneous role modeling of the outreach worker.

Obstacles that potentially impede the success of consumers and professionals working together are difficulties in separating the identity of a consumer "as patient" and "as mental health worker," reflected by consumers assuming the role of the mental health worker and losing their special value as a peer supporter (Davidson et al. 1999). The absorption of consumers as bona fide employees into mental health agencies is very new, so there is reason to be optimistic that the dilemmas noted above will eventually be resolved. Both professionals and peer supporters share a commitment to developing and maintaining relationships with patients that are infused with dignity, genuine concern, empathy, warmth, and unconditional regard.

New training programs for both peer supporters and mental health professionals will be needed. Efforts in this direction have begun. There are certification programs for training peer supporters to work in mental health agencies. Some such programs are offered by community colleges, with others offered by nonprofit organizations. NAMI families and consumers have begun to offer brief, recovery-oriented seminars for psychiatrists and other mental health professionals in hospitals, clinics, and mental health centers. NAMI also offers Family-to-Family educational seminars on serious mental illness that are led by family members who are certified after undergoing thorough training. Similarly, this ever-expanding organization trains individuals with mental disorders to lead Peer-to-Peer educational seminars in which consumers lead the groups. Individuals who have made reasonable recoveries from their schizophrenia and other serious disorders are given supervision to present a destigmatizing message, In Our Own Voice, to students and medical and mental health professionals and service agencies. They "voice" their own personal stories that emphasize not only how much they suffered from their illness but also how they found their pathway to recovery. Graduate school and continuing education programs for mental health professionals in psychiatric rehabilitation and recovery are clearly a development for the future, as little has been done up to the present.

INTEGRATING EVIDENCE-BASED PRACTICES INTO REHABILITATION

Listed in Table 10.5, evidence-based practices have been validated for their efficacy by research, expert consensus, and guidelines published by professional societies. Their demonstrable effectiveness has meant that recovery from serious mental illness is no longer a dream. Unfortunately, very few of these programs have been implemented in currently available mental health and rehabilitation services.

Integrating evidence-based practices with ongoing mental health services is a challenging endeavor. The competencies for community integration required by personal support specialists and multidisciplinary teams were described and graphically represented in Chapter 8 ("Vehicles for Delivering Rehabilitation Services"). Even with highly competent clinicians, there are many obstacles at the administrative, clinician, patient, and technique levels that interfere with the introduction of evidence-based practices into routine clinical practice (Isett et al. 2007). These include:

● **TABLE 10.5**

Evidence-based services for the seriously and persistently mentally ill

SINGLE-TREATMENT MODALITIES	MULTI-ELEMENT VEHICLES FOR SERVICE DELIVERY
Motivational interviewing	Assertive community treatment
Social skills training	Integrated services for the dually diagnosed
Supported employment	
Behavioral family management	Social learning therapy (token economy)
Cognitive-behavioral therapy	
Illness management	

- Inertia among mental health practitioners and agencies that continue to use services that have been in their repertoire for years and even decades.
- Difficulty in learning new procedures, especially when they are complex, require coordinated teamwork, and are discordant with existing practices.
- Reliance on publications, presentations, conferences, consultation, and other ineffective methods of dissemination.
- Absence of fidelity criteria for using evidence-based practices in agency job descriptions and performance standards.
- Lack of administrative, legal, social, or fiscal rewards or sanctions to motivate change in practices by clinicians and agencies.
- Use of training techniques that are based on written materials, watching videos, lectures and discussion, and other passive modes of learning.
- Slow penetration of evidence-based practices into the curricula of professional training programs.
- Failure of researchers and practitioners to share or understand each other's basic assumptions and clinical priorities in routine clinical practice.
- Failure of insurance firms and local, state, and federal agencies to make reimbursement and payment for services conditional upon use of empirically validated services.

DISSEMINATING AND ADOPTING INNOVATIONS IN MENTAL HEALTH

What then can be done to surmount these barriers to the professional adoption and integration of innovative and evidence-based practices for rehabilitation and recovery? Because experience is the best teacher, it is incumbent on those responsible for facilitating the implementation of evidence-based practices to learn from the know-how gained by other fields regarding adoption of innovations. For more than 100 years, commercial and industrial enterprises, as well as the nonpsychiatric fields of medicine, have learned to modernize their procedures and practices or else lose their competitive edge.

When a company or corporation has decided to upgrade or modernize its operations, it brings in an outside consulting group to help it with that process. Consultants work by 1) analyzing a company's operations and identifying avenues for change; 2) engaging the managers and employees of a firm in the change process of setting objectives, training goals, and methods; 3) conducting the training and then evaluating the impact of training on the

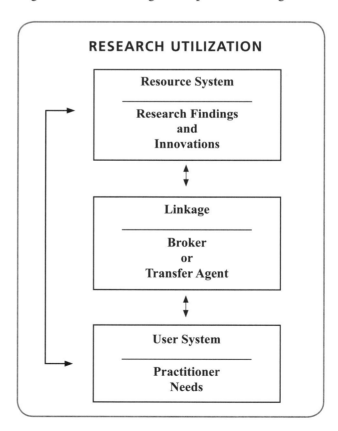

FIGURE 10.15 A linkage agent or broker for dissemination of clinical innovations connects researchers who develop innovations with mental health practitioners and administrators who must adopt the novel treatment techniques to improve prospects for recovery in their patients.

company's operations; and 4) maintaining a presence in the company until the new operations have solidly implanted with quality assurance procedures.

Consultants can be seen as *linkage agents* connecting the innovations with those agencies and people who are the designated recipients and users of the innovations. Linkage or technology change agents have been used with great effectiveness by the U.S. Farm Bureau, with experts who have worked for over a century with farmers to assist them in developing seeds for higher-yielding and more disease-resistant crops and using more efficient methods of planting, harvesting, irrigation, and cultivation. Other examples of consultants serving as linkage agents between the innovators and the prospective users of the innovations are architects, information technology consultants, pharmaceutical sales representatives, and technical support specialists introducing high-tech medical equipment into hospitals. Figure 10.15 illustrates how a linkage agent fosters integration of evidence-based practices in mental health.

By adapting the hard-earned principles of dissemination and adoption of innovations from these fields, rehabilitation should be able to accelerate its technological development. The result will be an enhanced capability for helping more people recover from serious and persisting mental illness. The principles enumerated in Table 10.6, drawn from decades of experience

● **TABLE 10.6**

Methods for promoting adoption and integration of evidence-based practices into customary care

1. Involve all stakeholders of the agency and community in planning for dissemination process.

    Obtain maximum involvement with clinicians, administrators, consumers, family members, and other interested parties. Engage stakeholders in a process whereby they feel ownership in the innovation and its successful adoption by the agency.

2. Present credible evidence of the value of the innovation through summarizing relevant research in ways that clinical staff and other stakeholders can readily understand.

3. Use a *clinical microsystem* approach whereby trainers and consultants meet with the "front-line" staff of each unit of an agency that provides direct service to patients and families:

    a. Inform them that, as they have the responsibility for providing the best-quality care, they know better than others what would be most important for them to improve, problem-solve, or analyze.

    b. Once they have identified a problem area to focus on, encourage them to work together as a team to generate alternative ideas that might be effective in reducing the problem and improving the quality of care.

(continued)

- **TABLE 10.6** (*cont'd.*)

c. Ask staff to monitor their relevant benchmark for signs of improvement.

d. Recommend that staff continue to search for alternative innovations that are evaluated by their capacity to improve the measurable benchmark.

4. Survey and talk with staff in groups and individually to fathom the perceived salience for them of the innovative, evidence-based practice.

5. Promote interpersonal contact between change agents and recipient clinicians, managers, and administrators, leavened by selecting and reinforcing one or more local "champions" or advocates for adopting the new practices.

   Regular telephone conferences, starting with collaborative planning for the training process, cost very little and can be used to develop ways of coping with the inevitable challenges posed by implementing an innovation.

6. Continue outside consultation and technical assistance for the adoption process itself.

   Technical assistance by credible experts should continue until the novel programs are adopted and the local clinicians are engaged in problem solving focused on their psychological resistances, administrative obstacles, and unintended side effects of the novel practices.

7. Enlist organizational support for the innovation by top and middle management.

   Support includes highly visible, substantive verbal and behavioral actions by managers; allocation of resources and scheduled time required by the new services; establishment of new job descriptions and performance standards for clinicians on staff; and changes in the mission statement and clinical ideology of the adopting agency that are consistent with the evidence-based practice.

8. Break down a complex evidence-based practice into its component parts so that the method can be taught in steps and it becomes more likely that competence will be acquired.

   Similarly, evidence-based practices can be "packaged" or organized in "user-friendly" workbooks, video-assisted manuals, and modules.

9. Use active-directive and experiential learning procedures when training clinicians in the evidence-based practices.

   This entails social modeling, role-playing, repeated practice to levels of competence, abundant reinforcement for approximating competence, corrective but not critical feedback, and implementation exercises outside of the training site.

10. Tailor the evidence-based practice and the training activities for its implementation so that they are compatible with the prevailing therapeutic ideology of the site that has agreed to adopt it.

    All stakeholders are involved in the planning and implementation of the novel practices so they gain a feeling of "ownership" of the innovations and can identify with them.

11. Encourage flexible adaptation of the evidence-based practice, as well as re-invention of spin-offs and derivatives, to fit the local patient population, unique clinical problems, and the strengths and constraints of personnel and resources at the adopting site.

in many fields, may foster the diffusion and implementation of innovations into the work of rehabilitation agencies and practitioners (Backer et al. 1986; Liberman, in press). A sine qua non for integrating an innovative practice into customary mental health services is the support of top and middle management. Training line-level staff members in the use of an evidence-based practice is doomed to failure without careful attention to the administrative provisions for visible and tangible support of the practice at all levels of the organization.

EXAMPLE

The importance of administrative support in bringing about adoption of an evidence-based practice was evident in a state psychiatric hospital where staff members were being asked to implement a novel mode of psychosocial rehabilitation (Smith 1998). The most numerous staffers by far in the hospital were nursing assistants with high school educations who subserved custodial functions. However, many of these employees possessed natural gifts for teaching skills to long-term patients; their personal qualities included enthusiasm, warmth, and spontaneity in their relationships with patients, a desire to see patients improve, and a desire to learn and improve themselves. The external consultants responsible for the dissemination of the new rehabilitation approach persuaded the director of the hospital and state-level personnel office to establish a new job title, with a modest salary increase, for those nursing assistants who demonstrated competence in using the evidence-based practice. Competence was measured by their meeting fidelity criteria during skills training sessions as part of their annual performance evaluations.

Other principles of effective dissemination used at this hospital were 1) cultivating a rehabilitation specialist as the local champion for the innovation; 2) reinforcing this person's active role as an advocate and trainer by promoting her to the position of director of rehabilitation; 3) publishing a monthly newsletter that highlighted the accomplishments of specific staff members in using the techniques; 4) attaining statewide recognition of the hospital's rehabilitation program as exemplary, offering second-generation training by hospital staff to other facilities and practitioners throughout the state; and 5) developing new programs to teach patients skills in new areas of functioning, using the format and basic principles of the original evidence-based practice.

Another important motivation for staff to "buy into" an evidence-based practice is for the innovator to gain credibility for the practice. Credibility can be obtained by conducting staff training using experiential and active learning principles: social modeling, role-playing, coaching, in vivo practice, and positive and corrective feedback. Training is done in the host work environment by the innovator or trainer who is attempting to change existing practices and introduce more effective methods. Credibility for the newly introduced techniques can be accomplished by having respected in-house colleagues "champion" the new technique and serve as role models and "influentials." Also, clinicians can actually see the new technique being used with the very patients who attend the program where in-service training is taking place. Unless these two modes of gaining credibility are present, it is very difficult to overcome the skepticism of clinicians who are being asked to change their practices and offer the technique to their own patients.

EXAMPLE

Six innovative and evidence-based modules, including modules for behavioral family interventions and social skills training for the seriously mentally ill, were disseminated to community mental health centers throughout the country. As a first step, directors of the mental health centers made written commitments to set aside time for staff to use the innovations once they were learned. Training of staff from the mental health centers was scheduled to take place at the local sites, but before the training occurred, each of the facilities had to identify a clinician from among the staff who 1) had previously reviewed the modules, 2) had agreed to serve as a local coordinator or advocate for the new modules, and 3) was respected by his/her colleagues for the quality of his/her clinical services. When the training commenced, demonstrations of each module were carried out by the visiting "change agents" with volunteer patients from each mental health center whom the local staff screened for their being typical of their clientele.

Nearly 1,000 therapists from 40 mental health centers were trained in the new procedures, and at the 12-month follow-up, two-thirds of the mental health centers reported that they had implemented one or more of the new services (Liberman et al. 1982).

INTEGRATING RESEARCH INTO REHABILITATION

Compared with research in other areas of psychiatry and neuroscience, the research being done on rehabilitation and recovery is scanty and methodologically weak. Theory-driven, hypothesis-testing research is almost non-existent, and there have been few examples of translating basic science from the lab to the clinic or community. This lack of adequate research has led to an unfortunate situation where psychiatric rehabilitation is not on the "radar screen" of mainstream psychiatry. The little research that is published tends to be sequestered in journals of lesser quality with inadequate peer review and limited circulation. To move forward, rehabilitation research will have to become more rigorous and visible. This will require the following efforts:

- *Closer liaison between rehabilitation practitioners and academic researchers.* This linkage will attract academic researchers to take on clinically important problems and challenges facing the field. In a reciprocal manner, researchers in basic fields such as cognitive neuroscience, learning theory, educational technology, and organizational psychology will need to acquaint rehabilitation practitioners with ways to translate their research to applied clinical problems.
- *Linkages between the rehabilitation field and granting agencies,* including advocacy for prioritizing rehabilitation as a prime area for studies. Most psychiatric researchers are unaware of funding agencies that already are devoted to supporting rehabilitation research—the National Institute on Disability and Rehabilitation Research, the Social Security Administration, and the Substance Abuse and Mental Health Services Administration.
- *Hypothesis-driven research on recovery from severe mental disorders.* Conducting hypothesis-driven research on recovery from severe mental disorders must be a major initiative in our field. Recovery as a guiding light for our field will extinguish unless energized by investigations of factors associated with recovery and intervention studies to test the utility and validity of these factors. Research should seek to understand the relationships between subjective factors related to the process of recovery (e.g., hope, empowerment, responsibility) and benchmarks of being in the state of recovery, as indicated by symptom remission, improved functional abilities, and participation in society.

Hypothesis-testing research on recovery can evaluate the extent to which evidence-based interventions presumed to be instrumental in promoting symptom remission and a functional life in the community actually achieve these outcomes. Do individualized, multi-element treatment programs utilizing social skills training, cognitive-behavioral therapy, rational psychopharmacology, assertive community treatment, integrated dual-diagnosis programs, supported employment, and family supports produce higher rates of recovery when offered continuously, competently, and flexibly according to the phase of each person's illness? To what extent do evidence-based services strengthen subjective values and indicators of the process of recovery: empowerment, hope, self-responsibility, and achievement of meaningful goals?

Can predictors of recovery be validated? Do good premorbid adjustment, less time without treatment, no substance abuse, normal cognitive functioning, family support marked by effective communication and problem solving, and favorable response to initial treatment with antipsychotic drugs predict recovery? For those factors that are documented as important for recovery, which are malleable and therefore potential "targets" for intervention studies?

How can investigators study the various factors that illuminate the *process of recovery* that is a central theme for consumers in their quest for better, dignified lives? For example, how can such factors as "growth," "dignity," "empowerment," "hope," and "self-responsibility" be measured and used as dependent or independent variables in hypothesis-generating and hypothesis-testing research? Can the scientific discipline of life-span developmental psychology contribute to these terms, such as "growth" of individuals with mental disorders through the life cycle?

INTEGRATING PRINCIPLES, VALUES, AND SKILLS IN THE REHABILITATION RELATIONSHIP

The basic principles of psychiatric rehabilitation, as described in Chapter 2 ("Principles and Practice of Psychiatric Rehabilitation"), are reliable guides for integrating the personal, professional, social, and political factors that influence our field. The principles are the source of our values and practices that affect our face-to-face, human encounters with our patients and co-workers. Wherever we work, whomever we help, and whatever our roles, the final common pathway from principles, practices, and values leads to the person-to-person contacts that we have each day in our professional activities. These contacts are where the integrated vision and mission of rehabilitation exerts its therapeutic effects. Our attention and concerns may be diverted to the larger stage of transforming systems of care, but we make a difference in the lives of our patients at the time and place of meeting with them. What we bring to those meetings and how we use our time together are decisive in improving their functioning, symptoms, cognitive capacities, and hope.

The point of contact between practitioner and patient is shown in Figure 10.16 as they meet on the road from disability to recovery. Their meeting is sheltered by the overarching framework of *rehabilitation principles* that gov-

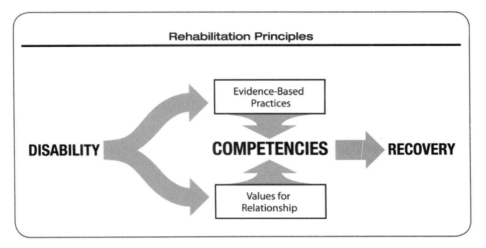

FIGURE 10.16 Conjoining of recovery values and evidence-based services in competent practitioners promotes rehabilitation and recovery for the seriously mentally ill.

ern how *evidence-based practices* can accelerate the recovery process. But within this framework, evidence-based practices intersect with the positive and sustaining *values* inherent in patients' desires for recovery: dreams and goals, hope, empowerment, self-responsibility, mutual respect, and a meaningful, purposeful life. Values without effective treatments are abstractions, glittering generalities, and rhetoric. Effective treatments without values are sterile and insignificant. Blending the humanistic values of psychiatric rehabilitation with effective treatments can generate *professional competencies* that determine whether practitioners make a difference in the lives of patients. *Values* and *evidence-based practices* determine whether rehabilitation services will be implemented and have their intended positive effects.

Figure 10.16 represents how the *values of recovery* meet *evidence-based practices* in the special and unique *relationship between patient and mental health professional.* The outcome of this encounter—which can be multiplied by thousands of interactions each month and year—is determined by the *competencies* of the professional in the realms of *values, attitudes,* and *proficiencies.* There is no separating the values, attitudes, and relationship from the proficiencies in functional assessment, illness management, social skills training, family education, or cognitive-behavioral therapy. These attributes blend to produce an integrated set of competencies for the mental health professional. Values, attitudes, and skills, sewn together in a common fabric, profoundly influence the process and outcome of treatment. These attributes of the practitioner and mental health team define the quality of psychiatric rehabilitation. The degree to which our patients move toward recovery from disability depends upon interactions between a patient and a competent practitioner. Forget about the statistically significant superiority of evidence-based treatments; recovery comes to each person, one by one.

A higher rate of recovery among the seriously mentally ill can be expected as we overcome obstacles that hinder the widespread use of evidence-based services. As with any biopsychosocial disorder, recovery from serious and disabling mental disorders occurs more readily when available services are delivered by agencies and practitioners using the 10 C's listed below:

- **Comprehensive** functional assessment as well as pharmacological and psychosocial services
- **Continuous** for as long as a person lives or needs the services
- **Coordinated** by all service providers but also by patient and family
- **Collaborative** with patients and families
- **Compatible** with the patient's culture and individualized needs
- **Consistent** with the patient's personally relevant goals
- **Connected** flexibly with phase of illness
- **Competency-based** with fidelity to the techniques of evidence-based practices
- **Cooperative** with community agencies
- **Compassionately consumer-oriented**

By organizing our services so they employ these clinical imperatives, we can increase the number of patients who recover from their disorder. *How* we use the best practices is just as important as the practices themselves.

Recovery from disabling mental illness should not be allowed to become a buzzword that is adopted by everyone who has a mental disorder, by their families, and by the mental health establishment. It is a truism that the process of recovering from a mental disorder depends on attitudes and beliefs of hope, self-responsibility for "getting a life," and a positive sense of self regardless of symptoms, stigma, and disability. It is also self-evident that practitioners can facilitate the empowerment of their patients by encouraging choices and active participation in the treatment enterprise. Personal growth is another important process in recovering, but of course everyone—disabled or not—strives for growth over the life span. Thus, we have two parallel and interacting ways to conceive of recovery. It is both:

1. A *process* that enables individuals to
   » set realistic, personally meaningful goals;
   » obtain the treatment they will find helpful and hope-inspiring;

» use natural supports that will protect against relapse and disability, such as positive family involvement and self-help groups; and

» bounce back from adversity to experience promise for a better future and a fulfilling and satisfying life.

2. A return to *reasonably normal functioning* by

» achieving their personally relevant goals for success in the multiple roles deemed important by them and their community;

» enjoying their choice for optimal involvement in work, education, friendships, family ties, independent living, and social and recreational activities in normative settings;

» gaining relief from symptoms that, through treatment, subside to a low enough level so as not to intrude on everyday life; and

» being accepted by society with dignity and participation as a contributing citizen.

These two conceptions of recovery reinforce each other. Good-quality treatment and rehabilitation can nourish the process of recovering—a process that is a never-ending story. Best practices of evidence-based biobehavioral therapy and psychosocial services, rooted in meaningful therapeutic relationships, can eliminate symptoms and restore psychosocial functioning. In turn, improved functioning empowers, raises self-acceptance, conveys hope, and permits individuals to take responsibility for their actions. It is not an accident that the leaders of the consumer-inspired recovery movement are individuals who have few symptoms and high levels of social role functioning.

Yes, all stakeholders in the mental health system—including the patient and family—are doing the very best they can to promote maximum improvement in symptoms, social functioning, quality of life, self-acceptance, and hope for the future. Differences among individuals are related to the inevitable limitations that influence the amount of progress toward recovery. These influences—for good or ill—include those imposed by the psychobiological nature of persons' vulnerability to a mental disorder and stressors and protective factors at the personal, family, community, and professional levels. Some examples of protective factors are:

• Good premorbid adjustment.

• Supportive family with members who are knowledgeable about the disorder and know how to cope effectively with its vicissitudes and advocate for quality care.

- Social skills and competence of the individual with the disorder—especially in using the skills to obtain everyday life needs and achieve one's personally relevant goals.
- A relationship with one or more helping persons—professional or natural supporter—that is imbued with hope and confidence that improvement and a better life will ensue.

But while everyone can endorse the importance of expanding the choices available to patients in setting their treatment goals and services, enhancing their active participation in treatment, and reducing stigma, a meaningful definition of recovery goes beyond the best efforts of individuals and their practitioners.

Empowerment, self-responsibility, self-management of illness, and a more fulfilling quality of life are achieved as patients progress toward their personally relevant goals, taking small but successful steps that are converted to improved self-esteem. By acquiring skills, recruiting supportive services, participating in normal community activities, and being integrated into the functional life of a citizen, patients move along the road to recovery. On the other hand, when *recovery* is used as a trendy term with razzmatazz that enables all patients to say, "I've recovered from mental illness," and every practitioner to boast, "We offer recovery-oriented services," it's the patients with mental disabilities who are cheated from the possibilities stemming from high-quality services.

When everyone can say that they have "recovered," the term loses its meaning. Overly inclusive self-satisfaction with one's personal station in life impedes motivation to build mutually respectful partnerships between patients and practitioners. Why invest the extraordinary time, effort, and money to achieve symptom remission, gain social competence, and participate in psychosocial services that can enhance independent living and a working life? It's much simpler to just talk about recovery and proclaim that one is growing and empowered to make a personal decision to terminate treatment.

Catchwords trump dry logic, dull evidence, and mere facts. A loosely used term of recovery disdains laboriously achieved professional standards of excellence in favor of what feels right. A word like *recovery* can take on a life of its own, divorced from the hard realities of treatment and rehabilitation. Gut thinking and conceptualizing pose another set of dangers to a scientific approach for psychiatric rehabilitation. All too often, wishful thinking and buzzwords bump into science, and when they do, they tend to win—at least in the short term. It is instructive to consider the independent living movement advocated by persons with physical disabilities such as paraplegics, amputees, and others with serious limitations of mobility. Their empowerment and growth came only when they won many "wars" to gain accommodations and supports that fostered their participating at a higher level of functioning through access to public services and achievement of personal goals for work, education, recreation, and independent living.

> "The human understanding resembles not a dry light, but admits of tincture of the will and passions, which generate their own system accordingly. For man always believes more readily that which he prefers. In short, his feelings imbue and corrupt his understanding in innumerable and sometimes imperceptible ways."
>
> SIR FRANCIS BACON, *NOVUM ORGANUM*

As we move forward in the twenty-first century, we must not become overly enamored of our current parade of evidence-based practices. Confident in our ability to make a real difference in the lives of our patients, we should retain humility for all that we do not know. In the decades to come, others will look back on our era, amused by our näiveté and simplistic methods. Treatments and services may change, but the essential integration of values with practices will always imbue the connection between patient and clinician.

Moving the field of rehabilitation forward requires increased integration and collaboration across many borders: professionals and consumers, administrators and practitioners, researchers and clinicians, basic scientists and treatment investigators, psychiatrists and psychologists, social workers and occupational therapists, nurses and rehabilitation counselors. Untapped sources for new treatments will be developed by professionals who cross disciplinary lines and technical boundaries. Discontent with present approaches of psychiatric rehabilitation brings with it an openness to change. "Nothing endures but change, and those who turn away from change lose the future" (Heraclitus, sixth century B.C.).

The field of psychiatric rehabilitation is maturing and becoming valued

> "I find the great thing in this world is not so much where we stand, as in what direction we are moving."
>
> OLIVER WENDELL HOLMES SR.

for its contributions to making recovery a reality for disabled patients. It has already made significant contributions to the well-being of patients with serious and disabling mental disorders. We can be certain that rehabilitation practitioners will multiply their therapeutic impact in the years to come. As progress continues, we will be able to refer less to the "seriously and persistently mentally ill" and more to those persons whose disability has ameliorated and who are well on their way to recovery with full and productive lives.

▶ Summary

The prospects for recovery from schizophrenia and other disabling mental disorders are brighter than ever. New and effective modes of treatment and rehabilitation are being developed and validated every year. One of these new treatments is *cognitive-behavioral therapy* for psychotic symptoms. Adapted from techniques that have been effective for anxiety and depression, cognitive-behavioral therapy has shown value in reducing the intrusiveness and disruption caused by hallucinations and delusions. Derived from cognitive neuroscience, and distinctly different from cognitive-behavioral therapy, *cognitive rehabilitation* represents an example of the translation of basic laboratory research to the clinical arena.

The plasticity of the central nervous system and the advent of computers permit the tireless repetition required for training the brain's neurocognitive functions. Cognitive rehabilitation, sometimes called *cognitive remediation,* uses programmed computers to do the training that would not be feasible if done by practitioners, whose efforts would rapidly become tiresome. Two innovations have improved the impact of cognitive rehabilitation on practical, everyday functioning: 1) motivating patients to perform the requisite computer drills by connecting the purpose of the laboratory practice sessions to each individual's personal goals; and 2) creating group or individually based, transitional treatment sessions that bring community-based learning opportunities closer to the computerized training. Both of these innovations amplify the generalization of cognitive rehabilitation from training the brain in the lab or clinic to using the newly trained neural circuits in everyday life.

Technological advances promise to speed up the benefits accruing from a wide range of skill-building and supportive services; for example, computer-based cognitive-behavioral therapy for psychotic, depressive, and anxiety symptoms is becoming more available. Internet chat rooms and other computer capabilities are bringing people together to learn how to cope with symptoms and disability while also benefiting from the mutual support of individuals with similar problems and experiences but differing ways of managing that can be shared with one another. Cell phones, telepsychiatry, and prompting devices will increase their utility as treatment-extenders in the coming decade by permitting more cost-effective services to reach patients who would not otherwise have access to higher and more flexible levels of intervention.

Prevention of disability and relapse through early intervention and better treatment programs is in the experimental stage at this time but spreading throughout the Western world. When young people are engaged soon after their first psychotic episode and remain in continuous, comprehensive, coordinated, collaborative, and evidence-based treatments, the vast majority go into almost complete remission of their symptoms, and over 90% are able to return to work or school. Since research programs are by their very nature time-limited, it will require public systems of care to maintain the progress made by these young patients through continuing care of high quality. When this happens, we will see increasing numbers of recovered patients in the community—further reducing stigma and granting the patients fulfilling lives.

Although capturing headlines, the experimental programs that attempt to prevent the onset of psychosis by engaging teenagers who have the prodromal symptoms of schizophrenia in treatment have not proven very effective. However, by adding more, highly individualized psychosocial services to the low-dose antipsychotic medications currently relied upon as the principal modality of preventive intervention, more successful results may begin to appear. The same model has been used very successfully for over 20 years in the prevention of depression in high-risk individuals, in which psychological and vocational services have been the mainstay of the programs.

Reduction of stigma is slowly picking up steam through public education campaigns. Surveys have shown that only 7% of the public views schizophrenia and bipolar disorders as personal weaknesses, not that far behind diabetes and cancer, which are rated as personal weaknesses by 4% and 5%, respectively. However, when asked, "Would you be comfortable telling a friend or co-worker that you had schizophrenia or bipolar disorder?" only 58% responded in the affirmative, in contrast with 97% who would self-disclose their diabetes or cancer. When recovered mentally ill persons discuss their experiences with students in elementary and secondary schools, the latter show a diminution in negative appraisals of the mentally ill. On the other hand, a majority of the public surveyed state that they would feel uncomfortable interacting with persons who have bipolar disorder or schizophrenia.

Consumer organizations such as the National Alliance on Mental Illness have begun experiential programs that bring recovered patients into psychiatric facilities to speak "In Our Own Voice." This brings psychiatrists and their professional colleagues to a compelling awareness that the psychotic and disabled patients they've been treating in the hospital represent only a small cross-section of the vast numbers of persons with psychotic disorders who slowly recover and are living full lives in the community. In the coming years, psychiatric training programs will require residents to follow their hospitalized patients into the community for long-term treatment. This will acquaint the residents with the myriad services in the community and family supports that enable patients to recover slowly and at their own pace. Another NAMI-sponsored program has opened the doors of hospitals and clinics for family members to offer seminars aimed at giving psychiatrists and mental health trainees a better understanding of how family members tend to "live on the edge" with their mentally ill offspring, how they have learned to cope, and what assistance and collaboration they desperately need from professional caregivers. In coming years, consumers will take increasing roles in meeting their needs through self-help programs. Of importance will be, for example, developing successful and profitable consumer-run businesses that will increase community integration, reduce stigma, and earn income for individuals often scraping by with minimal Social Security benefits.

The bottom line for the value of innovative treatments comes from a question: To what extent can new and promising treatments be disseminated and adopted by ordinary clinicians working in ordinary clinical facilities without the research assistants, grants, and other perks associated with academic research? A technology of transfer of new treatments from academia to customary clinical sites has begun to emerge in which journeyman practitioners ply their trades with unselected patients.

New in vivo training modes are a critical aspect of successful dissemination and adoption. Consultants who are experts in treatment teach clinicians in mental health centers and psychiatric hospitals directly on the wards and in the clinics with the very same patients who are receiving services there. This approach to direct training enables the "students" to participate in the treatment process as they learn it and to realize that the methods work even with their most difficult cases. Competency or fidelity scales for each new modality are available to determine when a clinician has gained mastery of the treatment technique. These scales can also be used to indicate which staff members should have primary leadership roles in using the novel treatments. Neophyte clinicians, who have just been trained, can compare their skills with the competencies of experienced trainers. By receiving positive feedback for gradual improvement in their skills, the trainees master the methods. In many places, the mastery of the new techniques brings enthusiasm that is shared with other clinicians working in mental health programs where training did not occur. We have seen an increasing number of first-generation trainees and facilities develop training teams to become second-generation training sites for other clinicians and facilities in their area (Liberman et al. 1982).

But we must temper our enthusiasm for what the future may bring with the ugly facts of today. Thousands of mentally disabled persons with untreated psychotic and mood disorders are behind bars in county jails and state and federal prisons. Thousands more live meager, impoverished, and unsanitary lives of vagrants in the streets of our major cities. In Los Angeles alone, surveys have found more than 90,000 homeless people, of whom one-third suffer from major mental disorders.

It would be a mistake to lay the blame for these social casualties on legislators and city, county, state, and federal administrators of health and mental health services. The responsibility for bringing evidence-based treatment to the full spectrum of mentally ill persons also falls into the bailiwick of those of us currently working in mental health facilities where we continue to use outdated, pallid, and suboptimal biobehavioral treatments, squandering precious time and resources that could achieve better results. Recovery from disability will become a reality for many more of our patients when we stop giving thousands of reasons why we cannot employ well-coordinated, consumer-oriented, evidence-based treatments continuously, comprehensively, and consistently and, instead, acknowledge that all we need is one good reason why we can and must.

▶ Key Points

- Optimism and hope for expanding the proportion of mentally disabled persons who recover and join their communities as participating citizens will depend upon the continuing development of evidence-based rehabilitation services. Our faith in a better future for our patients is bolstered by innovations that are moving from the horizon into present reality.

- Research is translating principles and technologies from behavioral and cognitive sciences into clinical use. Similarly, creative and novel designs for clinical services, propelled by unmet needs of the mentally disabled, are arising from practitioners who are dissatisfied with existing systems of service.

- The plasticity of the brain has enabled scientist-practitioners to develop a variety of modalities that have the capacity to improve the cognitive functioning of persons with serious and persisting mental disorders. Cognitive rehabilitation takes many forms: "training the brain" to directly improve cognition, errorless learning, and social and environmental strategies that compensate for neurocognitive impairments. Given the strong relationship between cognition on the one hand and functioning at work and in the community on the other, these new treatments are certain to increase the prospects for recovery from mental disabilities.

- Cognitive therapy, described in Chapter 9 ("Special Services for Special People"), focuses on modifying the deviations of "what" a person thinks, while cognitive remediation focuses on improving the mechanisms for "how" a person thinks.

- To ensure generalization of cognitive rehabilitation, practitioners are using existing evidence-based practices such as social skills training and assertive community treatment to serve as bridges from the computer lab where cognitive remediation takes place to the tasks and challenges of daily life in the community.

- Technology is making its contributions to rehabilitation by extending the reach of practitioners through electronically mediated contacts with patients in their natural environments. When cell phones, beepers, and the Internet are used, therapeutic interactions can be accomplished more frequently and with cost-effectiveness. For example, these technologies can be used to remind patients about attending appointments, promote medication adherence, monitor symptoms and social functioning, and prompt and reinforce homework assignments for community involvement. Internet chat rooms are being established for psychoeducation and consultation with families and primary caregivers. Telemedicine permits diagnostic and functional assessments from a distance, as well as therapeutics and social support.

  » Computer-driven, video-assisted training of social skills, cognitive capacities, and other abilities needed for recovery is being designed and shows promise for the future.

- Prevention of chronicity in schizophrenia and other mental disabilities has been shown to be feasible through early detection and intervention. Through education of the public and "gatekeepers" of the mental health system—such as primary care physicians, teachers, and clergy—more individuals showing the early signs of serious mental disorders can be identified and rapidly referred for treatment. With improved outcomes from early intervention, patients, their families, and the general public will adopt more optimistic views of mental disorders, thereby contributing to destigmatization.

- Recovery is becoming less a promise and more of a reality through integration of consumers or patients into service delivery. Consumers and patients are being trained to deliver specific types of interventions as well as serving as peer advocates. There has been slow but steady improvement in the dissemination and adoption of evidence-based best practices that will contribute to quality improvement of mental health services in years to come.

- Evidence-based practices are now intersecting with the positive and hopeful values inherent in patients' desires for recovery. Values without effective treatments are abstractions and rhetoric. Effective treatments without values are sterile and lack meaningfulness. Blending humanistic values with effective treatments can generate professional competencies in support of a person-centered, recovery-oriented collaboration between practitioners and their patients.

▶ Selected Readings

American Psychological Association: Training Grid Outlining Best Practices for Recovery and Improved Outcomes for People With Serious Mental Illness. Washington, DC, American Psychological Association, 2005

Brody R: Effectively Managing Human Service Organizations, 3rd Edition. Thousand Oaks, CA, Sage Publications, 2005

Chamberlain J, Rogers E, Ellison M: Self-help programs: a description of their characteristics and their members. Psychiatr Rehabil J 19:33–42, 1996

Clay S (ed): On Our Own Together: Peer Programs for People With Mental Illness. Nashville, TN, Vanderbilt University Press, 2005

Davidson L, Chinman M, Kloos B, et al: Peer support among individuals with severe mental illness: a review of the evidence. Clinical Psychology: Science and Practice 6:165–187, 1999

Davidson L, Harding C, Spaniol L (eds): Recovery From Severe Mental Illness: Research Evidence and Implications for Practice. Boston, MA, Boston Center for Psychiatric Rehabilitation, 2005

Falloon IRH, Montero I, Sungur M, et al: Implementation of evidence-based treatment for schizophrenic disorders: two-year outcome of an international field trial of optimal treatment. World Psychiatry 3:104–109, 2004

Glick I, Dixon L: Patient and family support organization services should be included as part of treatment for the severely mentally ill. J Psychiatr Pract 8:63–69, 2002

Humphreys K: Circles of Recovery: Self-Help Organizations. Cambridge, UK, Cambridge University Press, 2004

Kandel E: A new intellectual framework for psychiatry. Am J Psychiatry 155:457–469, 1998

Kurtz MM, Moberg PJ, Gur RC, et al: Approaches to cognitive remediation of neuropsychological deficits in schizophrenia: a review and meta-analysis. Neuropsychol Rev 11:197–210, 2001

Lefley H: Advocacy, self-help and consumer operated services, in Psychiatry, 2nd Edition. Edited by Tasman A, Kay J, Lieberman JA. Chichester, West Sussex, UK, Wiley, 2003, pp 2274–2288

Liberman RP: Cognitive remediation in schizophrenia, in Comprehensive Treatment of Schizophrenia: Linking Neurobehavioral Findings to Psychosocial Approaches. Edited by Kashima H, Falloon IRH, Mizuno M, et al. Tokyo, Springer-Verlag, 2002, pp 254–275

Maheu MM, Pulier ML, Wilhelm FH, et al: The Mental Health Professional and the New Technologies. Mahwah, NJ, Erlbaum, 2005

Marks IM, Mataix-Cols D, Kenwright M, et al: Pragmatic evaluation of computer-aided self-help for anxiety and depression. Br J Psychiatry 183:57–65, 2003

Medalia A, Revheim N: Computer-assisted learning in psychiatric rehabilitation. Psychiatric Rehabilitation Skills 3:77–98, 1999

New Freedom Commission on Mental Health: Achieving the Promise: Transforming Mental Health Care in America (DHHS Publ No SMA-03-3832). Rockville, MD, Department of Health and Human Services, 2003

Noordsy D, Schwab B, Fox L, et al: The role of self-help programs in the rehabilitation of persons with severe mental illness and substance use disorders. Community Ment Health J 32:71–81, 1996

Penn DL, Waldhete EJ, Perkins DO, et al: Psychosocial treatment for first-episode psychosis: a research update. Am J Psychiatry 162:2220–2232, 2005

Ralph RO: Consumer contributions to mental health: a report of the Surgeon General. Psychiatric Rehabilitation Skills 4:376–517, 2000

Resnick S, Rosenheck RA: Recovery and positive psychology: parallel themes and potential synergies. Psychiatr Serv 57:120–122, 2006

Ressler KJ, Rothbaum BO, Tannenbaum L, et al: Cognitive enhancers as adjuncts to behavior therapy. Arch Gen Psychiatry 61:1136–1144, 2004

Rogers EM: Diffusion of Innovations. New York, Simon & Schuster, 1995

Siegel DJ: The Developing Brain: Toward a Neurobiology of Interpersonal Experience. New York, Guilford, 1999

Silverstein SM, Wilkniss SM: The future of cognitive rehabilitation in schizophrenia. Schizophr Bull 30:679–692, 2004

Simpson E, House A: Involving users in the delivery and evaluation of mental health services. BMJ 325:1265–1270, 2002

Skilbeck C: Microcomputer-based psychiatric rehabilitation, in Microcomputers and Clinical Psychology: Applications and Future Directions. Edited by Ager A. New York, Wiley, 1991, pp 247–274

Taylor CE, LoPiccolo CJ, Eisdorfer C, et al: Reducing rehospitalization with telephonic, targeted care management in a managed health care plan. Psychiatr Serv 56:652–653, 2005

Twamley EW, Jeste DV, Bellack AS: A review of cognitive training in schizophrenia. Schizophr Bull 29:359–382, 2003

Wykes T: Cognitive remediation is better than cognitive behaviour therapy, in Schizophrenia: Challenging the Orthodox. Edited by McDonald C, Schulze K, Murray RM, et al. London, Taylor & Francis, 2004, pp 163–172

▶ References

Backer TE, Liberman RP, Kuehnel TG: Dissemination and adoption of innovative psychosocial interventions. J Consult Clin Psychol 54:111–118, 1986

Baxter LR Jr, Schwartz JM, Bergman KS, et al: Caudate glucose metabolic rate changes with both drug and behavior therapy for obsessive-compulsive disorder. Arch Gen Psychiatry 49:681–689, 1992

Bell MD, Bryson G, Greig TCC, et al: Neurocognitive enhancement therapy with work therapy: effects on neurocognitive test performance. Arch Gen Psychiatry 58:763–768, 2001

Brody AL, Saxena S, Silverman DH, et al: Brain metabolic changes in major depressive disorder from pre- to post-treatment with paroxetine. Psychiatry Res 91:127–139, 1999

Carlbring P, Bohman S, Brunt S, et al: Remote treatment of panic disorder: a randomized trial of Internet-based cognitive behavior therapy supplemented with telephone calls. Am J Psychiatry 163:2119–2125, 2006

Davidson L, Chinman M, Kloos B, et al: Peer support among individuals with severe mental illness: a review of the evidence. Clinical Psychology: Science and Practice 6:165–187, 1999

Gates LB, Klein SQ, Akabas SH et al: Outcomes-based funding for vocational services and employment of people with mental health conditions. Psychiatric Services 56:1429-1435, 2005

Glynn SM, Randolph ET, Lui A: Feasibility trial of a novel on-line intervention for families of persons with schizophrenia. Paper presented at the annual meeting of the Association for Behavioral and Cognitive Therapies, Chicago, IL, November 22, 2006

Green MF: Interventions for neurocognitive deficits. Schizophr Bull 25:197–200, 1999

Green MF, Ganzell S, Satz P, et al: Teaching the Wisconsin Card Sorting Test to schizophrenic patients. Arch Gen Psychiatry 47:91–92, 1990

Green MF, Marshall BD, Wirshing WC, et al: Does risperidone improve verbal working memory in treatment-resistant schizophrenia? Am J Psychiatry 154:799–804, 1997

Hogarty GE, Flesher S, Ulrich R, et al: Cognitive enhancement therapy for schizophrenia: effects of a 2-year randomized trial on cognition and behavior. Arch Gen Psychiatry 61:866–876, 2004

Institute of Medicine: Reducing Risks for Mental Disorders. Washington, DC, National Academies Press, 1994

Isett KIR, Burnam MA, Coleman-Beattie B, et al: The state policy context of implementation issues for evidence-based practices in mental health. Psychiatr Serv 58:914–921, 2007

Kern RS, Liberman RP, Kopelowicz A, et al: Applications of errorless learning for improving work performance in persons with schizophrenia. Am J Psychiatry 159:1921–1926, 2002

Kern RS, Green MF, Mitchell S, et al: Extensions of errorless learning for social problem-solving deficits in schizophrenia. Am J Psychiatry 162:573–579, 2005

Kopelowicz A, Liberman RP, Ventura J, et al: Neurocognitive correlates of recovery from schizophrenia. Psychol Med 35:1165–1172, 2005

Liberman RP: Dissemination and adoption of social skills training: social validation of an evidence-based treatment for the mentally disabled. Journal of Mental Health (in press)

Liberman RP, Robertson MJ: A pilot, controlled skills training study of schizotypal high school students. Verhaltenstherapie 15:176–180, 2005

Liberman RP, Eckman T, Kuehnel TG, et al: Dissemination of new behavior therapy programs to community mental health centers. Am J Psychiatry 139:224–226, 1982

Machon RA, Huttenen MO, Mednick SA, et al: Schizotypal personality disorder characteristics associated with second-trimester disturbance of neural development, in Schizotypal Personality. Edited by Raine A, Mednick SA. New York, Cambridge University Press, 1995, pp 43–55

Marks IM, Maitaix-Cols D, Kenright M, et al: Pragmatic evaluation of computer-aided self-help for anxiety and depression. Br J Psychiatry 183:57–65, 2003

McCrone P, Knapp M, Proudfoot J, et al: Cost-effectiveness of computerised cognitive-behavioural therapy for anxiety and depression in primary care: randomized controlled trial. Br J Psychiatry 185:55–62, 2004

McGlashan TH, Zipursky RB, Perkins DO, et al: Randomised, double-blind trial of olanzapine vs placebo in patients prodromally symptomatic for psychosis. Am J Psychiatry 163:790–799, 2006

McGorry PD, Yung AR, Phillips LJ, et al: Randomized controlled trial of interventions designed to reduce the risk of progression to first-episode psychosis in a clinical sample with subthreshold symptoms. Arch Gen Psychiatry 59:921–928, 2002

Mishara AL, Goldberg TE: A meta-analysis and critical review of the effects of conventional neuroleptic treatment on cognition in schizophrenia. Biol Psychiatry 55:1013–1022, 2004

Mohr DC, Hart SL, Julian L, et al: Telephone-administered psychotherapy for depression. Arch Gen Psychiatry 62:1007–1014, 2005

Olevitch BA, Hagan BJ: An interactive videodisc as a tool in the rehabilitation of the chronically mentally ill. Comput Human Beh 7:57–73, 1991

Proudfoot J, Ryden C, Everitt B, et al: Clinical efficacy of computerised cognitive-behavioural therapy for anxiety and depression in primary care. Br J Psychiatry 185:46–54, 2004

Schwartz JM, Stoessel PW, Baxter LR Jr, et al: Systematic changes in cerebral glucose metabolic rate after a successful behavior modification treatment of obsessive-compulsive disorder. Arch Gen Psychiatry 53:109–113, 1996

Silverstein SM, Wilkniss SM: The future of cognitive rehabilitation in schizophrenia. Schizophr Bull 30:679–692, 2004

Silverstein SM, Menditto AA, Stuve P: Shaping attention span: an operant conditioning procedure to improve neurocognition and functioning in schizophrenia. Schizophr Bull 27:247–257, 2001

Smith RC: Implementing psychosocial rehabilitation with long-term patients in a public psychiatric hospital. Psychiatr Serv 49:593–595, 1998

Spaulding WD, Fleming SK, Reed D, et al: Cognitive functioning in schizophrenia: implications for psychiatric rehabilitation. Schizophr Bull 25:275–289, 1999

Spek V, Cuijpers P, Nyklicek I, et al: Internet-based cognitive behaviour therapy for symptoms of depression and anxiety: a meta-analysis. Psychol Med 37:319–328, 2007

Twamley EW, Jeste DV, Bellack AS: A review of cognitive training in schizophrenia, Schizophrenia Bulletin 29:359–382, 2003

Van der Gaag M, Kern R, Van den Bosch RJ, et al: A controlled trial of cognitive remediation in schizophrenia. Schizophr Bull 28:167–176, 2002

Velligan DI, Bow-Thomas C, Huntzinger C, et al: Cognitive adaptive training as compensation for neurocognitive impairments in schizophrenia. Am J Psychiatry 157:1313–1323, 2000

Woodward ND, Purdon SE, Meltzer HY, et al: A meta-analysis of neuropsychological change to clozapine, olanzapine, quetiapine and risperidone in schizophrenia. Int J Neuropsychopharmacol 8:457–472, 2005

Index

Page numbers printed in **boldface** type refer to tables or figures.